Mental Health and Older People

Carolyn A. Chew-Graham • Mo Ray
Editors

Mental Health and Older People

A Guide for Primary Care Practitioners

 Springer

Editors
Carolyn A. Chew-Graham
Keele University
Newcastle Under Lyme
Staffordshire
UK

Mo Ray
Keele University
Newcastle Under Lyme
Staffordshire
UK

ISBN 978-3-319-29490-2   ISBN 978-3-319-29492-6   (eBook)
DOI 10.1007/978-3-319-29492-6

Library of Congress Control Number: 2016937415

© Springer International Publishing Switzerland 2016
This work is subject to copyright. All rights are reserved by the Publisher, whether the whole or part of the material is concerned, specifically the rights of translation, reprinting, reuse of illustrations, recitation, broadcasting, reproduction on microfilms or in any other physical way, and transmission or information storage and retrieval, electronic adaptation, computer software, or by similar or dissimilar methodology now known or hereafter developed.
The use of general descriptive names, registered names, trademarks, service marks, etc. in this publication does not imply, even in the absence of a specific statement, that such names are exempt from the relevant protective laws and regulations and therefore free for general use.
The publisher, the authors and the editors are safe to assume that the advice and information in this book are believed to be true and accurate at the date of publication. Neither the publisher nor the authors or the editors give a warranty, express or implied, with respect to the material contained herein or for any errors or omissions that may have been made.

Printed on acid-free paper

This Springer imprint is published by Springer Nature
The registered company is Springer International Publishing AG Switzerland

Foreword

It is a pleasure to have been asked to provide a foreword for this excellent book edited by Carolyn A. Chew-Graham and Mo Ray.

Mental health in older people is an important part of everyone's life. With an increasing age of the population and an increased number of older people (a great success story) come the challenges to maintain health and wellbeing as we age. Mental health is arguably the most important component of that. The explosion of interest recently in dementia is welcome, and Carolyn and Mo's contribution is a timely reminder that the important issues are not just around those organic dementias but the whole range of mental health difficulties which can affect older people.

This book attempts a lot but succeeds. It covers the full range of mental health difficulties in older people, it provides up-to-date evidence to support clinical decision-making, it offers specific guidance on clinical issues and, if that was not enough, it succeeds in emphasising the importance of integrating health and social care. In older people this is a priority. The eclectic nature of the choice of the authors strengthens the book considerably, and the range is impressive spanning details of the scale of the challenge, through detailed analyses of depression and anxiety to psychotic disorders and delirium and dementia. The range from early diagnosis to end of life care is covered admirably. With the increasing importance of care of older people and their mental wellbeing, this contribution is a landmark publication, and Carolyn and Mo are to be congratulated at bringing it together.

Alistair Burns
Professor of Old Age Psychiatry, University of Manchester
National Clinical Director for Dementia, NHS England
Consultant Old Age Psychiatrist, Manchester Mental Health and Social Care
Trust, Manchester, UK

Preface

We hope that this book will be a useful resource for anyone who works with, or is interested in, the mental health of older people.

We have attempted to adopt a broad approach, recognising the complexity of older people's lives, the interplay between the physical, psychological and social, and the need for integration between primary and specialist health care, specialist health care and social care and the voluntary ('third') sector.

Our aim is that this book will appeal to students in health and social care professions, general practitioners and primary care nurses, social workers, clinicians in specialist care and practitioners in the voluntary sector.

We, and our contributors, have drawn from their professional experiences in writing the chapters. We have used 'cases' to illustrate the concepts and topics, which reflect contributors' work and expertise. We have also included suggestions for personal reflection and audit, in order to challenge the reader into thinking how what they have read will impact on their practice.

We hope that this text will contribute to increased recognition of mental health problems in older people and an improvement in their care.

Keele, Staffordshire, UK   Carolyn A. Chew-Graham, MD, FRCGP
                                                              Mo Ray, PhD

Contents

Part I Introduction

1. **Setting the Context** 3
   Carolyn A. Chew-Graham and Mo Ray

2. **Resilience and Well-Being** 9
   Jane C. Richardson and Carolyn A. Chew-Graham

3. **Living Well with Loss in Later Life** 19
   Bernadette Bartlam and Linda Machin

4. **Policy Context for Mental Health and Older People** 29
   Mo Ray

Part II Depression and Anxiety

5. **Anxiety and Depression in Older People: Diagnostic Challenges** 45
   Carolyn A. Chew-Graham

6. **Social Participation, Loneliness and Depression** 57
   Heather Burroughs and Ross Wilkie

7. **Link Between Anxiety and Depression and Pain and Sleep Disruption** 67
   John McBeth

8. **The Management of Depression and Anxiety in Older People: Evidence-Based Psychological Interventions, Stepped Care and Collaborative Care** 79
   Simon Gilbody

9. **Pharmacological Management of Anxiety and Depression in Older People** 93
   Philip Wilkinson and Sophie Behrman

10. **Depression and Anxiety: Admission and Discharge** 115
    Alan Thomas

11	Depression and Anxiety: The Role of the Third Sector............	121
	Christopher Dowrick and Susan Martin	
12	Creativity and the Arts for Older People Living with Depression...	133
	Mo Ray	
13	Depression in Care Homes..................................	145
	Alisoun Milne	

Part III Delirium

14	Delirium...	163
	Rashi Negi and Valentinos Kounnis	

Part IV Psychosis

15	Psychosis in the Elderly	181
	Salman Karim and Kimberley Harrison	

Part V The Dementias

16	Dementia: Introduction, Epidemiology and Economic Impact	197
	Perla Werner, George M. Savva, Ian Maidment, Jochen René Thyrian, and Chris Fox	
17	Timely Diagnosis of Dementia in Ireland: Recent Policy Developments..	211
	Suzanne Cahill	
18	Person-Centred Care and Dementia...........................	219
	Mo Ray	
19	Identification and Primary Care Management	229
	Eugene Yee Hing Tang and Louise Robinson	
20	Psychotherapy Interventions with People Affected by Dementia ...	241
	Richard Cheston	
21	'They Are Still the Same as You on the Outside Just a Bit Different on the Inside': Raising Awareness of Dementia Through the School Curriculum	253
	Teresa Atkinson and Jennifer Bray	
22	Mum and Me, a Journey with Dementia: A Personal Reflection....	257
	Jackie Jones and Mo Ray	

| 23 | Role of Specialist Care in Dementia | 267 |

Chris Fox, Andrea Hilton, Ken Laidlaw, Jochen René Thyrian, Ian Maidment, and David G. Smithard

| 24 | Living with Dementia in a Care Home: The Importance of Well-Being and Quality of Life on Physical and Mental Health | 283 |

Lynne Phair

| 25 | Communication with People with Dementia | 293 |

Louise McCabe

| 26 | The Dementias: Risks to Self and Others | 301 |

Steve Iliffe and Jill Manthorpe

| 27 | The Dementias: Mental Capacity Act and Legal Aspects | 309 |

Jill Manthorpe and Steve Iliffe

| 28 | Caring for People with Dementia Towards, and at, the End of Life | 319 |

Louise Robinson and Eugene Yee Hing Tang

Part VI Conclusions/Summary

| 29 | Enhancing Older People's Mental Wellbeing Through Research: A Case Study | 331 |

Denise Tanner and Rosemary Littlechild

| 30 | Interprofessional Working | 341 |

Jon Glasby

| 31 | Challenges and Opportunities | 347 |

Carolyn A. Chew-Graham and Mo Ray

Appendix 1: GAD-7 Anxiety ... 351

Appendix 2: PHQ-9 Depression ... 353

Index ... 355

Contributors

Teresa Atkinson, BSc Psy, MSc C.Neuropsychiatry Association for Dementia Studies, University of Worcester, Worcester, UK

Bernadette Bartlam, MA, PhD Research Institute for Primary Care and Health Sciences, Keele University, Keele, Staffordshire, UK

Sophie Behrman, BA, BMBCh, MRCPsych Department of Psychiatry, Warneford Hospital, Oxford, Oxfordshire, UK

Jennifer Bray, BSc French and Mathematics Association for Dementia Studies, University of Worcester, Worcester, UK

Heather Burroughs, BSocSci, MPhil, PhD Research Institute for Primary Care and Health Sciences, Keele University, Keele, Staffordshire, UK

Suzanne Cahill, B.Soc.Science, M.Soc.Science, PhD The Dementia Services Information and Development Centre, St. James's Hospital and Trinity College Dublin, Dublin, Ireland

Richard Cheston, MA, PhD, Dip C Psychol Department of Health and Social Sciences, University of the West of England, Bristol, UK

Carolyn A. Chew-Graham, MD, FRCGP Research Institute, Primary Care and Health Sciences, Keele University, Keele, Staffordshire, UK

Christopher Dowrick, BA, MSc, MD Department of Psychological Sciences, University of Liverpool, Liverpool, UK

Chris Fox, MB, BS, Mmedsci, MRCPsych MD Department of Clinical Psychology, Norwich Medical School, Norwich, Norfolk, UK

Simon Gilbody Mental Health and Addictions Research Group, Department of Health Science, University of York, York, UK

Jon Glasby, PhD, MA/DipSW, PG Cert (HE), BA Health Services Management Centre, University of Birmingham, Birmingham, West Midlands, UK

Kimberley Harrison, MBBS, BSc, MRCPsych Royal Bolton Mental Health Unit, Old Age Psychiatry, Hazelwood Ward, Royal Bolton Hospital, Bolton, Lancashire, UK

Andrea Hilton, BPharm (Hons), MSc, PhD Faculty of Health and Social Care, University of Hull, Hull, UK

Steve Iliffe, MBBS, FRCGP Research Department of Primary Care and Population Health, University College London, London, UK

Jacqueline Jones Stoke-on-Trent, Staffordshire, UK

Salman Karim, MBBS, MSc, MD, FCPS Central Lancashire Memory Assessment Service, Lancashire Care NHS Trust, Preston, Lancashire, UK

Valentinos Kounnis, MD, MSc, PhD Department of Oncology, Oxford University Hospitals NHS Foundation Trust, University of Oxford, Oxford, Oxfordshire, UK

Ken Laidlaw, MA (Hons), MPhil., PhD, C.Psychol. Department of Clinical Psychology, Faculty of Medicine and Health Sciences, Norwich Medical School, University of East Anglia, Norwich, UK

Rosemary Littlechild, Msoc Sci, Bsoc Sci, CQSW Institute of Applied Social Studies, University of Birmingham, Birmingham, West Midlands, UK

Linda Machin, MA, PhD Research Institute for Social Sciences, Keele University, Keele, Staffordshire, UK

Ian Maidment, PhD School of Life and Health Sciences, Aston University, Birmingham, UK

Jill Manthorpe, MA Social Care Workforce Research Unit, Kings College London, London, UK

Susan Martin, BA, MSc, PhD Netherton Feelgood Factory, Liverpool, UK

John McBeth, MA, PhD Centre for Musculoskeletal Research, Arthritis Research UK Centre for Epidemiology, The University of Manchester, Manchester, UK

Louise McCabe, MA, MPhil, PhD School of Social Sciences, University of Stirling, Stirling, UK

Alisoun Milne, BA, CQSW/Diploma ASS, MA, PhD Sociology and Social Research, School of Social Policy, University of Kent, Chatham Maritime, Kent, UK

Rashi Negi, MBBS, MD, MRCPsych, MSc Med Department of Old Age Psychiatry, South Staffordshire and Shropshire Foundation Trust, Lichfield, Staffordshire, UK

Lynne Phair, MA, BSc (Hons), Nursing RMN, RGN Lynne Phair Consulting Ltd, Heathfield, East Sussex, UK

Mo Ray, PhD Gerontological Social Work and Programme, School of Social Science and Public Policy, Keele University, Keele, Staffordshire, UK

Jane C. Richardson, BA (Hons.), MSc, PhD Research Institute for Primary Care and Health Science, Keele University, Keele, Staffordshire, UK

Louise Robinson, MBBS, MRCGP, MD Newcastle University Institute for Ageing and Institute of Health and Society, Newcastle University, Newcastle upon Tyne, UK

George M. Savva, PhD School of Health Sciences, University of East Anglia, Norwich, UK

David G. Smithard, BSc, MBBS, MD, FRCP Department of Clinical Gerontology, King's College Hospital NHS Foundation Trust, Princess Royal University Hospital, Farnborough, Kent, UK

Eugene Yee Hing Tang, MBChB, BSc, MRCSEd, MSc, PGDip. Newcastle University Institute for Ageing and Institute of Health and Society, Newcastle University, Newcastle upon Tyne, UK

Denise Tanner, PhD, MSocSc, BSc, CQSW Institute of Applied Social Studies, University of Birmingham, Birmingham, West Midlands, UK

Alan Thomas, MRCPsych, PhD Institute of Neuroscience, Newcastle University, Newcastle upon Tyne, UK

Jochen René Thyrian, PhD, Dipl-Psych Site Rostock/Greifswald, German Center for Neurodegenerative Diseases (DZNE), Greifswald, Germany

Perla Werner, PhD Department of Community Health, University of Haifa, Haifa, Israel

Ross Wilkie, BSC, PhD Research Institute for Primary Care and Health Sciences, Keele University, Keele, Staffordshire, UK

Philip Wilkinson, BM, BS, FRCPsych Department of Psychiatry, Warneford Hospital, Oxford, Oxfordshire, UK

Part I
Introduction

Setting the Context

Carolyn A. Chew-Graham and Mo Ray

1.1 What Is Older Age?

'Older age', although lacking a clear definition, represents an important period of life in which health and social care needs rise substantially and in which multiple mental and physical health problems are common and interacting, often compounded by social isolation.

'Older age' generally encompasses two broad transitions [1]:

- The predominantly social transition from working life to retirement – not only capturing a constellation of potential life changes, e.g. in a person's perceived role, daily routine, income level and social environment, but also reflecting a time when patterns and lifestyles are set up which may have important longer-term implications, e.g. financial planning, patterns of family and social relationships and choice of housing.
- The potential transitions of later 'old age', which include the accumulation of health conditions and increasing physical frailty, the consequent or threatened loss of independence, social isolation potentially accompanying loss of independence, compounded by bereavements and movement to institutional or other supported accommodations.

C.A. Chew-Graham, MD, FRCGP (✉)
Research Institute, Primary Care and Health Sciences,
Keele University, Keele, Staffordshire ST5 5BG, UK
e-mail: c.a.chew-graham@keele.ac.uk

M. Ray, PhD
Gerontological Social Work and Programme, School of Social Science and Public Policy,
Keele University, Keele, Staffordshire, UK
e-mail: m.g.ray@keele.ac.uk

© Springer International Publishing Switzerland 2016
C.A. Chew-Graham, M. Ray (eds.), *Mental Health and Older People: A Guide for Primary Care Practitioners*, DOI 10.1007/978-3-319-29492-6_1

1.2 The Ageing Population

According to demographic statistics, the population of the United Kingdom is becoming increasingly older [Office for National Statistics (ONS), 2010]. At the turn of the twentieth century, only 5 % of the UK population, then totalling 32.5 million people, were aged 65 years or more. In contrast, the equivalent data for the turn of the twenty-first century estimated that 16 % of a population, which by then accounted for 52 million, was over 65 years of age (Census, 2001). Current projections for the year 2050 suggest that 25 % of the UK population, which by then is estimated to be in excess of 75 million, will be aged 65 years or more [2]. Moreover, the life expectancy at birth for the UK population is now around 82 years of age for females and 78 for males; over a century ago, life expectancies for women and for men were below 50 years of age. The population trend in the United Kingdom is also occurring on an international scale in developing and developed countries.

When the National Health Service was founded in 1948, 48 % of the population died before the age of 65; that figure has now fallen to 14 %. Life expectancy at 65 is now 21 years for women and 19 years for men, and the number of people over 85 has doubled in the past three decades [3, 4]. By 2030, one in five people in England will be over 65 [5].

This success story for society, and for modern medicine, has transformed our health and social care needs. Many people stay healthy, happy and independent well into old age, and there is mounting evidence that tomorrow's older people will be more active and independent than today's [6]. However, as people age, they are progressively more likely to live with complex co-morbidities, disability and frailty. People aged over 65 years account for 51 % of gross local authority spending on adult social care, and two-thirds of the primary care prescribing budget, while 70 % of health and social care spend is on people with long-term conditions. There is evidence that mental health services for older people are underfunded. Achieving parity in service provision for adults aged 55–74 with those aged 35–54 would require a 24 % increase in NHS mental health spending [7].

1.3 Health and Social Care

In the United Kingdom, primary care services are an integral part of the National Health Service (NHS) in which general practitioners (GPs) work as independent contractors. People are required to register as patients with a general practice; currently a practice determines its boundaries and only accepts patients who reside within this area. The GP is a generalist and provides personal, primary and continuing care to individuals, families and a practice population, irrespective of age, gender, ethnicity and problem.

GPs increasingly work with a range of healthcare professionals in a multidisciplinary primary healthcare team. The team includes a practice manager and administrative staff, practice nurses and nurse practitioners or specialist nurses. Community nurses, such as district nurses, active case managers and McMillan nurses, and health visitors may be co-located or linked with a group of practices. Increasingly social workers are also linked with a group of practices. Multidisciplinary team working is essential in order to manage the complex demands placed on general practice, which are partly due to caring for an increasingly ageing population with chronic and multiple health problems. The greater emphasis on preventative care, the transfer of clinical responsibility for some chronic diseases from secondary to primary care and the shift in service provision in order to deliver care closer to patients' homes have contributed to these demands [8].

The implementation of a new General Medical Services (GMS) Contract in 2004, which is updated each year, [9] fundamentally changed the way in which general practitioners work in the United Kingdom. The Contract defines essential primary care services and optional enhanced services that are additionally remunerated. The Contract links achievements in clinical and non-clinical care quality to financial rewards, through a Quality and Outcomes Framework derived from evidence-based care, and encourages the delivery of optimum care in clinical domains, with emphasis on chronic disease management [10]. The recently published Primary Care Workforce Commission [11] recommends that practices should develop a stronger population focus and an expanded workforce. Many existing healthcare professionals will develop new roles, and patients will be seen more often by new types of healthcare professional such as physician associates, practice nurses with special interests and pharmacists. It is suggested that such roles would specifically support the management of older people and those with complex problems. Integrating third sector services within the broader primary care teams suggested by the Commission document would provide innovative, accessible services, again, particularly relevant to older people.

Social care covers a range of services and support to help people maintain their health and independence in the community. Such services may include home care (personal care, meals, laundry, shopping), day services and respite care. The current direction of social care policy suggests that funded residential or nursing home care should only be available for those people with the most complex needs who cannot receive adequate care at home or in alternative forms of housing, such as extra care housing [5]. In England, the Care Act (2014) highlights the expectation that care is integrated and personalised [12]. Initiatives include a continued emphasis on developing integrated care and identifying good practice examples, coordinating care and support effectively and providing clear information about health and care needs. The role of personal budgets in personalised care, whereby people who require social care can opt to receive payments directly and purchase services themselves, continues to have a central role in care policy. Positive outcomes such as promoting independence and choice, in the use of personal budgets, have been reported for younger adults with physical or learning disabilities [13], but evidence relating to positive outcomes for older people is less clear. The national evaluation of pilot sites highlighted a negative impact on psychological well-being and little evidence of heightened levels of control amongst older people in receipt of personal budgets

[14]. The ability of direct payment arrangements to be responsive to fluctuating and uncertain conditions also remains an issue. Social work and social care services have a key safeguarding role with older people, and this is likely to be especially relevant when those people lack decision-making capacity.

1.4 Inequity of Access to Care

Health and care services have failed to keep up with the dramatic demographic shift.

The NHS has designed hospital medical specialties around single organ diseases. Primary care consultations and payment systems do not lend themselves to treating patients with multiple and complex conditions [15, 16]. Common conditions of older age receive less investment, fewer system incentives and lower-quality care than general medical conditions prevalent in midlife [17]. Local governments have experienced significant funding cuts over the past 4 years which has impacted on adult social care with an estimated funding gap of 4.3 billion by the end of the decade [18].

There is substantial evidence of ageism and age discrimination in health and care services, ranging from perceived patronising attitudes and behaviours to poorer access to treatment [19–21]. Older people may have access to primary care, but their mental health problems may not be recognised or addressed [22, 23].

1.5 Recent Policies to Address Inequity of Access

The strategy *'No Health Without Mental Health'*, published in 2011 (HM Government 2011) [24], perfectly captures the ambitious aim to mainstream mental health in England, with a clear statement that there should be so-called parity of esteem between mental and physical health services. The document emphasises the importance of addressing mental health problems in older people, particularly when there are co-morbid physical health problems, and the importance of social inclusion in this population.

Similarly, the publication *'No decision about me, without me'* [25] stressed the governing principle that people who use services should be at the centre of everything that is done in the health services and that care should be personalised to reflect the person's needs, not those of the professional or the system. The need for people to have access to information and support to make informed choices about both provider of care and treatment or management is central to this policy document. In addition, the aim was to empower local organisations and practitioners to have the freedom to innovate and to drive improvements in services that deliver support of the highest quality for people of all ages and all backgrounds and cultures.

The Health and Social Care Act 2012 [26] profoundly altered the structure and management of the National Health Service in England, putting patients 'at the centre of the NHS' and changing the emphasis of measurement to clinical outcomes and empowering health professionals, in particular GPs who would play a key role

Table 1.1 Parity of esteem

Parity of esteem means that, when compared with physical healthcare, mental health care is characterised by:
Equal access to the most effective and safest care and treatment
Equal efforts to improve the quality of care
The allocation of time, effort and resources on a basis commensurate with need
Equal status within healthcare education and practice
Equally high aspirations for service users
Equal status in the measurement of health outcomes

in commissioning local services for local populations. One main stated aim of this Act is to facilitate health and social care services to work more closely together, with responsibility for health promotion activities, and commissioning, given to health and well-being boards.

The Health and Social Care Act also secured explicit recognition of the Secretary of State for Health's duty towards both physical and mental health. In conjunction with a clear legislative requirement to reduce inequalities in benefits from the health service, these place an obligation on the Secretary of State to address the current disparity between physical and mental health.

The Department of Health therefore asked the Royal College of Psychiatrists to establish an expert working group to consider the issues in detail, to develop a definition and vision for 'parity of esteem' and to produce recommendations for how to achieve parity of esteem between mental and physical health in practice.

The published report [27] makes key recommendations for how parity for mental health might be achieved in practice and includes a set of commitments to actions they will be taking to help achieve parity of esteem. In essence, 'parity of esteem' is best described as 'Valuing mental health equally with physical health' (Table 1.1).

So, it is against this background that older people with symptoms which may suggest mental health problems negotiate the health and social care systems in order to access care.

References

1. Public mental health priorities: investing in the evidence. Annual Report of the Chief Medical Officer 2013. https://www.gov.uk/government/uploads/system/uploads/attachment_data/file/351629/Annual_report_2013_1.pdf. Accessed 14th Nov 2014.
2. Sunak R, Rajeswaran S. A portrait of modern Britain. Policy Exchange. 2014.
3. Office for National Statistics. 2011 census – population and household estimates for England and Wales, March 2011. London: Office for National Statistics; 2012.
4. Office for National Statistics. What does the 2011 Census tell us about the 'oldest old living in England & Wales? London; 6 Dec 2013. www.ons.gov.uk/ons/dcp171776_342117.pdf.
5. House of Lords. Ready for ageing? HL Paper 140. London: House of Lords Select Committee on Public Service and Demographic Change. Report of Session 2012–13. 2013.
6. Spijker J, MacInnes J. Population ageing: the timebomb that isn't? BMJ. 2013;347:f6598. doi:10.1136/bmj.f6598.

7. Beecham J, Knapp M, Fernández J-L, Huxley P, Mangalore R, McCrone P, Snell T, Winter B, Wittenberg R. Age discrimination in mental health services. PSSRU Discussion Paper 2536. May 2008. http://kar.kent.ac.uk/13344/1/dp2536.pdf.
8. Department of Health. Our health, our care, our say: a new direction for community services. London: Department of Health; 2006.
9. Department of Health. General Medical Contract. Available at: www.nhsemployers.org/GMS2014-15. Accessed 10 Jan 2015.
10. Lester H, et al. The quality outcomes framework of the GMS Contract. Br J Gen Pract. 2006;56:245–6.
11. Primary Care Workforce Commission. The future of primary care: creating teams for tomorrow. London: Higher Education England; 2015. [Online] Available from: http://hee.nhs.uk/wp-content/blogs.dir/321/files/2015/07/The-future-of-primary-care.pdf. Accessed 15th Aug 2015.
12. Department of Health. Care Act 2014: statutory guidance for implementation. London: Department of Health; 2014. https://www.gov.uk/government/publications/care-act-2014-statutory-guidance-for-implementation.
13. Leece D, Leece J. Direct payments: creating a two-tiered system in social care? Br J Soc Work. 2006;36(8):1379–93.
14. Netten A, Jones K, Knapp M, Fernandez J, Chalis D, Glendinning C, Jacobs S, Manthorpe J, Moran N, Stevens M, Wilberforce M. 'Personalisation through individual budgets: does it work and for whom? Br J Soc Work. 2012;42:1556–73.
15. Beales D, Tulloch A. Community care of vulnerable older people: cause for concern. Br J Gen Pract. 2013;63:615. pp 549–50.
16. Roland M. Better management of patients with multimorbidity. Br Med J. 2013;346:f2510.
17. Steel N, Bachmann M, Maisey S, Shekelle P, Breeze E, Marmot M, Melzer D. Self reported receipt of care consistent with 32 quality indicators: national population survey of adults aged 50 or more in England. Br Med J. 2008;337:a957.
18. Local Government Association. State of the Nation Report: 2014. London: Local Government Association; 2014. http://www.local.gov.uk/documents/10180/5854661/Adult+social+care+funding+2014+state+of+the+nation+report/e32866fa-d512-4e77-9961-8861d2d93238.
19. Centre for Policy on Ageing. Ageism and age discrimination in mental health care in the United Kingdom: a review from the literature. London: Centre for Policy on Ageing; 2009.
20. Centre for Policy on Ageing. Ageism and age discrimination in primary and community health care in the United Kingdom: a review from the literature. London: Centre for Policy on Ageing; 2009.
21. Centre for Policy on Ageing. Ageism and age discrimination in secondary health care in the United Kingdom: a review from the literature. London: Centre for Policy on Ageing; 2009.
22. Chew-Graham C, Kovandžić M, Gask L, Burroughs H, Clarke P, Sanderson H, Dowrick C. Why may older people with depression not present to primary care? Messages from secondary analysis of qualitative data. Health Soc Care Community. 2011;20(1):52–60.
23. Gask L, Bower P, Lamb J, Burroughs H, Chew-Graham C, Edwards S, Hibbert D, Kovandžić M, Lovell K, Rogers A, Waheed W, Dowrick C, and the AMP group. Improving access to psychosocial interventions for common mental health problems in the United Kingdom: review and development of a conceptual model. BMC Health Serv Res. 2012;12:249. doi:10.1186/1472-6963-12-249.
24. Department of Health. No health without mental health: a cross-government mental health outcomes strategy for people of all ages. London; 2011.
25. Department of Health. Liberating the NHS: no decision about me, without me. 2012. http://www.dh.gov.uk/en/Publicationsandstatistics/Publications/PublicationsPolicyAndGuidance/DH_11735.
26. Department of Health. Health and Social Care Act. 2012. https://www.gov.uk/government/publications/health-and-social-care-act-2012-fact-sheets.
27. Royal College of Psychiatrists. Whole person-care: from rhetoric to reality. Achieving parity between mental and physical health. Occasional Paper OP88. http://www.rcpsych.ac.uk/policyandparliamentary/whatsnew/parityofesteem.aspx. 2014.

Resilience and Well-Being

Jane C. Richardson and Carolyn A. Chew-Graham

> *The world breaks everyone, and afterward, some are strong at the broken places.*
>
> (Ernest Hemingway, A Farewell to Arms, 1929)

2.1 Introduction

The need to improve the treatment and management of long-term conditions is one of the most important challenges facing the NHS [1]. The idea of 'resilience' represents a paradigm shift to a treatment model that promotes positive adaptation, using an asset-based model of resilience, in the context of long-term health issues [2].

2.2 What Is Resilience?

In 2002, Ganong and Coleman suggested that we have entered the 'age of resilience' [3]. Indeed the term appears to have proliferated over the last 10–15 years: a quick Internet search reveals, for example, psychological resilience, ecosystem resilience and resilience in relation to peak oil, to the ability of a city to resist a terrorist attack and to a number of organizations dedicated to promoting resilience of individuals, cities and systems. A search for well-being produces similar, although perhaps not as prolific, results. Resnick et al. draw attention to the value of resilience as espoused through traditional adages and mythology [4], and, we would add, through now ubiquitous phrases that have entered popular culture (e.g. 'Keep calm and carry on'), that also espouse resilience.

Resnick et al. suggest that the popularity of the concept is due to the prospect that resilience can be fostered. (In fact, they go one step further and suggest that fostering of resilience can be used for primary prevention of chronic illness in at-risk

---

J.C. Richardson, BA (Hons.), MSc, PhD (✉) • C.A. Chew-Graham, MD, FRCGP
Research Institute for Primary Care and Health Sciences, Keele University,
Keele, Staffordshire, UK
e-mail: j.c.richardson@keele.ac.uk; c.a.chew-graham@keele.ac.uk

populations.) [4] It is also likely that the proliferation of interest in resilience and well-being, at least in the developed world, is linked to demographics: larger numbers of people living longer, with greater expectations of their health, coupled with a decrease in public services, makes an emphasis on resilience and well-being very timely. A critical approach to resilience and well-being, however, means that there must be caution about blaming victims if they do not exhibit resilience and resisting the romanticization of resilience:

> How can we celebrate an individual's accomplishments and well-being in adverse situations without either blaming those whose lives show less cause for celebration, or dropping the critique of the contextual structures that promote the adversity. [5]

Given this background, the remainder of this chapter aims to provide a brief overview of resilience and well-being in the context of older people in primary care.

2.3 The 'Disability Paradox'

Many older people with chronic conditions describe themselves as healthy. General Household Surveys in the UK, for example, have found that although 60 % of those aged over 65 report some form of chronic illness or disability, less than a quarter rate their health as poor [6], sometimes referred to as the 'disability paradox' [7]. At the same time, doctors are generally working within a pathogenic paradigm, which emphasizes burden, disease and decline [8]. This tension has the potential to adversely influence consultations between doctors and older patients [9].

A salutogenic approach enables these paradoxes to be explored [10]. In the salutogenic approach, wellness (absence of morbidity) and illness (presence of morbidity) are seen as a continuum rather than a dichotomy; the focus is on factors that support health rather than factors that cause disease, and questions such as why some people manage better than others can be explored. Research adopting this perspective sometimes uses the idea of people 'beating the odds' or 'punching above their weight' (metaphors also used for resilience) [11–13]. Previous studies exploring why some people do better than others have compared, for example, healthy and unhealthy 'agers' in deprived areas (where no differences were found in terms of life histories and current circumstances) [14] or people whose self-reported health status differed from that predicted by a model derived from questionnaire responses [15]. The salutogenic approach thus has great potential for exploring health in later life [6].

An assumption is often made that resilience contributes to well-being; however, 'The Wellbeing and Resilience Paradox' report [16] suggests that this relationship is not always straightforward. The authors make a useful distinction between well-being as a complex concept that captures a 'psychological state at a point in time' and resilience, while no less complex, as being more dynamic and incorporating aspects of the past and future. Well-being is strongly related to resilience, and there is overlap in the factors that influence both, but there are also individuals and communities for whom well-being is high but resilience is low. Communities with high well-being but low resilience tend to have larger numbers of older people. The authors suggest that the individuals and communities who exhibit this paradox are particularly vulnerable but perhaps not so easily identifiable as other groups, which has implications for health care for older people.

2.4 Definitions and Dimensions of Resilience and Well-Being

The 'salutogenic umbrella' incorporates a number of resilience-related psychological and sociological concepts, including resilience and well-being, for example, hardiness, assets, inner strength and coping [17]. The concept of resilience is increasingly used in the field of gerontology but lacks consistency in definition and use [18]. It has had numerous meanings in the literature, but generally refers to a pattern of functioning indicative of positive adaptation in the context of significant risk or adversity [19]. But beyond that common understanding, there are different views on (a) whether resilience is a personality trait or a process, (b) the dimensions of resilience, (c) the validity of resilience as a concept and its consistency over time and (d) the relationships of resilience with adaptation and whether it adds something new in developmental and life course theories [20]. Research into resilience was originally developed in the domain of developmental psychology, dealing with childhood and adolescence, and has only recently been extended to other periods of the lifespan, including old age.

Looking in more detail at the construct of resilience, two dimensions have been proposed – exposure to adversity and showing signs of positive adaptation to this adversity [20, 21]. According to this definition, identifying resilience requires two judgements: is there now or has there been a significant risk of adversity to be overcome and is the person 'doing okay'? In many studies, 'doing okay' is measured by assessing mood, well-being or quality of life before and after being exposed to adversity [22–24]. Maintained or increased psychosocial well-being and quality of life are indicative that the person is doing okay and is therefore resilient.

Those with resilient outcomes to adverse situations have been reported to draw on a broader range of social and individual resources than those with vulnerable outcomes. As a consequence, these people were better able to maintain continuity of their previous lives and were more in control and, therefore, more able to transform an adverse event into a benign one [25]. Drawing on previous experiences of loss and coping to create a sense of oneself as resilient has been found to help women deal with challenges from current ill-health [26].

Kuh makes a case for studying not only physiological but also social and psychological resilience alongside frailty in older people, raising the prospect of being able to be physically frail but psychologically and socially resilient [27]. This suggests that resilience may offer an appropriate framework for understanding wellness and well-being in the context of older age and/or chronic conditions. This also comes across in Windle's proposed definition of resilience, developed from a review and concept analysis:

> Resilience is the process of effectively negotiating, adapting to, or managing significant sources of stress or trauma. Assets and resources within the individual, their life and environment facilitate this capacity for adaptation and 'bouncing back' in the face of adversity. Across the life course, the experience of resilience will vary. [28]

In this definition, 'bouncing back' and adaptation are both seen as part of resilience, which, I would suggest, make it more appropriate to older people. Adaptation also distinguishes resilience from stoicism, which, although often lauded as a positive response, has no elements of flexibility, which are key to resilience [29].

However, the notion of bouncing back, at least in the context of older people with chronic conditions, could also be seen as flawed. Chronic conditions, by definition, persist and might get worse rather than better, and resilience here may mean that a person 'keeps going' despite the adversity, rather than returning to a pre-adversity state. Some research uses comparison of measures such as well-being and quality of life before and after adversity to determine resilience, with the focus on bouncing back rather than keeping going. It is difficult to measure adversity 'objectively', and people may experience the same adversity differently. This demonstrates the importance of looking at older people's own definitions of adversity, well-being and resilience [18]. These are important because they will shape the actions they take, and have taken, over their lifetime. It is important for healthcare professionals to consider older people's own definitions of resilience (or perhaps rather 'keeping going') as part of a patient-centred approach.

2.5 Measuring Resilience

The measurement of resilience is problematic: a recent review of resilience scales found no current 'gold standard' amongst 15 measures of resilience [30]. This review reported that a number of scales are in the early stages of development, but all require further validation work. The authors identify the lack of attention paid to family and community resources as a major weakness of existing attempts to create a valid measure of the concept. A further problem, particularly for those wanting to adopt a salutogenic approach, is that measures for older people often focus on deficits, such as challenges of living with chronic illness, pain, loss and loneliness [31]. The growing literature on optimal ageing [32] yields more positive measures, for example, Wagnild and Young developed a resilience scale measuring positive attributes (including equanimity, perseverance, self-reliance, existential aloneness and spirituality/meaningfulness) through interviews with 'resilient' individuals [33].

Other examples of measuring resilience include Martens et al., who used 'mastery' as a proxy measure, or marker, of resilience [34] and measured it using the 'Personal Mastery Scale' [35]. They suggest that having a high level of mastery helps older people to cope with and adapt to living with a chronic condition. They also suggest that further longitudinal research is necessary to unravel the long-term effects of mastery, income and social support on 'relatively successful functioning' in chronically ill patients. Lamond et al. suggest that the CD-RISC is an internally consistent scale for assessing resilience amongst older women and that greater resilience as assessed by the CD-RISC related positively to key components of successful ageing [36]. The strongest predictors of CD-RISC scores in this study were higher emotional well-being, optimism, self-rated successful ageing, social engagement and fewer cognitive complaints. Janssen et al. conducted a qualitative study and suggest that the main sources of strength ('to improve resilience') identified amongst older people were constituted on three domains of analysis; the individual, interactional and contextual domain and thus proactive interactions need to help older people build on the positive aspects of their lives [37].

This resonates with Wild et al.'s [18] model (Fig. 2.1) of the different levels of resilience, including individual, family and community [18].

2.6 Alternatives to Resilience

The salutogenic umbrella can also be referred to as an 'asset-based approach' – identifying the protective factors that create health and well-being and in contrast with the deficit-based approach described earlier. Resilience can be seen as an asset. Clearly in health care, a deficit model is necessary to identify need, priorities and so on, but an asset-based approach would seem more acceptable as a complement to this deficit-based approach. However, as with resilience, the focus of much research in this area has been personal factors and cognitive resources, and there is a need to

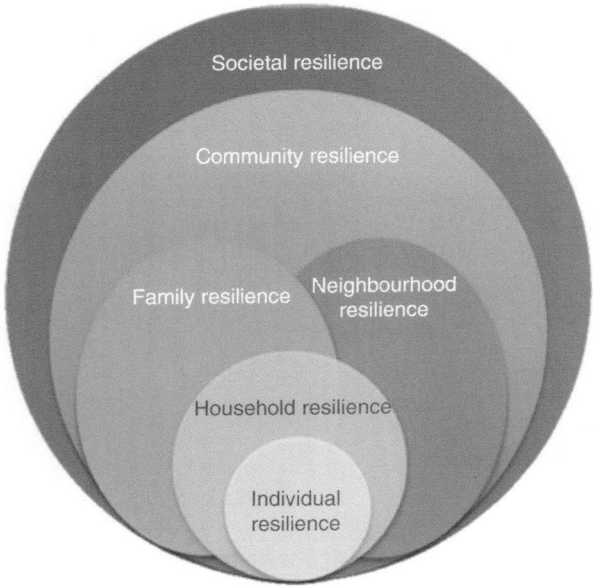

Fig. 2.1 Levels of resilience (From: Wild et al. [18] with permission)

extend this further. The scales of resilience (individual, household, family, neighbourhood, community, societal), seen in Fig. 2.1, can also be applied to an asset-based approach, as can the different domains of resilience, shown in the second model above, for example, financial, environment, physical, social, psychological, mobility and so on.

2.7 The Importance of Resilience in Context

Wild et al. acknowledge the potential for applying the concept of resilience to older people, acknowledging as they do that it can incorporate and balance vulnerability alongside strength across a wide range of contexts [18]. Locating resilience within these broader contexts removes the focus from individual characteristics and the associated blame for those who do not 'achieve resilience' [18]. The model also acknowledges that people may be resilient in one area but not in others (Fig. 2.2).

Older people, particularly those with chronic conditions, might not consider themselves to have a medical condition but simply to be getting older; nevertheless, they have to face up to changes in their physical abilities and their perception of themselves. Being 'resilient' (in the sense suggested by Wild et al. [18] and Windle [28] above) means being able to accommodate and adapt to physical changes and fluctuations in health and well-being in order to sustain what is important in life and for a valued sense of self.

Windle draws attention to the 'normal, everyday' nature of resilience, echoing Masten's evocative phrase 'ordinary magic' and suggesting that 'the opportunity for positive adaptation should be an option for everyone' [28]. Perfect physical health

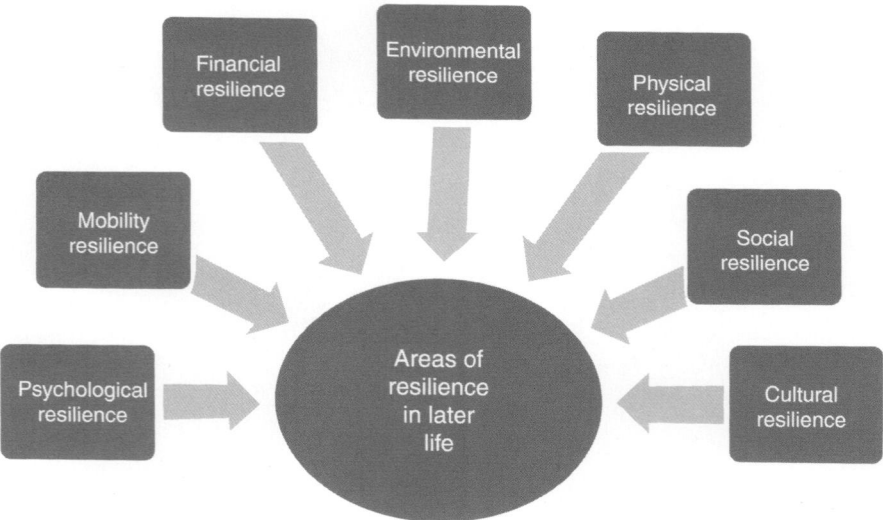

Fig. 2.2 Areas of resilience (From: Wild et al. [18] with permission)

is neither necessary nor sufficient for successful ageing as defined by the older adults themselves. Their holistic self-appraisal involves strong emphasis on psychological factors such as resilience, optimism and well-being, along with an absence of depression.

2.8 Implications of Taking Account of Resilience

Most of the public discourse on population ageing involves dire predictions and negative stereotypes. This negative view of old age has been contrasted by empirical research on older adults who continue to function well and are ageing 'successfully'.

Health and welfare services may be part of the environment of many older people, particularly those with chronic conditions, but those who provide care need to appreciate that a frail body is not indicative that the cared-for person lacks a resilient sense of self or is not able to draw on other domains or levels to achieve resilience.

Clinicians can help reduce societal ageism through their optimistic approach to the care of seniors. Treating the frail body should not come at the expense of undermining an older person's sense of self. In order to balance professional perceptions of an individual's 'frailty' with an individual's embodied and lived experience, we suggest that health and social care providers take an individual's own approach to managing their condition as the starting point for any support.

Further research on how older adults develop and maintain positive self-appraisals in the presence of biological decline may also inform similar adaptations across the lifespan.

2.9 Suggested Activity

Think about a particular patient using a salutogenic approach and using the models shown above. Is it possible to identify different levels of resilience that the patient can draw on/could be helped to draw on, outside of his/herself? Are there other domains in which the patient is resilient that can be used to support an area of difficulty? Does the patient have valued activities? How can they be supported to continue with these? How could any treatment given to a patient be used to support rather than undermine a positive sense of self? Are there opportunities for fostering resilience in older people with current high levels of well-being?

References

1. Coulter A, Roberts S, Dixon A. Delivering better services for people with long-term conditions. London: The King's Fund; 2013.
2. Jeste DV, Palmer BW. A call for a new positive psychiatry of ageing. Br J Psychiatry. 2013;202:81–3.

3. Ganong LH, Coleman M. Family resilience in multiple contexts. J Marriage Fam. 2002;64(2): 346–8.
4. Resnick B, Gwyther LP, Roberto KA, editors. Resilience in aging: concepts, research and outcomes. New York: Springer; 2011.
5. Massey S, Cameron A, Ouellette S, Fine M. Qualitative approaches to the study of thriving: what can be learned? J Soc Issues. 1998;54(2):337–55.
6. Sidell M. Older people's health: applying Antonovsky's salutogenic paradigm. In: Douglas S, Earle S, Handsley S, Lloyd CE, Spurr S, editors. A reader in promoting public health. 2nd ed. London: Sage; 1995/2010. p. 27–32.
7. Albrecht G, Devlieger PJ. The disability paradox: high quality of life against all odds. Soc Sci Med. 1999;48(8):977–88.
8. Bowling A. Lay perceptions of successful ageing, findings from a national survey of middle aged and older adults in Britain. Eur J Ageing. 2006;3:123–6.
9. Bowling A, Dieppe P. What is successful ageing and who should define it? BMJ. 2005; 331(7531):1548–51.
10. Antonovsky A. Health, stress and coping. San Fransisco: Jossey-Bass; 1979.
11. Bartley M. (Undated, accessed online July 2012). Capability and resilience, beating the odds. ISBN 0-9527377-9-5 ISBN 978-0-9527377-9-7. www.ucl.ac.uk/capabilityandresilience.
12. Dupre ME, George LK. Exceptions to the rule, exceptional health among the disadvantaged. Res Aging. 2011;33:115–44.
13. Canvin K, Marttila A, Burstrom B, Whitehead M. Tales of the unexpected? Hidden resilience in poor households in Britain. Soc Sci Med. 2009;69:945–54.
14. Gilhooly M, Hanlon P, Mowat H, Cullen B, Macdonald S, Whyte B. Successful ageing in an area of deprivation, part 1 – a qualitative exploration of the role of life experiences in good health in old age. Public Health. 2007;121:807–13.
15. Bryant LL, Corbett KK, Kutner JS. In their own words, a model of healthy aging. Soc Sci Med. 2001;53:927–41.
16. Mguni N, Bacon N, Brown JF. The wellbeing and resilience paradox. London: The Young Foundation; 2012.
17. Lindström B, Eriksson M. The Hitchhiker's guide to salutogenesis. Salutogenic pathways to health promotion. Helsinki: Folkhälsan Research Center; 2010.
18. Wild K, Wiles JL, Allen RES. Resilience: thoughts on the value of the concept for critical gerontology. Aging Soc. 2013;33(1):137–58.
19. Schoon I. Risk and resilience. Adaptation in changing times. Cambridge: Cambridge University Press; 2006.
20. Luthar S, Cichetti D, Becker B. The construct of resilience: a critical evaluation and guidelines for future work. Child Dev. 2000;71(3):543–62.
21. Masten A. Ordinary magic. Resilience processes in development. Am Psychol. 2001;56(3): 227–38.
22. Netuveli G, Wiggins RD, Montgomery SM, Hildon Z, Blane D. Mental health and resilience at older ages: bouncing back after adversity in the British Household Panel Survey. J Epidemiol Commun Health. 2008;62(11):987–91.
23. Hildon Z, Montgomery SM, Blane D, Wiggins RD, Netuveli G. Examining resilience of quality of life in the face of health-related and psychosocial adversity at older ages: what is "right" about the way we age? Gerontologist. 2010;50:36–47.
24. Windle G, Woods RT, Makland DA. Living with ill-health in older age: the role of a resilient personality. J Happiness Stud. 2009;11(6):763–77.
25. Hildon Z, Smith G, Netuveli G, Blane D. Understanding adversity and resilience at older ages. Sociol Health Illn. 2008;30(5):726–40.
26. Gattuso S. Becoming a wise old woman: resilience and wellness in later life. Health Sociol Rev. 2003;12(2):171–7.
27. Kuh D, the New Dynamics of Ageing (NDA) Preparatory Network. A life course approach to healthy aging, frailty and capability. J Gerontol: Med Sci. 2007;62A(7):717–21.

28. Windle G. What is resilience? A review and concept analysis. Rev Clin Gerontol. 2011;21(2): 152–69.
29. Moore A, Grime J, Campbell P, Richardson J. Troubling stoicism: sociocultural influences and applications to health and illness behaviour. Health (London). 2013;17(2):159–73.
30. Windle G, Bennett KM, Noyes J. A methodological review of resilience measurement scales. Health Qual Life Outcomes. 2011;9:8. doi:10.1186/1477-7525-9-8.
31. Langer N. Resilience and spirituality: foundations of strengths perspective counseling in the elderly. Edu Gerontol 2004;30(7):611–17.
32. Baltes PB, Baltes MM, editors. Successful aging: perspectives from the behavioral sciences. New York: Cambridge University Press; 1990.
33. Wagnild GM, Young HM. Development and psychometric evaluation of the resilience scale. J Nurs Meas. 1993;1(2):165–78.
34. Martens VC, Bosma H, Groffen DAI, van Eijk JTM. Good friends, high income or resilience? What matters most for elderly patients? Eur J Public Health. 2011;22(5):671–6.
35. Pearlin LI, Schooler C. The structure of coping. J Health Soc Behav. 1978;24:2–15.
36. Lamond AJ, Depp CA, Allison M, Langer R, Reichstadt J, Moore DJ, Golshan S, Ganiats TG, Jeste DV. Measurement and predictors of resilience among community-dwelling older women. J Psychiatr Res. 2008;43(2):148–54. Epub 2008 May 1.
37. Janssen BM, Van Regenmortel T, Abma T. Identifying sources of strength: resilience from the perspective of older people receiving long-term community care. Eur J Ageing. 2011;8(3): 145–56.

Living Well with Loss in Later Life

Bernadette Bartlam and Linda Machin

The concept of living well with loss in later life is consistent with contemporary, critical perspectives on ageing. Such perspectives challenge traditional notions of ageing as problematic and burdensome and support the growing awareness of older people as assets and contributors to the societies in which they live [1, 2]. They also challenge us to understand more fully the nature of losses over the life course and their consequences in later life and, in so doing, to identify more effective strategies for countering them and enhancing quality of life as we age. Within that context, this chapter has three aims: to explore contemporary understandings of loss and grief over the life course, to examine how these can contribute to improvements in outcomes for older people and to identify the implications for practice.

3.1 Loss and the Life Course

Human lives are shaped by a diverse range of factors, some of which are relatively fixed (e.g. gender, ethnicity) whilst others may change over the life course (e.g. health and disability, socio-economic status, sexual orientation), with the physical environment, economic upheavals and social change also having cumulative effects in later life [3–5]. Grief is commonly seen as the response to bereavement, which 'confronts people with some of the most stressful adaptational challenges that humans experience' [6]. Where grief is complicated, it is said to be characterized by difficulty in

---

B. Bartlam, MA, PhD (✉)
Research Institute for Primary Care and Health Sciences, Keele University,
Keele, Staffordshire, UK
e-mail: b.bartlam@keele.ac.uk

L. Machin, MA, PhD
Research Institute for Social Sciences, Keele University, Keele, Staffordshire, UK
e-mail: l.machin@keele.ac.uk

© Springer International Publishing Switzerland 2016
C.A. Chew-Graham, M. Ray (eds.), *Mental Health and Older People:
A Guide for Primary Care Practitioners*, DOI 10.1007/978-3-319-29492-6_3

functioning in work and in social relationships, a sense of meaninglessness, prolonged yearning for the deceased and disruption in personal beliefs. It also carries an increased risk of depression, generalized anxiety and panic disorder, alcohol abuse and use of medications, sudden cardiac events and suicide [7, 8]. Yet loss and change over the life course are intrinsic to the human condition, and grief responses can be triggered by a wide variety of circumstances and events, not just bereavement. The timing and nature of events can either support or disrupt the expected flow of life across age stages [2, 4]. For example, particular individual experiences of loss may result from broken or damaged relationships such as divorce; abuse; illness; disability (chronic or acute); disappointment in unfulfilled ambitions, e.g. childlessness; and bereavement through traumatic or untimely death [9]. All of these experiences occur within a wider social, economic and political environment which itself may provide supportive and fulfilling life opportunities or may generate other losses such as poverty, poor housing or unemployment [10, 11]. Acquiring a capacity to cope with significant life changes demands an acceptance of the implicit losses and the feelings associated with them along with appropriate adjustment to altered social circumstances. Evidence of effective coping demonstrates resilience and is characterized by positive self-esteem, courage, flexibility, optimism and finding meaning within the experience of loss and change (see Fig. 3.1) [9].

For older people, loss and change will have shaped past experience, and current losses may be multiple and complex, in particular the prevalence of ill-health and long-term conditions increases with advancing age [12]. Such loss experiences may promote psychological and behavioural competence within an individual or be accrued as unresolved developmental tasks [13].

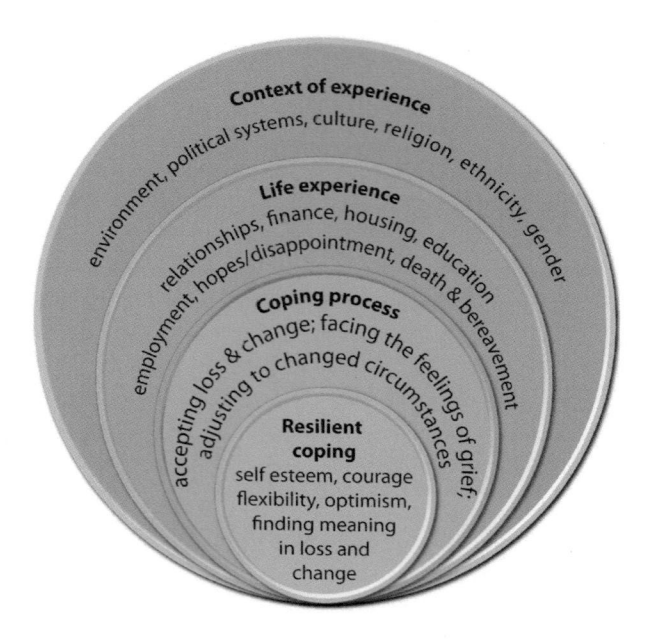

Fig. 3.1 Ageing well with loss

3.2 The Challenge for Practice

Losses such as these have potential implications for mental health as individuals react to them and seek to cope with their consequences. The Mental Health Strategy for England (2011) emphasizes the importance of addressing mental health problems, particularly when these are co-morbid with physical health problems [14]. Having a long-term condition can bring with it various losses, and depression and anxiety are more common in such individuals for whom it worsens the prognosis, and psychological health outcomes and adversely affects overall quality of life [15–17]. Depression and loneliness are strongly associated, and longitudinal work has reported loneliness as an independent risk factor for future depression [18, 19]. It is associated with a high degree of morbidity including poor physical and mental health/function and also with increased mortality, whilst those with adequate social relationships have a 50 % greater likelihood of survival compared to those with poor or insufficient social relationships [20–23]. Loneliness is often a consequence of bereavement, particularly in spousal bereavement or divorce, and loneliness and low social interaction are predictive of suicide in older age [24]. Loneliness is associated with increased health and social services utilization, with lonely people more likely to visit their GP and have higher use of medication, higher incidence of falls and increased risk factors for long-term care, including early entry into residential or nursing care [20, 25, 26].

3.3 Ageing Well in the Face of Cumulative Losses: The Range of Response to Loss Model

In the light of such evidence, and given the changing demography in terms of ageing populations (see Chap. 1), developing theoretical and practical frameworks that can both identify how an individual is dealing with loss and support them in the assimilation of inevitable, cumulative and complex losses into positive later life experiences, rather than them being accepted as an inevitable and negative consequence of ageing, is a critically important challenge. The Range of Response to Loss (RRL) model offers one such theoretical framework [9, 27]. The Adult Attitude to Grief (AAG) scale, which reflects the concepts in the RRL model, offers a tool for practitioners and patients to identify both core reactions and dominant coping responses in the face of loss(es) [9, 28] and consider the most appropriate intervention to enhance coping and improve outcomes.

The RRL model conceptualizes grief as a two-dimensional interactive process made up of, first, core reflexive reactions to loss and, second, coping responses made in the active management of loss and its consequences [29, 30]. In the RRL model, these dimensions are represented by a spectrum of contrasting characteristics (see Fig. 3.2).

Core reactions are represented on a spectrum of a state of being *overwhelmed* in which the distress of grief is dominant to a *controlled* state in which the instinct to suppress expressions of grief dominates. *Coping responses* can be seen in a range from vulnerable to resilient. Most people will be vulnerable immediately after a significant

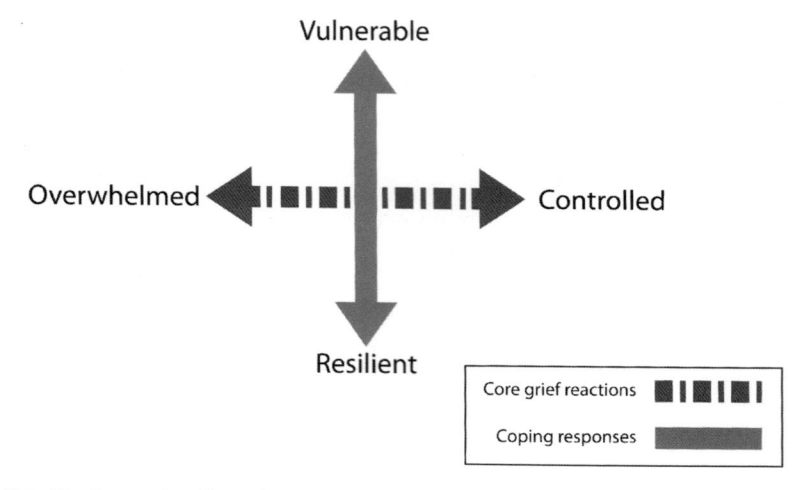

Fig. 3.2 The interacting dimensions of the range of response to loss model

loss as their own resources and those of supportive others may not yet be operationalized. However, when there is an increased capacity to acknowledge and accept those things which are irreversibly changed and those things which can be actively pursued in managing the loss and its consequences, living well with loss becomes possible.

3.4 Developing a Practice Tool: The Adult Attitude to Grief Scale

The AAG self-report scale provides a clear profile of the overwhelmed or controlled grief reactions and the vulnerable or resilient responses to loss (see Table 3.1). The scale consists of nine items devised to test the validity of the categories initially making up the RRL model – overwhelmed, controlled and balance/resilience. The items are scored on a Likert scale of 5 categories from 'strongly agree' to 'strongly disagree'. In addition to supporting the factor structure of the RRL model, research suggested the practical potential of the AAG, based on its capacity to profile the combination of factors unique to an individual and their experience of grief and its face validity for both practitioners and patients [9, 31].

With the development of the RRL model to include vulnerability as the spectrum opposite to resilience, research validated the use of the AAG to calculate an indication of this new component, by reversing the resilient item scores and adding them to the overwhelmed and controlled item scores, gives a range from 0 to 36: O + C   R = V [28]. The research determined statistically the optimum cut-off scores on the scale for the classification of different levels of vulnerability:

Severe vulnerability	>24
High vulnerability	21–23
Low vulnerability	<20

Table 3.1 Adult attitude to grief scoring and comment sheet

Client number   Date   Session number

Vulnerability indicator scores: R = Resilient C= Controlled O = Overwhelmed

Adult attitude to grief scale	Strongly agree	Agree	Neither agree nor disagree	Disagree	Strongly disagree	Additional responses/comments
R 1. I feel able to face the pain which comes with loss	0	1	2	3	4	
O 2. For me, it is difficult to switch off thoughts about the person I have lost	4	3	2	1	0	
R 3. I feel very aware of my inner strength when faced with grief	0	1	2	3	4	
C 4. I believe that I must be brave in the face of loss	4	3	2	1	0	
O 5. I feel that I will always carry the pain of grief with me	4	3	2	1	0	
C 6. For me, it is important to keep my grief under control	4	3	2	1	0	
O 7. Life has less meaning for me after this loss	4	3	2	1	0	
C 8. I think its best just to get on with life and not dwell on this loss[a]	4	3	2	1	0	
R 9. It may not always feel like it but I do believe that I will come through this experience of grief	0	1	2	3	4	

©Linda Machin 2010

[a]Modified 2013 (resilient scores reversed to allow for a simple addition) Vulnerability indicator scores = total score for the 9 items

Additionally, cross-tabulation of the AAG scores with the demographic and clinical research data provided an indication of the characteristics associated with severe and high vulnerability. The following key factors were identified:

- Age under 25 and over 76
- Loss of a child
- Grief reactions: inability to accept the death, powerful distress/despair and difficulty in day-to-day functioning
- Coping responses: difficulty dealing with one's own feelings and difficulty dealing with the meaning of loss
- Complicating factors: mental health problems and financial problems
- Social factors: isolation

These findings are consistent with established risk factors for morbidity and mortality in grieving people and link with other specific studies relating to mental health issues in later life [32].

3.5 Implications for Practice

Widening access to appropriate mental health care is a public health policy priority in the UK [33]. However, a major concern in the study of grief throughout most of the twentieth century has been with the complicated psychological consequences of bereavement [34–39]. More recently the focus has moved to recognition of the huge variability in grief reactions and evidence that the majority of grieving people demonstrate resilience and satisfactorily adjust to loss [40–42]. This rise in positive psychology has provided a less pathological perspective on grief and one which suggests that resilience is more universal than previous theories of grief might have suggested [43, 44]. The focus on resilience within the RRL, therefore, not only gives a less pessimistic view of loss and grief but an important therapeutic focus when addressing vulnerability. These are hugely encouraging factors when thinking about loss in later life.

'The family physician is the only specialist who, through his or her position in the health system and in the community, can give emotional support to the bereaved and simultaneously deal with the health problems associated with the process' [45]. This is true of non-bereavement losses also. Moreover, failure to intervene appropriately with those who are most vulnerable results in an increased demand for health and social care resources, and mitigating the negative outcomes of loss and bereavement is, therefore, a significant issue for public and personal health [8]. Finally, recent review of the literature highlighted the importance of ensuring that more intensive interventions are targeted at those with greatest need and who are most likely to benefit [46].

Matching health and social care resources to individual loss needs requires careful assessment and review. At the time of writing, the Patient Health Questionnaire and the General Anxiety Disorder scale are commonly used in primary care in the UK to assess the severity of depression and anxiety, respectively [47, 48]. Whilst depression and anxiety can be important consequences of loss, neither of these scales captures the individual expression and experiences of grief more widely evident in bereaved people. Current research and practice experience suggest that the AAG offers practitioners a concise and easy-to-use tool that does exactly that, and, in doing so, both empower patients (by offering insight) and enable practitioners to target appropriate resources to those most in need. Moreover, it facilitates the comprehensive, holistic person-centred approach to care that has been identified as best practice [49]. Given the growing population with more complex needs and the importance of tailoring interventions to meet the individual needs and preferences of patients, the full range of support available should be considered, from voluntary sector befriending and social interventions to specialist mental health services [50, 51].

3.6 Practice Audit

To remain responsive to diverse and changing populations of older people, we need to understand how our existing services can better tailor mental health treatments. With that in mind, a number of audit opportunities present themselves:

- Using the AAG to facilitate practitioner-patient dialogue and understanding of the impact of particular loss(es)
- Using the AAG as a baseline from which to identify vulnerability and refer onto other services
- Follow-up use of the AAG to indicate change over time and establish whether the intervention has resulted in increased resilience
- Identifying the acceptability of the AAG to patients
- Identifying the acceptability of any resulting referral intervention to patients and what other sources of support might be helpful

3.7 Next Steps

Whilst bereavement is associated with significant morbidity and mortality, the evidence on which health and social care practitioners can base their practice remains limited [52]. The situation holds true also when working with older people experiencing multiple losses, of which bereavement may be just one. Existing practice use of the AAG scale suggests that it is simple to use and has face validity, i.e. patients are able to relate their own grief to the items in the scale and experience it as providing some normality for the sense of emotional and mental turmoil generated by their loss [31]. It has the potential to provide practitioners with a tool able to distinguish those most in need of support either within the context of primary care or for referral on to other services, as well as identifying change over time. Interest and enthusiasm for the model and the scale have been reflected in their adoption in palliative and bereavement care contexts and in the recognition given to their contribution to contemporary theories of bereavement needs assessment [53–55].

Supported by the expertise of CORE Information Management Systems (CORE ims)[1] in routine outcome measurement, plans are being made for the wider use of the AAG. Part of this cooperative development with CORE aims to establish a learning collaborative across the bereavement care sector as the catalyst and context for further research and enhanced professional practice. It is anticipated that a learning collaborative will contribute to a growing evidence base on the use of the AAG in a wide variety of settings and amongst different population experiences a range of losses.

In reflecting the concepts in the RRL model, the AAG provides a profile of the psychological distress prompted by the loss(es) experienced, identifies the possibilities that may positively counter any negative consequences and can provide the basis for exploring the resources needed to face the pain and harness of such possibilities. By recognizing that grief is not only a reaction to loss but is a process of actively coping with its consequences, the RRL, and with it the AAG, points to the multi-factored possibilities for living well with loss.

References

1. Baars J, Dannefer D, Phillipson C, Walker A. Aging, globalization, and inequality: the new critical gerontology. Baywood Pub., 2006; eScholarID:188594.
2. Phillipson C. The political economy of longevity: developing new forms of solidarity for later life. Sociol Q. 2015;56(1):80–100. doi:10.1111/tsq.12082. eScholarID:236924.
3. Elder Jr GH. The life course in time and place. In: Heinz, Marshal, editors. Social dynamics of the life course: transitions, institutions and social relations. New York: Walter de Gruyter; 2003. p. 57–72.
4. Walker A, editor. Understanding quality of life in old age. Maidenhead: Open University Press/McGraw Hill; 2005.
5. Phillipson C. Ageing. Cambridge: Wiley; 2013. eScholarID:185275.
6. Folkman S. Revised coping theory and the process of bereavement. In: Stroebe MS, Hansson RO, Stroebe W, Schut H, editors. Handbook of bereavement research. Washington: American Psychological Association; 2001. p. 563–84.
7. Parkes CM, Weiss RS. Recovery from bereavement. New York: Basic; 1983.
8. Stroebe W, Stroebe MS. Bereavement and health. Cambridge: Cambridge University Press; 1987.
9. Machin L. Working with loss and grief. 2nd ed. London: Sage; 2014.
10. Carr D, Jeffreys JS. In: Neimeyer RA, Harris DL, Winokeur HR, Thornton GF, editors. Spousal bereavement in later life in grief and bereavement in contemporary society: bridging research and practice. New York: Routledge; 2011. p. 81–91.
11. O'Rand AM, Isaacs K, Roth L. In: Dannefer D, Phillipson C, editors. Age and inequality in global context in the sage handbook of social gerontology. Los Angeles: Sage; 2013. p. 127–36.
12. Age UK. Healthy ageing evidence review. Available on-line at: 2010. http://www.ageuk.org.uk/Documents/EN-GB/For-professionals/Health-and-wellbeing/Evidence%20Review%20Healthy%20Ageing.pdf?dtrk=true.
13. Erikson EH. Identity and the lifecycle: a reissue. New York: W. W. Norton; 1980.

---

[1] CORE ims is a not-for-profit leader in the field of routine outcome measurement in mental health psychological therapies, which delivers and supports validated, reliable routine measurement tools (http://www.coreims.co.uk).

14. Department of Health. No health without mental health. 2011. https://www.gov.uk/government/uploads/system/uploads/attachment_data/file/213761/dh_124058.pdf.
15. Anderson R, Freedland K, Clouse R, Lustman P. The prevalence of comorbid depression in adults with diabetes: a meta-analysis. Diabetes Care. 2001;24:1069–78.
16. Katon W, Ciechanowski P. Impact of major depression on chronic medical illness. J Psychosom Res. 2002;53:859–63.
17. Mercer SW, Gunn J, Wyke S. Improving the health of people with multimorbidity: the need for prospective cohort studies. J Comorbidity. 2011;1(1):4–7. http://www.jcomorbidity.com/index.php/test/article/view/10.
18. Heikkinen RL, Kauppinen M. Depressive symptoms in late life: a 10-year follow-up. Arch Gerontol Geriatr. 2004;38:239–50.
19. Cacioppo JT, Hughes ME, Waite LJ, Hawkley LC, Thisted RA. Loneliness as a specific risk factor for depressive symptoms: cross-sectional and longitudinal analyses. Psychol Aging. 2006;21(1):140–51.
20. O'Luanaigh CO, Lawler BA. Loneliness and the health of older people. Int J Geriatr Psychiatry. 2008;23:1213–21.
21. James BD, Wilson RS, Barnes LL, Bennett DA. Late-life social activity and cognitive decline in old age. J Int Neuropsychol Soc. 2011;17(6):998–1005. http://www.ncbi.nlm.nih.gov/pubmed/22040898.
22. Lyyra T-M, Heikinnen RL. Perceived social support and mortality in older people. J Gerontol. 2006;61B(3):S147–52.
23. Holt-Lunstad J, Smith TB, Layton JB. Social relationships and mortality risk: a meta-analytic review. PLoS Med. 2010;7(7):e1000316. http://www.plosmedicine.org/article/fetchObject.action?uri=info%3Adoi%2F10.1371%2Fjournal.pmed.1000316&representation=PDF.
24. O'Connell H, Chin A, Cunnigham C, Lawlor B. Recent developments: suicide in older people. Br Med J. 2004;29:895–9.
25. Cohen GD, Perstein S, Chapline J, Kelly J, Firth KM, Simmens S. The impact of professionally conducted cultural programs on the physical health, mental health, and social functioning of older adults. Gerontologist. 2006;46(6):726–34. doi:10.1093/geront/46.6.726.
26. Russell DW, Cutrona CE, de la Mora A, Wallace RB. Loneliness and nursing home admission among rural older adults. Psychol Aging. 1997;12(4):574–89 [PubMed].
27. Machin L. Exploring a framework for understanding the range of response to loss; a study of clients receiving bereavement counselling. Unpublished PhD thesis: Keele: Keele University; 2001.
28. Sim J, Machin L, Bartlam B. Identifying vulnerability in grief: psychometric properties of the adult attitude to grief scale. Qual Life Res. 2013. doi:10.1007/s11136-013-0551-1.
29. Attig T. How we grieve: relearning the world. revisedth ed. New York: Oxford University Press; 2011.
30. Stroebe MS, Folkman S, Hansson RO, Schut H. The prediction of bereavement outcome: development of an integrative risk factor framework. Soc Sci Med. 2006;63:2440–51.
31. Machin L, Spall R. Mapping grief: a study in practice using a quantitative and qualitative approach to exploring and addressing the range of response to loss. Couns Psychother Res. 2004;4:9–17.
32. Sanders CM. Risk factors in bereavement outcome. In: Stroebe MS, Stroebe W, Hansson RO, editors. Handbook of bereavement. Cambridge: Cambridge University Press; 1993. p. 255–67.
33. Department of Health. Closing the gap: priorities for essential change in mental health. London: Department of Health; 2014.
34. Parkes CM. Bereavement: studies of grief in adult life. London: Routledge; 1972/1989/1996.
35. Raphael B. The anatomy of bereavement. London: Unwin Hyman; 1984.
36. Mikulincer M, Florian V. The relationship between adult attachment styles and emotional and cognitive reactions to stressful events. In: Simpson JA, Rholes WS, editors. Attachment theory and close relationships. New York: Guilford Press; 1998. p. 143–65.
37. Cassidy J, Shaver PR, editors. Handbook of attachment: theory, research and clinical application. New York: Guilford Press; 1999.

38. Fraley RC, Shaver PR. Loss and bereavement: attachment theory and recent controversies concerning grief work and the nature of detachment. In: Cassidy J, Shaver PR, editors. Handbook of attachment: theory, research, and clinical applications. New York: Guilford; 1999. p. 735–59.
39. Parkes CM. Love and loss – the roots of grief and its complications. London: Routledge; 2006.
40. Stroebe M. Coping with bereavement: a review of the grief work hypothesis. Omega. 1992/1993;26:19–42.
41. Stroebe M, Schut H. The dual process model of coping with bereavement: rationale and description. Death Stud. 1999;23:197–224.
42. Bonanno GA. Loss, trauma and human resilience. Am Psychol. 2004;59(1):20–8.
43. Seligman MEP. Building human strength: psychology's forgotten mission. Am Psychol Assoc Monit. 1998;29:1.
44. Bonanno GA, Papa A, O'Neill K. Loss and human resilience. Appl Prev Psychol. 2002;10:193–206.
45. Garcia-Garcia JA, Landa V. The provision of grief services by primary care physicians. Eur J Palliat Care. 2006;13(4):45.
46. Arthur A, James M, Stanton W, Seymour J. Bereavement care services: a synthesis of the literature. London: Department of Health; 2010. https://www.gov.uk/government/uploads/system/uploads/attachment_data/file/215799/dh_123810.pdf.
47. Kroenke K, Spitzer RL. The PHQ-9: a new depression and diagnostic severity measure. Psychiatr Ann. 2002;32:509–21.
48. Spitzer RL, Kroenka K, Williams J. A brief measure for assessing generalised anxiety disorder. The GAD –7. Arch Intern Med. 2006;166:1092–7.
49. Royal College of General Practitioners. The GP consultation in practice. 2010. http://www.gmc-uk.org/2_01_The_GP_consultation_in_practice_May_2014.pdf_56884483.pdf.
50. National Health Service England. Improving general practice: a call to action. 2013. http://www.england.nhs.uk/wp-content/uploads/2013/09/igp-cta-evid.pdf.
51. Lovell K, Gask L, Bower P, Waheed W, Chew-Graham C, Aseem S, Beatty S, Burroughs H, Clarke P, Dowrick A, Edwards S, Gabbay M, Lamb J, Lloyd-Williams M, Dowrick C. Development and evaluation of culturally sensitive psychosocial interventions for under-served people in primary care. BMC Psychiatry. 2014;14:217. doi:10.1186/s12888-014-0217-8.
52. Nagraj S, Barclay S. Bereavement care in primary care: a systematic literature review and narrative synthesis. Br J Gen Pract. 2011;61(582):e42–8. doi:10.3399/bjgp11X549009.
53. Relf M, Machin L, Archer N. Guidance for bereavement needs assessment in palliative care. London: Help the Hospices; 2008/2010.
54. Brocklehurst T, Hearnshaw C, Machin L. Bereavement needs assessment – piloting a process. Prog Palliat Care. 2014;22(3):143–9.
55. Agnew A, Manktelow R, Taylor BJ, Jones L. Bereavement needs assessment in specialist palliative care: a review of the literature. Palliat Med. 2009;24:46–59.

Policy Context for Mental Health and Older People

Mo Ray

4.1 Introduction

The 'problem' of old age dominated post-war old age policy and practice, and for years after its abolition in 1948, the Poor Law continued to exert a considerable influence on progress in policy and practice. Expectations about the care of older people were low, fuelled by assumptions of inevitable decline, and institutional care continued to be the assumed means by which formal care was provided. At the time of publication of Townsend's study 'The Last Refuge' [1], three fifths of elderly people admitted to residential care were accommodated in buildings originally commissioned as public assistance institutions. Accommodation and care were characterised by impoverished environments and harsh, institutional regimes. Other older people in institutional care were accommodated in long-stay hospitals, or hospital wards.

The aspiration to close long-stay institutions and hospital wards and to develop community responses for people in need of formal care, including older people, was a sustained political aspiration from the 1950s. 'Care in the Community', as it became known, was generally considered to be less expensive than long-stay institutional care and, at the same time, was seen as a humane and sensitive, if poorly fleshed out, policy [2]. But despite successive attempts to accelerate deinstitutionalisation and develop more comprehensive and imaginative community-based services for older people, progress over the next two decades remained very slow (for a full analysis and discussion, refer to Means et al. [3]). Residential care continued to occupy a central and assumed supremacy in the care of older people. It is against this backdrop that subsequent policy has attempted to modernise

M. Ray, PhD
Gerontological Social Work and Programme, School of Social Science and Public Policy,
Keele University, Keele, Staffordshire, UK
e-mail: m.g.ray@keele.ac.uk

services for older people with care needs and, specifically, with mental health problems.

Policy is not developed and implemented as a rational, linear progression but is, rather, developed incrementally, and its progress is shaped and influenced by numerous factors [4]. Political ideology, views about the role of the state in funding care for older people, the economy, the state of knowledge about what 'works' best or is considered most desirable and the ways in which older people are perceived and the priority they are accorded against other priority groups are just some examples of potential barriers or facilitators to policy development. Health and welfare policy for older people with mental health problems illustrates the incremental, fragmented and often slow nature of policy development. Considerable distance frequently exists between policy rhetoric, on the one hand, and the practical realities of service development and delivery, on the other [5]. As awareness of the mental health needs of older people grew, it was realised that policy and practice had paid insufficient attention to older people who were living with dementia, with depression and anxiety and complex needs surrounding co-existing, long-term physical and mental health needs [6]. Despite a considerable growth in policy over the past 20 years, espousing the development of comprehensive, accessible and coordinated mental health services for older people as a priority, the impact of factors such as the priority older people with mental health problems was accorded, age-based discrimination, and low expectations have been pervasive features inhibiting its development.

This chapter reviews some of the key policy developments in mental health for older people over the past 15 years which is arguably when a greater focus on mental health and old age policy became evident. The focus here is on public policy rather than on the significant legislative changes that have taken place over a similar period which are more fully addressed in Chap. 27.

4.2   Policy and Older People's Mental Health

Older people were not included in the National Service Framework (NSF) for Mental Health [7] which arguably confirmed the relative marginalisation of older people against other people with mental health problems. Prior to the publication of the National Service Framework for Older people [8], an Audit Commission report [9] evidenced a number of fundamental gaps in policy and practice in mental health services for older people. Recommendations for improvement included the implementation of a full range of accessible, community- and home-based services, improvements in access to a full range of therapeutic interventions, which at the time were almost non-existent for older people, and addressing significant geographical disparities in service provision. The report urged the development of a coherent service model which was acknowledged to be fragmented, uncoordinated and variable in quality. The National Service Framework for Older People [8] included a standard addressing mental health and core priorities across all areas of service delivery (e.g. recognition that mental health promotion was as crucial for older people as people across the rest of the life course, the under detection of mental health problems such as depression, improving diagnosis for people with cognitive impairment, access to therapeutic interventions and access to appropriate occupational opportunities for people living in care homes). Many of these priorities evidenced the significant gaps in older persons' mental health services and drew attention to the underpinning goal of the NSF which was to remove age-based discrimination and offer high-quality and equitable services based on need.

Subsequent policies continued to reflect the challenge of modernising services and to highlight the need for investment to bring about the levels of improvement that were needed [e.g. 10, 11]. The report 'Everybody's Business' [11] and a number of subsequent policies [12, 13] endorsed the service model proposed in the NSF and confirmed a number of core principles central to successful modernisation of mental health services:

- The involvement of service users and carers in service development, delivery and evaluation
- Person-centred planning
- Integrated, accessible and culturally appropriate services
- Basing service development on what works
- Workforce development
- A whole system approach to integrated services ranging from preventative, mental health promotion to inpatient care
- Equitable services – No services should exclude a person on the basis of their age, gender, sexual orientation or race

Despite the plethora of policies highlighting the importance of modernising mental health services and ending age-based discrimination, *Living Well in Later Life* [14] commented that an exception to the decline in age discrimination in health services was mental health. Here, it was argued, the organisational division between mental health service for adults of working age, and older people, continued to result in an unfair system.

By the end of the period between 2000 and 2010, a welter of policies, including the 'New Horizons' shared vision for mental health [15], presented overwhelming evidence of age-based discrimination in mental health services, persistent variations in the quality and availability of a full range of accessible services and poor awareness of mental health needs in older age [15–18]. The Centre for Policy on Ageing comments that 'the ten years from 1999 to 2009 has seen an increased focus on older people's issues. Concern at the state of mental health services for older people in the UK has been reflected in the publication of a large number of key reports relating to older people's mental health services, identifying the need to address age discrimination and to bring about significant improvements in service provision' [19].

Superseding the 'New Horizons' strategy, a cross-government strategy, taking a life course approach, focused on mental health outcomes for people of all ages [20]. The strategy defined six key objectives:

- More people will have good mental health.
- More people with mental health problems will recover.
- More people with mental health problems will have good physical health.
- More people will have positive experiences of help and support.
- Fewer people will suffer avoidable harm.
- Fewer people will experience stigma and discrimination.

Similar strategy documents address the mental health and wellbeing of populations in Scotland [21], Wales [22] and Northern Ireland [23].

4.2.1 Together for Mental Health: A Strategy for Mental Health and Wellbeing in Wales (2015) [22]

- The mental health and wellbeing of the whole population is improved.
- The impact of mental health problems and/or mental illness on individuals of all ages, their families and carers, communities and the economy more widely, is better recognised and reduced.
- Inequalities, stigma and discrimination suffered by people experiencing mental health problems and mental illness are reduced.
- Individuals have a better experience of the support and treatment they receive and have an increased feeling of input and control over related decisions.
- Access to, and the quality of preventative measures, early intervention and treatment services are improved and more people recover as a result.
- The values, attitudes and skills of those treating or supporting individuals of all ages with mental health problems or mental illness are improved.

All of the strategic documents recognise the importance of social determinants and life course inequality on mental health and wellbeing. The English strategy document, for example, included a focus on the prevalence and continued under-recognition of older people living with depression and associated risk factors. The experience of social isolation as a social determinant of mental ill health was cited as an example of a significant risk factor for some groups of older people. Older people were identified in the strategy as a priority group for further investment in psychological therapies with the intention of monitoring their access to those services.

The visibility and priority of older peoples' mental health was further supported by a growing number of practice guidance documents with evidence-based recommendations for driving up standards in practice and improving care. For example, the Social Care Institute for Excellence (SCIE) published extensive guidance on assessment practices with older people with mental health problems [24] and supporting positive and inclusive communication with people with dementia [25]. The NICE/SCIE guideline in supporting people with dementia and their carers in health and social care [26] provided a detailed and comprehensive evidence-based guideline based on the whole person. The Royal College of General Practitioners [27] developed guidance for practitioners to raise awareness of the importance of detecting depression amongst older people, and NICE [28] has produced a quality standard to support and promote good mental health and wellbeing amongst older people living in care homes.

Nevertheless, from a public policy perspective, a review by the National Audit Office [29] concluded that dementia services in England were not providing value for money to taxpayers or people with dementia. Nor had dementia been accorded the same priority as other conditions, such as cancer and heart disease, and thus had not had the same opportunity for improvement. The Department of Health subsequently identified dementia as a national health and social care priority [30], which ultimately led to the development of the first national Dementia Strategy for England [31]. The devolved nations of Great Britain have also developed dementia strategies to reflect the needs of their countries and communities [32–35] but with substantial overlap in terms of core priorities for development.

4.3 Policy Focus on Dementia

The vision underpinning the English dementia strategy made clear that its achievement would support and enable people living with dementia to 'live well'. Comprehensive recommendations included: improvement in dementia awareness, challenging stigma, improving diagnosis and early detection and developing effective and integrated improvements in treatment and interventions.

Subsequently, and in response to growing concerns about its (mis)use [36], an investigation into the use of antipsychotic (AP) medication with people with dementia was commissioned [37]. The investigation concluded that the use of antipsychotic medication was frequently and inappropriately used as a first line of intervention when other approaches should be used. The adverse effects and risks associated with AP medication for many people outweighed the benefit. With the overarching aim of reducing inappropriate prescribing, the report made a number of recommendations including providing specialist services to support primary care practitioners and care teams in residential and nursing homes working with people with complex needs and improving assessment and intervention skills in primary care, home settings and in hospital. Crucially, the report prioritised the importance of developing the evidence based on the use of nonpharmacological interventions and particularly highlighted older people living in care homes and their need for improved psychosocial intervention and sustained and valued occupational opportunity and engagement in day-to-day life.

Despite the apparent prominence given to the publication of the dementia strategy, evidence suggests that at its inception, it was insufficiently embedded as a core priority for improvement [38]. The National Audit Office [29] concluded that local leadership and joined up working was slow to develop and patchy and that there was much to do to 'ignite passion, pace and drive'. Steps to prioritise dementia in national outcomes frameworks such as the Commissioning for Quality and Innovation (CQUIN), the appointment of a national clinical leader for dementia, national awareness campaigns and the Prime Minister's challenge are examples of initiatives that have contributed to maintaining a focus on dementia. For example, the number of people being assessed by memory clinics has increased fourfold since 2010. An audit on the prescribing of AP medication for people with dementia demonstrated a reduction of 52 % between 2008 and 2011. The Royal College of Psychiatrists [39] audited the care of people with dementia in hospital and identified some improvement including growth in the number of hospitals with named dementia champions, some improvement in recording that a patient has dementia and information which may assist in providing appropriate care (e.g. communication, personal preferences, significant people).

The English dementia strategy ran its course and the All Parliamentary Group on dementia have called for a second strategy. Despite evidence of improvement in dementia care and support, there are still very significant areas for development, and the group cites the need for improved post-diagnostic support, advice and information; dementia leadership, the need to develop quality of life measures for dementia; and the continued need for culture change towards dementia and people living with the condition, their carers and professionals in the field of dementia care.

The Prime Minister's 'dementia challenges' [40, 41] received significant national and international attention and initially focused on priorities identified in the dementia strategy (e.g. developing awareness, receiving early diagnosis and appropriate support and living well with dementia). The subsequent challenge focused on research, meaningful care and support following diagnosis and growth in the number of people identified as dementia friends and the number of dementia-friendly communities.

4.3.1 Dementia-Friendly Communities and Places: Practice Examples

The Alzheimer's Society as part of their 5-year strategy will work with people living with dementia and their supporters to define and develop dementia-friendly communities (http://www.alzheimers.org.uk/site/scripts/documents_info.php?documentID=1843) [42].

Dementia Without Walls – Joseph Rowntree Foundation – this initiative has three main strands:

- Strengthening the voice of people living with dementia.
- Thinking and talking differently about dementia.

- Supporting the development of dementia-friendly communities. This element of the project has commissioned projects in Northern Ireland, Scotland, Wales and England and hosts a variety of resources related to dementia-friendly design and development as well as a number of legacy projects emanating from the 'Dementia Without Walls' initiative (http://www.jrf.org.uk/topic/dementia-without-walls) [43].

Design at the Dementia Services Development Centre, Stirling – the Design Centre aims to improve design for people with dementia (work includes design in hospitals, care homes, communities, housing) and provides bespoke advice, design services and training and professional development (http://dementia.stir.ac.uk/design) [44].

Dementia-Friendly Wales – with funding from the Welsh Government Intermediate Care Fund, a project has developed to raise awareness of dementia and make the environment dementia friendly (http://www.dementiafriendlybrecon.org.uk/welsh_government_funding_for_dementia_friendly_powys) [45].

Enhancing the healing environment at the Kings Fund – Multidisciplinary teams worked in partnership with service users to improve the environment where care was delivered. A number of resources are available to enable hospitals, care homes, primary care premises and specialist housing providers to become more dementia friendly. The project worked with over 250 organisations and has a completed project directory (http://www.kingsfund.org.uk/projects/enhancing-healing-environment/completed-projects) [46].

The Enhancing Healing Environments initiative is now completed at the Kings Fund and has transferred to the Association for Dementia Studies at Worcester University (http://www.worcester.ac.uk/discover/ads-enhancing-the-healing-programme.html) [47].

Dementia-Friendly Northern Ireland with joint funding from the Northern Ireland government and the charitable trust Atlantic Philanthropies, the Dementia Services Development Centre is focusing on improving the lives of people living with dementia by promoting dementia-friendly communities and the implementation of the Northern Ireland Regional Dementia Strategy. http://dementia.stir.ac.uk/communities/dementia-friendly-northern-ireland [48].

The Debenham Project – recognised as the UK's foremost rural dementia-friendly community providing a wide range of help and support, dementia-friendly and accessible resources (http://www.the-debenham-project.org.uk/index.html) [49].

The UK used its presidency of the G8 (eight nations comprising France, Germany, Italy, the United Kingdom, Japan, the United States, Canada and Russia, who take turns to host an annual meeting to promote understanding and consensus on issues of global significance) to host a dementia summit [50]. The summit focused on three areas of discussion: improving life and care for people living with dementia and their carers, preventing and delaying dementia and social adaptation to dementia. A number of aspirations were identified by the summit which included the development of disease-modifying or curative treatment by 2025, an increase in the amount spent on dementia research, the recruitment of a global envoy for dementia innovation, the development of an international agenda for research and sharing information and data on research across G8 countries.

Reviewing plans in 11 countries, Alzheimer's Disease International and BUPA [51] have published a distillation of approaches in the development of national dementia plans. The authors argue that a national dementia plan is the most powerful tool to improve dementia care and support and identify best practice in content, development and implementation of plans. The Organisation for Economic Cooperation and Development (OECD) [52] has highlighted the imperative for global policy action on dementia, and the World Health Organisation (WHO) hosted their first ministerial conference on dementia in 2015 [53]. The subsequent call for action claimed that global efforts to support people living with dementia and a raft of associated measures should be accorded the highest priority.

4.4 Discussion

This chapter has briefly reviewed some of the very considerable array of public policy that has been published over the past two decades with the specific purpose of improving mental health services for older people. Persistent messages in mental health policy have focused on an urgent need to develop coherent, accessible and comprehensive services (see Sect. 4.3.1). Crucially, evidence that the progress and development of mental health services has been fundamentally influenced by age-based discrimination has led to a welter of policy calling for its removal from service development and delivery. Similarly, the need to address the stigma that is often associated with older age and older people living with mental health problems or dementia is also persistently argued.

Improvements in mental health services for older people are evident. The attention directed towards dementia and the priority that it has been accorded has seen significant and positive change in commissioning, service development, design and delivery. Nevertheless, it is clear that despite improvement, there is still a lot of work remaining. Research with carers of people living with dementia starkly illustrated the difficulties that people experience in accessing much needed advice and information [54]. All too often, research participants likened their struggles to metaphors associated with the battlefield. Thus, initial focus on detection and early diagnosis is of little use to many people living with dementia and their carers without benefit of comprehensive, accessible and timely advice and information and access to support services or signposting to appropriate services.

The focus on dementia clearly reflects a priority of paramount importance, but it is important that other mental health problems experienced by older people are not sidelined or overlooked. Living with depression continues to remain a significant area of health improvement and concern for those older people at particular risk – including older people living with dementia. Other areas of mental ill health continue to merit attention including suicide prevention and substance misuse, older people with learning disabilities and mental health problems and older people from black and minority ethnic groups. Detection and treatment are priorities but so too is the primary role of mental health promotion in older age. The multifaceted nature of mental health promotion involves working across and joining up various aspects of policy (e.g. arts and creativity, sport and recreation, education, housing, education, employment and transport) in order to develop coherent life course approaches which properly include later life.

Ageing is not a static experience, and mental health policy and practice must be responsive to diversity and change. For example, evidence demonstrates that older people with high support and complex needs are too often marginalised from meaningful participation in decisions about their own care and support; the potential risk of multiple disadvantage, inequitable access to mental health services and persistent concerns about poorer outcomes are evident for older people from black and minority ethnic groups. Older people who are asylum seekers or refugees constitute a small but significant presence in the UK and are described as some of the most marginalised of people. Lived experiences which may involve trauma, torture, imprisonment and stress associated with living in and leaving their country of origin, living in unsettled and unfamiliar conditions and anxieties associated with loss and separation suggest that asylum seekers and refugees are at an increased risk of developing mental health problems across the life course and including older age. As the so-called boomer generation continue to age, changes in behaviour such as the growth of late-life divorce will have potential implications for housing, financial stability in older age, social networks, increased likelihood of living alone and social isolation [55].

The persistence of ageism and stigma associated with mental health remains a pervasive challenge. Drawing attention to the existence of endemic age-based discrimination in policy is important, but unsurprisingly, arguing the case for its removal does not of itself address the problem. Action on all fronts is called for. The voice of older people living with high support needs remains significantly marginalised, and there is a continued need to find ways to enable those people to have a voice in their experience as patients and users and in the development and evaluation of services. Work by the Joseph Rowntree Foundation has highlighted this as a priority [56]. Examples such the user-led organisation the Scottish Dementia Working Group illustrate the tremendous achievements that can be made when people who use services are more fully involved in partnerships with other stakeholders traditionally responsible for strategy and service development and delivery.

The contemporary welfare policy focus is primarily concerned with notions of active ageing, independence and self-responsibility. Combined with the dichotomy that, on the one hand, practitioners must give person-centred care and, on the other, respond to increasing demands for efficiency and efficiency savings runs the risk that the space which older people with complex mental health problems can legitimately occupy becomes more tenuous. Lloyd [57] argues that how older people live towards the end of their lives is not well understood by researchers, policy makers and service providers. Developing theoretical understanding of ageing with complex needs is crucial to older people on the receiving end of care as well as those people and services who are responsible for giving care. Research exploring the role of dignity and care, for example, affirms the hard work and investment that older people make to maintain their health and independence in the face of challenges to their sense of self caused by the impact of illness [58]. Support and care sensitive to older peoples' individual experience is most likely to be care which enhances personal dignity. In her work on transitions and the life course, Grenier [59] argues that 'linking the social, cultural, psychological and personal processes that occur in relation to continuity and change could inform policy and practice for ageing and late life. The challenge at this point is whether governments and policy makers are open to hearing such detailed accounts that may profoundly challenge professional and standard accepted understandings of transition in late life'.

4.5 Questions for Reflection

- To what extent do you think your work environment provides a 'dementia-friendly' environment? What strategies and approaches could you use to develop projects which enhance the environment for people living with dementia?
- How are older people with mental health problems currently involved in service development and evaluation in your area? How might this be improved or developed and what would you need to think about to support those developments?
- In what ways does your organisation set about challenging age-based discrimination in mental health service development and delivery and what impact does it have?

4.6 Appendix 4.1 Useful Resources/Further Reading

Kings Fund Centre 'Enhancing the Healing Environment' (http://www.kingsfund.org.uk/projects/enhancing-healing-environment/completed-projects)

Resources and information to support the development of positive environments in collective care settings. Website includes material on dementia-friendly design.

Mental Health Foundation (2013) *Getting on… with life*: *Baby boomers, mental health and ageing*, London, Mental Health Foundation http://www.mentalhealth.org.uk/publications/getting-on-full-report/

Mind Matters Mental Health and Older People Future Focus Films limited https://www.youtube.com/watch?v=63f0lRvdB5s

Twenty-minute DVD raising awareness of mental health and wellbeing for older people. Interviews with older people experience psychological and emotional distress, their experience of illness and service use.

References

1. Townsend P. The last refuge: a survey of residential institutions and homes for the aged in England and Wales. London: Routledge, Kegan, Paul; 1962.
2. Parker R. Elderly people and community care: the policy background. In: Sinclair I, Parker R, Leat D, Williams J, editors. The kaleidoscope of care: a review of research and welfare provision for elderly people. London: National Institute of Social Work; 1990. p. 5–22.

3. Means R, Richards S, Smith R. Community care policy and practice. 3rd ed. Basingtoke: Palgrave Macmillan; 2003.
4. Davies C. Understanding the policy process. In: Fraser S, Matthews S, editors. The critical practitioner in social work and health care. London: Open University/Sage; 2008. p. 203–21.
5. Lester H, Glasby J. Mental health policy and practice. Basingstoke: Palgrave Macmillan; 2006.
6. Hurst P. What do you expect at your age? In: Williamson T, editor. Older people's mental health today: a handbook. London: Mental Health Foundation; 2009.
7. Department of Health. National service framework for mental health: modern standards and service models. London: Department of Health; 1999.
8. Department of Health. National service framework for older people. London: Department of Health; 2001.
9. Audit Commission. Forget me not: mental health services and older people. London: Audit Commission; 2000.
10. Department of Health. Securing better mental health in older adults. London: Department of Health; 2005.
11. Department of Health. Everybody's business: integrated mental health services for older adults: a service development guide. London: Department of Health; 2005.
12. Department of Health. A new ambition of old age: next steps in implementing the national service framework. London: Department of Health; 2006.
13. Care Services Improvement Partnership. A supplementary guidance for older people's mental health services. London: CSIP; 2007.
14. Commission for Social Care Inspection, Audit Commission and Health Care Commission. Living well into later life. London: CSCI, Audit Commission, Health Care Commission; 2006.
15. Department of Health. New horizons. London: Department of Health; 2009.
16. Health Care Commission. Equality in later life. London: Health Care Commission; 2009.
17. Mental Health Foundation. All things being equal: age equality in mental health care for older people in England. London: Mental Health Foundation; 2009.
18. Royal College of Psychiatrists. Age discrimination in mental health services: making equality a reality. (Royal College of Psychiatrists' position statement PS2/2009). 2009. http://www.mentalhealthequalities.org.uk/silo/files/age-discrimination-in-mental-health-services.pdf.
19. Centre for Policy on Ageing. Ageism and age discrimination in mental health care in the UK: a review from the literature. London: Centre for Policy on Ageing; 2009.
20. Department of Health. No health without mental health. London: Department of Health; 2011.
21. Scottish Government. Mental Health Strategy for Scotland 2012–2015. Edinburgh: Scottish Government; 2012. scotland.gov.uk/Publications/2012/08/9714/downloads#res398762.
22. Welsh Assembly Government. Better together for mental health: a strategy for mental health and wellbeing in Wales. 2012. http://gov.wales/docs/dhss/publications/130328mhsummaryen.pdf.
23. Department of Health, Social Services and Public Safety. Service framework for mental health and well being. Northern Ireland: Department of Health, Social Services and Public Safety; 2012. http://gov.wales/docs/dhss/publications/130328mhsummaryen.pdf.
24. Social Care Institute for Excellence. Assessing the mental health needs of older people. London: SCIE; 2006.
25. Social Care Institute for Excellence. Aiding communication with people with dementia: research briefing 3. London: Social Care Institute for Excellence; 2004. http://www.scie.org.uk/publications/briefings/briefing03/.
26. National Institute Clinical Excellence/Social Care Institute Excellence. Guideline on supporting people with dementia and their carers in health and social care: guideline 42. London: NICE/SCIE; 2007.
27. Royal College of General Practitioners. Management of depression in older people: why this is important to primary care. London: Royal College of General Practitioners; 2011.
28. National Institute for Health and Care Excellence. Mental well being in older people in care homes: quality standard 50. London: NICE; 2013.
29. National Audit Office. Improving dementia services in England: an interim report. London: NationalAuditOffice;2010.http://www.nao.org.uk/report/improving-dementia-services-in-england-an-interim-report/.

30. NHS Operating Framework. 2008. http://webarchive.nationalarchives.gov.uk/+/www.dh.gov.uk/en/publicationsandstatistics/publications/publicationspolicyandguidance/dh_081094.
31. Department of Health. Living well with dementia: a national dementia strategy. London: Department of Health; 2009.
32. Alzheimer's Society. National dementia vision for wales. 2009. http://www.wales.nhs.uk/healthtopics/conditions/dementia.
33. Scottish Government. Scotland's national dementia strategy. 2010. Edinburgh: Scottish Government.
34. Scottish Government. Scotland's national dementia strategy: 2013–16. 2013. Edinburgh: Scottish Government. http://www.gov.scot/Topics/Health/Services/Mental-Health/Dementia.
35. Department of Health. Ireland's national dementia strategy. Dublin: Department of Health; 2014. http://www.atlanticphilanthropies.org/sites/default/files/uploads/Irish-National-Dementia-Strategy-Eng.pdf.
36. All Party Parliamentary Group on Dementia. Always as a last resort: inquiry into the prescription of antipsychotic drugs to people with dementia in care homes. 2008. https://www.alzheimers.org.uk/site/scripts/download_info.php?fileID=322.
37. Banerjee S. The use of antipsychotic medication for people with dementia: time for action. London: Department of Health; 2009. https://www.rcpsych.ac.uk/pdf/Antipsychotic%20Bannerjee%20Report.pdf.
38. All Party Parliamentary Group on Dementia. A misspent opportunity? Inquiry into the funding of the NDS. 2010. https://www.alzheimers.org.uk/site/scripts/documents_info.php?documentID=1583&pageNumber=4.
39. Royal College of Psychiatrists. National Audit of Dementia. 2010. http://www.rcpsych.ac.uk/workinpsychiatry/qualityimprovement/nationalclinicalaudits/dementia/nationalauditofdementia.aspx.
40. Department of Health. Prime minister's challenge on dementia: delivering major improvements in dementia care and research by 2015. London: Department of Health; 2012.
41. Department of health. Prime minister's challenge on dementia: delivering major improvements in dementia care and research by 2020. London: Department of Health; 2015.
42. Alzheimer's Society. Building dementia friendly communities: a priority for everyone. 2013. https://www.alzheimers.org.uk/site/scripts/download_info.php?downloadID=1236.
43. Joseph Rowntree Foundation. Dementia without walls. 2012. http://www.jrf.org.uk/topic/dementia-without-walls.
44. Dementia Centre – Design. Dementia design centre, stirling, Stirling University. (undated) http://dementia.stir.ac.uk/design.
45. Dementia Friendly Brecon. Making Brecon a dementia friendly community. 2014. http://www.dementiafriendlybrecon.org.uk/.
46. Kings Fund. Enhancing the healing environment: environments of care for people with dementia. (undated). http://www.kingsfund.org.uk/projects/enhancing-healing-environment/ehe-in-dementia-care.
47. Association for dementia studies. Enabling environments programme. 2014. http://www.worcester.ac.uk/discover/ads-enhancing-the-healing-programme.html.
48. Dementia Centre. Dementia friendly Northern Ireland. 2012. http://dementia.stir.ac.uk/communities/dementia-friendly-northern-ireland.
49. The Debenham Project. (undated). http://www.the-debenham-project.org.uk/.
50. Department of Health. G8 summit: global action against dementia. London: Department of health; 2013.
51. Alzheimer's Disease International and BUPA. Ideas and advice on developing and implementing a national dementia plan. 2013. http://www.alz.co.uk/sites/default/files/pdfs/global-dementia-plan-report-ENGLISH.pdf.
52. OECD. Addressing dementia: the OECD response. 2015. http://www.oecd.org/health/addressing-dementia-9789264231726-en.htm.

53. World Health Organisation. First ministerial conference on global action against dementia. 2015. ww.who.int/mediacentre/events/meetings/2015/global-action-against-dementia/en.
54. Harding R, Peel E. It's a huge maze, the system, it's a terrible maze: dementia carers' constructions of navigating health and social care services. Dementia. 2013. doi:10.1177/1471301213480514. online publication date: July 3 2013.
55. Mental Health Foundation. Getting on ... with life. London: Mental Health foundation; 2013. http://www.mentalhealth.org.uk/publications/getting-on-summary-report/.
56. Blood I. Older people with high support needs: a round up of evidence. York: Joseph Rowntree Foundation; 2010.
57. Lloyd L. The individual in social care: the ethics of care and the 'personalisation agenda' in services for older people in England. Ethics Soc Welf. 2010;4(2):188–99.
58. Lloyd L, Calnan M, Cameron A, Seymour J, Smith R, White K. Maintaining dignity in later life: a longitudinal qualitative study of older people's experience of support and care. New Dynamics Ageing Find. 2011; 8. http://www.newdynamics.group.shef.ac.uk/assets/files/NDA%20Findings_8.pdf.
59. Grenier A. Transitions and the life course: challenging constructions of 'growing old'. Bristol: Policy Press; 2012.

Part II
Depression and Anxiety

Anxiety and Depression in Older People: Diagnostic Challenges

Carolyn A. Chew-Graham

This chapter considers the presentation of anxiety and depression in older people and explores the challenges clinicians face in making a diagnosis in the face of multiple health problems. Depression is a major global public health threat, and by 2030, depressive disorders are predicted to be the second leading cause of disease burden and disability worldwide [1]. Reducing the burden of depressive disorders is recognised as a major public health priority [2]. Anxiety and depression commonly overlap or coexist.

Depression severe enough to warrant intervention is one of the commonest mental health problems facing older people, affecting more than one in ten older people in the community. Demographic changes mean that even if prevalence rates were to remain stable, the growing numbers of older people will translate into large increases in the demand for treatment for these disorders in this population [3]. This is likely to place an increasing burden on health and social care. Untreated anxiety and depression leads to increased use of health and social care services and raised mortality [4]. Depression and anxiety are more prevalent in people with long-term physical conditions: prevalence of depression in people with diabetes may be as high as 30 % [5], and prevalence of anxiety in people with chronic obstructive pulmonary disease (COPD) is up to 25 % [6]. Depression is more than seven times more common in those with two or more chronic physical conditions [5]. Thus, mental and physical health problems tend to become entwined and manifest in complex co-morbidity) [7]. As co-morbidities are common in later life (36 % of people aged 65–74 and 47 % of those aged 75 and over have a limiting chronic illness), they constitute a serious risk factor for developing depression and/or anxiety. Treatment of depression has the potential to improve outcomes of diabetes [8] and to improve mortality from all causes in older adults [9].

C.A. Chew-Graham, MD, FRCGP
Research Institute, Primary Care and Health Sciences, Keele University, Staffordshire, UK
e-mail: c.a.chew-graham@keele.ac.uk

© Springer International Publishing Switzerland 2016
C.A. Chew-Graham, M. Ray (eds.), *Mental Health and Older People:
A Guide for Primary Care Practitioners*, DOI 10.1007/978-3-319-29492-6_5

Loneliness and depression are strongly associated in older people [10], and loneliness is an independent risk factor for depression [11].

5.1 Anxiety, Depression and Long-Term Conditions

Depression is associated with disability; increased mortality, including from suicide; poorer outcomes from physical illness; and increased use of primary and secondary and social care resources. Major depression is a recurring disorder, and older people are more at risk of recurrence than the younger population. The aetiology of depression in older people is illustrated in Table 5.1.

There are a number of risk factors for depression, which clinicians need to be aware of (Table 5.2), and some of these are also risk factors for anxiety, particularly chronic physical conditions and loneliness.

Anxiety disorders are also common in older people. 'Anxiety' covers the terms generalised anxiety disorder (GAD) and panic and phobic disorders. GAD is a common disorder, of which the central feature is excessive worry about a number of different events associated with heightened tension. Anxiety and depression often

Table 5.1 Aetiology of depression in older people

Structural brain changes: atrophy
Vascular hypothesis: apathy and retardation, reduced depressive symptoms, reduced insight, more cognitive impairment, poorer recovery
Neurodegenerative disorders: Alzheimer's disease, Parkinson's disease, vascular dementia, multiple sclerosis
Physical illnesses: endocrine abnormalities, anaemia, cancer (lung, pancreas), tuberculosis, neurosyphilis

Table 5.2 Risk factors for depression in older people

Physical factors
Chronic disease: diabetes, ischaemic heart disease, chronic obstructive pulmonary disease, inflammatory arthritis
Organic brain disease: dementia, Parkinson's disease, cerebrovascular disease
Endocrine/metabolic disorders: hypothyroidism, hypercalcaemia
Malignancy
Chronic pain
Psychosocial factors
Social isolation
Loneliness
Being a carer
Loss: bereavement, income, social status
History of depression
Being in institutional care

coexist (or overlap) in older people and may also be co-morbid with physical conditions (leading to poorer outcomes in those conditions).

5.2 Presentation of Anxiety and Depression

Older people with depression may present with a variety of symptoms (Table 5.3).

Other clinical features often found in older people with depression include somatic preoccupation, hypochondriasis and the morbid fear of illness, which are more common presentations than the complaint of low mood or sadness. In addition, physical symptoms, in particular seemingly disproportionate pain, are common, and the primary care clinician may feel they represent organic disease. This can cause problems for the GP, as a depressed patient's hypochondriacal complaints can be quite different from the bodily symptoms one might expect from knowledge of the patient's medical history. Subjective memory disturbance may be a prominent symptom and lead to a differential diagnosis of dementia, but true cognitive disturbance is also common in late-life depression.

People with anxiety disorders may complain of worry, irritability, tension, tiredness or 'nerves', but older people may present, instead, with somatic symptoms that may cause diagnostic difficulty for the GP and (if not identified) may result in unnecessary investigations for the patient – with the resultant worries about the possibility of physical illness aggravating the depression or anxiety symptoms. The GP needs to be aware of the link with alcohol misuse and anxiety and should always explore alcohol consumption in older people who present with symptoms of depression or anxiety.

5.3 Diagnostic Challenges

Depression and anxiety in older people are poorly detected and managed in primary care [12], particularly in people with chronic physical ill health where symptoms may be 'normalised' [13]. Older adults may have beliefs that prevent them from seeking help for mental health problems, such as a fear of stigmatisation or concern that antidepressant medication is addictive. They may not consider themselves candidates for care because of previous experience of help-seeking. In addition, older people may be reluctant to recognise and name 'depression' as a specific condition that legitimises attending their GP, or they may misattribute symptoms of major depression for 'old age', ill health or grief and use normalising attributional styles

	Emotional – sadness, anhedonia, worthlessness
	Cognitive – self-blame, self-dislike, guilt
	Motivational – low energy, lack of drive
	Neurovegetative – change in appetite, sleep
Table 5.3 Clinical features of depression	Psychotic – delusions, hallucinations

that see their depression as a normal consequence of ill health, of difficult personal circumstances or even of old age itself.

Depression in older people (particularly when there is no history of depression earlier in the patient's life) is associated with increased risk of subsequently developing a 'true' dementia. Lastly, a persistent complaint of loneliness in an older person (even when that person is known to live with others) should prompt enquiry into mood, feelings and views on the future and a more systematic enquiry about biological symptoms of depression, along with a formal assessment, including a risk assessment.

Clinicians may lack the necessary consultation skills and confidence to correctly diagnose depression in older people, and anxiety is particularly underdiagnosed. Clinicians may also be wary of opening a 'Pandora's box' in time-limited consultations and instead collude with the patient in what has been called 'therapeutic nihilism' [14]. Additionally, a lack of congruence between patients' and professionals' conceptual language about mental health problems, along with deficits in communication skills on the part of both patients and professionals, can lead to uncertainty about the nature of the problem and reduce opportunities to talk about appropriate management strategies [13].

Because of the risk of depression and anxiety in people with long-term conditions, clinicians should consider using case-finding questions in consultations to opportunistically identify depression or anxiety (Tables 5.4a and 5.4b).

Asking the patient 'Is this something you want help with?' is thought to be a useful third question to take the discussion further and enable the patient to explore their problems with the clinician.

Primary care clinicians may have difficulty asking these case-finding questions of patients with long-term conditions due to lack of skill in making full assessment of mood and, at least partly, due to lack of referral options [15].

To make the diagnosis of depression, it is important to ask about the two key symptoms in the DSM 5 (Diagnosis and Statistical Manual), followed by the

Table 5.4a Case-finding questions for depression

During the past month, have you often been bothered by feeling down, depressed, or hopeless?
During the past month, have you often been bothered by having little interest or pleasure in doing things?
A 'yes' to either question is considered a positive test. A 'no' response to both questions makes depression highly unlikely

Table 5.4b Case-finding questions for anxiety

Over the last 2 weeks, have you often been bothered by the following problems?
Feeling nervous, anxious or on edge
Not being able to stop or control worrying
A 'yes' to either question is considered a positive test. A 'no' response to both questions makes GAD highly unlikely

associated symptoms; in addition, the NICE guidelines for depression, and depression in people with chronic physical health problems [16, 17], stress the important of a thorough assessment of duration and severity of symptoms (Table 5.5).

There has been considerable emphasis on encouraging GPs to improve their skills in the diagnosis and management of depression, yet anxiety disorders have been relatively neglected [18]. Anxiety symptoms are more common than those of depression in the community and may be accompanied by significant morbidity.

When an anxiety disorder is suspected, the patient's symptoms should be explored in detail to establish the diagnosis (Table 5.6).

It is important to elicit a history of previous similar problems – this will affect a patient's understanding of their problems and impact on management decisions, particularly previous treatments and response to antidepressants. It is important to take an accurate drug history and ensure that the patient is not taking medication which could be contributing to a mood disorder. Enquiry into alcohol and non-prescribed drug use (particularly St John's wort, over-the-counter analgesics and illicit drugs such as benzodiazepines which can be obtained over the internet) is vital and often forgotten in older people. The clinician should ask about feelings of loneliness, social context and support, and the impact of symptoms on self-care and activities of daily living (e.g. motivation to shop and cook may be affected by low mood or panic attacks).

Where possible and with the patient's consent, a collateral history from a family member or other carer can provide important information, particularly about ability to cope at home (Table 5.7).

Table 5.5 Making the diagnosis of depression

Key symptoms	
	Persistent sadness or low mood
	Marked loss of interest or pleasure
At least one of these, most days, most of the time for at least 2 weeks	
	If any of above present, ask about associated symptoms
	Disturbed sleep (decreased or increased compared to usual)
	Decreased or increased appetite and/or weight
	Fatigue or loss of energy
	Agitation or slowing of movements
	Poor concentration or indecisiveness
	Feelings of worthvlessness or excessive or inappropriate guilt
	Suicidal thoughts or acts
Assess	
	Symptoms
	Duration of episode
	Course of illness
	Severity of symptoms

Table 5.6 Making the diagnosis of anxiety

The diagnostic criteria for generalised anxiety disorder (GAD) include
Excessive anxiety and worry (apprehensive expectation), occurring more days than not for at least 6 months, about a number of events or activities
The individual finds it difficult to control the worry
The anxiety and worry are associated with three (or more) of the following six symptoms (with at least some symptoms having been present for more days than not over the past 6 months)
Restlessness or feeling keyed up or on edge
Being easily fatigued
Difficulty concentrating or mind going blank
Irritability
Muscle tension
Sleep disturbance (difficulty falling or staying asleep, or restless, unsatisfying sleep)
The anxiety, worry or physical symptoms cause clinically significant distress or impairment in social, occupational or other important areas of functioning
The disturbance is not attributable to the physiological effects of a substance (e.g. alcohol drugs or medication) or another medical condition (e.g. hyperthyroidism)
The disturbance is not better explained by another mental disorder

Table 5.7 Holistic assessment of an older person

The following specific information should be obtained during the assessment of an older person with suspected mental health problems
Timing of onset of symptoms and their subsequent course
Any previous similar episodes
A description of behaviour over a typical 24 h (from patient and collateral history if possible)
Previous medical and psychiatric history (including previous intellectual ability and personality characteristics)
Accurate drug history
Family history of mental health problems
Living conditions
Financial position
Ability for self-care, shopping, cooking, laundry
Ability to manage finances and deal with hazards such as fire
Any behaviour that may cause difficulties for carers or neighbours
The ability of family/neighbours/friends to offer support
Other services already involved in the patient's care

The clinician should assess memory using the CG-COG and the Abbreviated Mental Test or asking the patient to name 15 animals (which is an excellent test for cognitive impairment and probably as useful as the Mini Mental State Examination or MMSE).

The NICE guidelines for anxiety (CG 113) [19] and depression (CGs 90 and 91) [16, 17] suggest that severity should be assessed using the GAD-7 [20] and PHQ-9

Table 5.8 Suggested investigations in suspected anxiety and/or depression in older people

FBC, U&E, liver and thyroid function tests, vitamin B_{12} and folate, HbA1C, bone profile, and any further tests dictated by clinical presentation

[21], respectively, in order to guide management (see Appendix 1 and 2 and chapters on managing anxiety and depression, Chaps. 8 and 9).

In older people, it is advisable for the clinician to exclude organic causes for change in mood and to organise for the patient to undergo a number of blood tests (Table 5.8).

5.4 Risk Assessment

Assessment of risk is important in any patient who is depressed, and older men are at particular risk of suicide. Apart from the risk of self-harm and suicide, the clinician should explore the risk of self-neglect, particularly when motivation is affected (Table 5.9).

A *normalising* approach may feel more comfortable to the patient and clinician than the more direct approach '*do you feel you would be better off dead?*' or '*have you been thinking of harming yourself?*' Thus, saying '*some people may feel like harming themselves when they feel down, as you tell me you do – do you ever feel like this?*' may be a useful approach.

It is important for the clinician to enquire about 'protective factors': does the patient have anything that stops them acting on thoughts of self-harm? Such factors might be faith, family, pets or an event to look forward to. If there are no protective factors, the risk of completed suicide is high.

Suicide mitigation is a vital role that primary care clinicians play as only 25 % of those who kill themselves are in contact with specialist mental health services. Contrary to some clinicians' worries, asking about suicide does not increase risk (actually reduces risk of self-harm and suicide). Clinicians should remember that if a patient is distressed, it is important *always* to explore thoughts of self-harm and to always document discussion. Similarly, it is important always to respond with compassion and maintain hope, and after managing the crisis, to ensure that the clinician himself or herself has support and supervision to talk through the consultation.

As well as agreeing a safety plan (developing strategies to remain safe, build up social network and utilise professional help including third sector services) and a crisis plan (agreed actions when suicidal thoughts increase or become persistent, how to access help, particularly out of hours) (http://www.connectingwithpeople.org/sites/default/files/SuicideMitigationInPrimaryCareFactsheet_0612.pdf).

Risk should always be managed through a team approach, whether this is within the primary care team or shared across the primary care/specialist care interface.

Management of anxiety and depression will be discussed in Chaps. 8 and 9.

Table 5.9 Assessment of risk

The following prompts may be helpful to encourage the patient to talk about self-harm and suicide
How do you see the future
Have there been times when you felt you had wanted to get away from everything
Sometimes when people are low, they feel like harming themselves*....do you ever feel like this? If yes, when? How often? Are these thoughts persistent? How easy is it to resist them
Have you made any plans? What have you considered
What has stopped you from carrying this out? What are the things that you still look forward to
The clinician needs to be alert to the following 'red flags'
Well-formed suicidal plans and preparations: recent worsening in intensity, persistence with distress
Hopelessness: especially if persistently hopeless, and/or only able to see a brief future, no plans beyond the consultation or in the days ahead, 'nothing to live for', expressions of guilt, 'I'm a burden'
Ambivalence
Rigid thinking
Distressing psychotic phenomena: persecutory and nihilistic delusions, command hallucinations perceived as omnipotent
Sense of 'entrapment'
Impulsivity
Pain and/or chronic medical illness
Lack of social support: no confidants, major relationship instability, recently bereaved

5.5 Case Studies

5.5.1 Case Study 1: Hidden Anxiety (Peter C)

Peter, 80, lives with his 78-year-old wife in a terraced house. Their two sons and daughter live in towns more than 40 miles away, all in different directions.

Peter has COPD and is finding that he is increasingly breathless on very minor exertion. His wife is fit and well, apart from some knee pain due to arthritis, and she takes tablets for high blood pressure. Her sister died of breast cancer 4 years ago, and Peter worries all the time that she might get cancer. Sometimes the worry takes over and he can't sleep at night. He then starts to panic, feels breathless and has to get up and walk around. In the night, he worries what will happen when he can no longer manage the stairs.

He has started to drink a small whiskey every night to help him get off to sleep, but his wife grumbles at him, so he now drinks it in secret.

He doesn't feel he can talk to anyone about how he feels and is not sure what might be available to help him.

Peter's problems are suggestive of an anxiety disorder. Anxiety can occur in up to 40 % of people with COPD [22] and increases the risk of health and social care use [23] as well as poorer patient outcomes. Depression is also common in people

5 Anxiety and Depression in Older People: Diagnostic Challenges

with COPD, so anxiety and depression may be co-morbid in a patient like Peter. People with anxiety may use alcohol to manage their anxiety, and the clinician should always explore alcohol use.

Peter is likely to consult his general practice about 12 times a year and is likely to see a practice nurse (PN) or GP for review of his COPD and medication. It is likely that Peter might be unwilling to disclose symptoms of anxiety, but these routine consultations offer an opportunity for opportunistic case-finding for anxiety and depression, using the case-finding questions (Tables 5.4a and 5.4b). If Peter responds positively to any of the case-finding questions, then the clinician can explore symptoms further and assess severity using the GAD-7 or PHQ-9 (see Appendix 1 and 2), in addition to exploring risk and managing appropriately.

Peter may not be happy about a label of anxiety or depression – this may not fit with his model of illness [13], or he may feel stigmatised by the suggestion that he has a mental health problem or that his symptoms are to be expected given his age and COPD [14]. The clinician's role is to find an explanation of Peter's symptoms that is understandable and acceptable, so that a discussion about management may be had. This may need to be over a number of consultations, and the clinician may need to use patient-information leaflets to support their discussion. Peter could be referred to a third sector service, if acceptable to Peter, at this stage, and he should be offered review.

Further management of a patient like Peter, with anxiety, will be described in Chap. 8.

5.5.2 Case Study 2: Diabetes and Depression (Afzal K)

Mr K is 75 years old and lives with his eldest son, who works as an accountant, daughter-in-law and their four children. His wife died suddenly 2 years ago following a subarachnoid haemorrhage. He stopped working in the family shop following his bereavement and gave the business to his second son. He has had diabetes since the age of 50 and tries hard to watch his diet; he usually takes his medication regularly but struggles to know what to do during Ramadan. His son has just been told he, too, has diabetes, and now the family meals are more focused on ensuring that all the family eat plenty of fruit and vegetables. Mr K rarely attends his general practice, except when he is told to make an appointment for an annual review with the practice nurse.

Mr K tries to speak to his grandchildren, who are teenagers, but they all seem so busy, so he spends a lot of time on his own. He goes to the Mosque but, otherwise, rarely leaves the house.

Sometimes he wishes he didn't wake up in a morning, but feels guilty about this.

From the above history, Mr K is likely to have a depressive illness. Depression is common in patients with diabetes and worsens outcomes from both the diabetes and depression [5], whilst Katon et al. (2012) demonstrated that actively managing both depression and diabetes can improve outcomes in both conditions [24]. As Mr K does not attend the general practice very often, when he does attend, the clinician could usefully ask the case-finding questions for depression (see Table 5.4a), followed up by a broader exploration of symptoms, duration, severity (including use of PHQ-9 – Appendix 2) and impact. An older person with depression is at risk of self-harm and completed suicide, particularly an older male. Thus, the clinician should gently explore risk, with an explanation of why (s) he is asking these questions and what protective factors stop Mr K from acting on thoughts of harming himself. His faith might play an important role in this, and the clinician should be aware of culturally sensitive services that are available locally, which Mr K might be prepared to consider trying out. Such services might also address Mr K's loneliness. This case serves to remind us that people can be lonely even if they do not live alone, and any patient complaining of feeling lonely is at risk of depression.

Further management of a patient like Mr K, with depression, is discussed in Chaps. 8 and 9.

5.6 Suggested Activities

Reflect on:

How recently have you suspected that a patient or client might have anxiety or depression? How do you confirm this? What role do you have in management?

When a patient has multiple physical health problems, how often do you think about their mood? Do you use the depression and/or anxiety case-finding questions?

What support do you need in managing people with anxiety or depression? Do you have regular supervision?

Do you know what third sector services are available in your locality, and what services are provided for older people?

> **Key Points**
> - Depression and anxiety are common in older people, particularly where there is physical co-morbidity.
> - Clinicians should consider case-finding for depression and anxiety in patients with long-term physical health problems.
> - Making a diagnosis of depression or anxiety in older people can be challenging, and a collateral history can be helpful.
> - Depression in older people is a risk factor for suicide, and a risk assessment should always be conducted when depression is suspected.

References

1. Mathers CD, Loncar D. Projections of global mortality and burden of disease from 2002 to 2030. PLoS Med. 2006;3(11):e442.
2. Ferrari AJ, Charlson FJ, Norman RE, Patten SB, Freedman G, Murray CJL, et al. Burden of depressive disorders by country, sex, age, and year: findings from the Global Burden of Disease Study 2010. PLoS Med. 2013;10(11):e1001547.

3. Laidlaw K, Pachana N. Ageing, mental health and demographic change: challenges for psychotherapists. Prof Psychol Res Pract. 2009;40(6):601–8.
4. Blazer D. Protection from late life depression. Int Psychogeriatr. 2010;22(2):171–3.
5. Moussavi S, Chatterji S, Verdes E, Tandon A, Patel V, Ustun B. Depression, chronic disease and decrements in health. Results from the world health surveys. Lancet. 2007;370:851–8.
6. Zhang MWB, Ho RCM, Cheung MWL, Fu E, Mak A. Prevalence of depressive symptoms in patients with chronic obstructive pulmonary disease: a systematic review, meta-analysis and meta-regression. Gen Hosp Psychiatry. 2011;33:217–23.
7. Katon W, Ciechanowski P. Impact of major depression on chronic medical illness. J Psychosom Res. 2002;53(4):859–63.
8. Katon WJ, Lin EH, Von Korff M, Ciechanowski P, Ludman E, Young B, Peterson D, Rutter CM, McGregor M, McCulloch D. Collaborative care for participants with depression and chronic illness. N Engl J Med. 2010;363:2611–20.
9. Gallo JJ, Morales KH, Bogner H, Raue PJ, Zee J, Bruce M, Reynolds C. Long term effects of depression care management on mortality in older adults: follow-up of a cluster randomized clinical trial in primary care. BMJ. 2013;346:f2570.
10. Heikkinen RL, Kauppinen M. Depressive symptoms in late life: a 10-year follow-up. Arch Gerontol Geriatr. 2004;38:239–50.
11. Cacioppo JT, Hughes ME, Waite LJ, Hawkley LC, Thisted RA. Loneliness as a specific risk factor for depressive symptoms: cross-sectional and longitudinal analyses. Psychol Aging. 2006;21(1):140–51.
12. Chew-Graham CA, Burns A, Baldwin RC. Treating depression in later life: we need to implement the evidence that exists. BMJ. 2004;329:181–2 [Invited Editorial].
13. Coventry P, Hays R, Dickens C, Bundy C, Garrett C, Cherrington A, Chew-Graham CA. Talking about depression: barriers to managing depression in people with long term conditions in primary care. BMC Fam Pract. 2011;12:10.
14. Burroughs H, Morley M, Lovell K, Baldwin R, Burns A, Chew-Graham CA. "Justifiable depression": how health professionals and patients view late-life depression; a qualitative study. Fam Pract. 2006;23:369–77.
15. Maxwell, et al. A qualitative study of primary care professionals' views of case finding for depression in patients with diabetes or coronary heart disease in the UK. BMC Fam Pract. 2013;14:46.
16. National Institute for Health and Clinical Excellence. Depression: the treatment and management of depression in adults (update) CG90. London: National Institute for Health and Clinical Excellence; 2009.
17. National Institute for Health and Clinical Excellence. Depression in adults with a chronic physical health problem. CG91. London: National Institute for Health and Clinical Excellence; 2009.
18. Buszewicz M, Chew-Graham CA. Improving detection and management of anxiety disorders in primary care. BJGP. 2011;589:489–90 [Invited Editorial].
19. National Institute for Health and Clinical Excellence. Generalised anxiety disorder and panic disorder (with or without agoraphobia) in adults: management in primary, secondary and community care. CG113. London: National Institute for Health and Clinical Excellence; 2011.
20. Spitzer RL, et al. A brief measure for assessing generalized anxiety disorder: the GAD-7. Arch Intern Med. 2006;166(10):1092–7.
21. Kroenke K, Spitzer RL, Williams JB. The PHQ-9: validity of a brief depression severity measure. J Gen Intern Med. 2001;16(9):606–13.
22. Eisner MD, et al. Influence of anxiety on health outcomes in COPD. Thorax. 2010;65(3):229–34.
23. Coventry PA, Gemmell I, Todd CJ. Psychosocial risk factors for hospital readmission in COPD patients on early discharge services: a cohort study. BMC Pulm Med. 2011;11:49.
24. Katon W, Russo J, Lin EHB, Schmittdiel J, Ciechanowski P, Ludman E, et al. Cost-effectiveness of a multicondition collaborative care intervention: a randomized controlled trial. Arch Gen Psychiatry. 2012;69(5):506–14.

Social Participation, Loneliness and Depression

Heather Burroughs and Ross Wilkie

6.1 Introduction

Retirement from paid employment and other changes in role can, for some older people, lead to a decline in social participation. A lack of social participation can cause loneliness, but the two states are not synonymous. Loneliness is emotional distress [1]; it has been described as a mismatch between the social relationships people desire and those that they actually have [2]. It can manifest in different forms – it can be a longing for the company of a particular person or it can be a generalised desire for a wider social circle. By widening the social circle and increasing social participation, there is some evidence that loneliness can be reduced [3].

Indeed, there is a body of research suggesting that participation in social activities is important in maintaining mental and physical well-being [4–7]. Numerous studies suggest that social participation can lead to an increase in physical exercise, social support and the sharing of health information [8–10]. In addition, social participation helps to maintain a sense of identity and can provide a sense of satisfaction and mastery [8].

6.2 Loneliness Is Linked to Depression

There are around 3.8 million people over the age of 65 living alone [11], and loneliness is common – it can be chronic or sporadic or manifest at particular times such as anniversaries or holidays. The prevalence of severe loneliness is up to 10 % [12].

H. Burroughs, BSocSci, MPhil, PhD (✉) • R. Wilkie, BSC, PhD
Research Institute for Primary Care and Health Sciences, Keele University,
Keele, Staffordshire, UK
e-mail: h.burroughs@keele.ac.uk; r.wilkie@keele.ac.uk

© Springer International Publishing Switzerland 2016
C.A. Chew-Graham, M. Ray (eds.), *Mental Health and Older People:
A Guide for Primary Care Practitioners*, DOI 10.1007/978-3-319-29492-6_6

Loneliness is thought to have negative consequences for humans because we are social beings and perceived isolation provokes feelings of being unsafe [13].

As a concept, loneliness can be divided into two categories – *social* loneliness, which is when one has a lack of social contacts, and *emotional* loneliness, when one is lacking a key emotional relationship [14]. Differentiating these two types of loneliness helps to explain why some people with a large number of social contacts or a non-satisfying quality of contacts consider themselves to be lonely, whereas others in a similar situation do not.

Loneliness is a normal part of human experience, but when it occurs for long periods or frequently and is felt very severely, then it becomes a cause for concern. Loneliness has been strongly associated with depression [15–17], and longitudinal work has reported loneliness to be an independent risk factor for future depression amongst older adults [18]. Cacioppo describes depressive symptomatology and loneliness as having a 'synergistic effect', mutually reinforcing one another to diminish well-being.

As well as common mental health problems such as depression, loneliness is predictive of more severe problems such as suicide in older age groups [19]. Further, loneliness has been found to be a precursor of dementia and cognitive decline [20], being a better predictor of such conditions than depression.

Cacioppo [12] argues that the chronically lonely become hypervigilant for signs of threat in the environment and over time cognitive biases colour perceptions so that the world is viewed in a more dangerous and negative light. The expectation of threat and negative interactions can become a self-fulfilling prophecy. In this way, the prospect of social interaction becomes a source of anxiety and is avoided.

Loneliness is linked not only to mental health problems – it predicts physical morbidity [21–23] increased health services utilisation [24] and increased mortality. It also slows recovery from illness [25], and its effects can be as detrimental as smoking [26].

6.3 Measuring Loneliness

There are existing tools that could be used to identify adults who are lonely and may benefit from interventions. The three-item loneliness scale (Table 6.1) [27] can be used through face-to-face and telephone interview in research and practice. The response options for all three items, 1 = hardly ever, 2 = some of the time and 3 = often, are summed with increasing scores indicating increasing loneliness. This correlates with the UCLA Loneliness Scale [28] which is used widely. To score, the Oftens = 3, the Sometimes = 2, the Rarelys = 1, and the Nevers = 0. In the United States, the ten-item version of the UCLA Loneliness Scale is offered by the American Association of Retired Persons to allow individuals to self-assess their level of loneliness and to seek intervention.

Table 6.1 The three-item loneliness scale

	Hardly ever	Some of the time	Often
'How often do you feel you lack companionship?'			
'How often do you feel left out?'			
'How often do you feel isolated from others?'			

From Hughes et al. [27] with permission

Table 6.2 The De Jong Gierveld Scale

1. There is always someone I can talk to about my day-to-day problems
2. I miss having a really close friend
3. I experience a general sense of emptiness
4. There are plenty of people I can lean on when I have problems
5. I miss the pleasure of the company of others
6. I find my circle of friends and acquaintances too limited
7. There are many people I can trust completely
8. There are enough people I feel close to
9. I miss having people around me
10. I often feel rejected
11. I can call on my friends whenever I need them

From De Jong Gierveld and Van Tilburg [14] with permission

The De Jong Gierveld [14] measure is based on the cognitive theory of loneliness, and it emphasises the discrepancy between the social contact a person desires and what they are actually experiencing. This scale is probably the most commonly used in research and clinical practice (Table 6.2). The scale should be scored as follows: yes! (emphatic); yes; more or less; no; no! (emphatic).

6.4 Social Participation as an Intervention to Reduce Loneliness

In terms of quantifiable social participation as opposed to loneliness, half of older adults report that they are not taking part in at least one aspect of the social participatory activities they would like [29]. Reporting one in five reports that he/she is in contact with family, friends and neighbours less than once a week, and one in ten is in contact less than once a month [30]. Also, two fifths of older people (about 3.9 million) describe the television as their main company [31].

Public health authorities and local government have become increasingly concerned about the problem of loneliness and the detrimental effects amongst the growing population of older adults. Unfortunately there is no one simple solution – older people are not a homogenous group – and the self-reinforcing spiral of depression, ill-health and isolation makes a difficult problem that needs an individually tailored response.

In terms of evidence, the best work is from the United States [32] which suggests that there is a potential benefit from group social or educational activities in specific groups. Evidence from a systematic review [33] suggests that the most successful interventions for loneliness, measured by improvement in the domains of physical, mental and social health, tend to be group based, participatory and offering some activity [34–36]. Such community-based interventions have been shown to have additional benefits in terms of social inclusion and social cohesion [37–39].

With regard to older adults, creativity has been argued to be a critical element to ageing well [40], which is thought to enhance health and well-being as well as increase and sustain social interactions amongst older people [32, 41]. Indeed, aside from the social benefits, it has also been argued that creative activity is therapeutic in itself [42], and a number of community-based 'art for health' initiatives have been created in the United Kingdom [43]. However, it is clear that better designed studies, and in particular randomised controlled trials, are needed to improve the evidence base [28].

The problem with group-based participatory activities is that, although they may work to encourage social participation, reduce loneliness and alleviate depression for those who can be reached, there are several barriers inherent within them for this population: older people may have difficulties with transport; they may feel unwilling to walk into an established group alone, especially if they are depressed; they may need some one-to-one therapeutic input to even begin to think about increasing their social participation; and they may need some guidance to think about what type of group activity they might find meaningful.

In the light of these barriers, a reasonable way of approaching the Gordian knot of depression, anxiety, ill-health and loneliness might be individualised therapeutic input with an emphasis on behavioural activation followed by practical assistance to attend a meaningful group activity. Further high-quality research in this area would be welcomed.

6.5 Measuring Social Participation

In clinical practice, the assessment and monitoring of social participation may be useful to inform clinical decisions (e.g. by identifying low or restricted social participation) and to evaluate the effectiveness of interventions. Measurement of social participation is in its infancy. There have been a number of reviews [44–47] that have highlighted instruments for use in research and to evaluate practice. Wilkie and colleagues in their review [46] highlighted instruments that have been designed to exclusively measure social participation in adult populations (and therefore provide a score specific for social participation), can be obtained easily, are free of charge and have some reported evidence of their ability to measure social participation to support their use (Table 6.1). None of these instruments as yet have been shown to have a clear advantage over the others. Selection of an instrument to measure social participation will depend on how the instrument measures social participation (e.g. frequency or as people would like) or the number of items, which will impact on responder burden and also on the detail of social participation that is measured. Each of the selected instruments in Table 6.1 is designed to measure participation in a different way; the Impact on Participation and Autonomy measures choice and control (i.e. the possibility to do the things the way you want) [48], the Keele Assessment of Participation measures performance in participation 'as and when you want', [28], Participation Measure for Post-Acute Care (PM-PAC) [49] measures limitation, Participation Objective, Participation Subjective (POPS) [50] measures objective (i.e. frequency) and subjective (i.e. satisfaction) participation, Rating of Perceived Participation measures the individual's perceived and desire to change [51] and the Participation Scale [52] measures participation compared to a 'peer norm'. All of the instruments measure participation in mobility, self-care, domestic life, interpersonal interaction and relationships, major life (e.g. work, education) and community and social life, except POPS which does not measure aspects of self-care. The instruments contain a varying number of items (range: 11–78); this is linked to the detail of participation measured (e.g. KAP contains the fewest items and measures participation broadly at domain level (i.e. measures participation in a number of activities in one item); POPS and ROPP contain the greatest number of items and provide greater detail by measuring participation in specific life situations).

At the moment, there are no instruments which have a proven ability to measure change in social participation, which is important for examining the impact of interventions and how participation may change over time. The health benefits gained from social participation will be through actual participation, and this may be the target for intervention studies. Currently there is a need to develop an instrument that measures actual participation in older adults that is responsive to change. This may require a better understanding of what social participation is in older adults which will facilitate development of the conceptual model for measurement, but it is crucial to identify links with loneliness. It is unknown whether loneliness may be linked more so with the quality of perceived participation (e.g. participating 'as and when they want') than with the amount of participation (Table 6.3).

Table 6.3 Summary of the characteristics of examples of instruments designed to measure participation and social function

Name of measure/scale	Purpose/content	Method of administration	Respondent burden (time to complete)	Administration burden	Interpretation of scores
Impact on Participation and Autonomy	23 items. Measures choice and control of participation	Self-complete questionnaire	30 min	Minimal	Higher score = greater perceived participation restriction
Keele Assessment of Participation	11 items. Measures person-perceived performance in participation tasks	Self-complete questionnaire	3 min. 98.2 % completion rate	Minimal	Range: 0–11, higher score = more restrictions
Participation Objective, Participation Subjective (POPS)	78 items. Measures objective and subjective participation in 26 activities	Self-complete or interview	No information	Minimal	Range for subjective participation: −4 to 4. Range objective participation: −3 to 3. Higher scores = greater participation
Rating of Perceived Participation	66 items. Measures perceived level, satisfaction and need for support to change the level of participation in 22 activities	Self-complete questionnaire	15–30 min	Minimal	Range: 0–88, Higher score = greater participation restriction
The Participation Scale	18 items. Compare an individual's participation to a 'peer norm'	Interview	20 min	20 min to administer	Range: 1–5, higher score = greater restriction. Arbitrary severity categories provided

6.6 Implications for Practice

Loneliness is a serious predicament that can have severely detrimental effects on mental and physical well-being to such an extent that it is increasingly being seen as a public health issue. The good news is that loneliness can be identified by using the correct tools, and there is evidence that interventions which facilitate meaningful social participation can be helpful.

6.7 Suggested Activities

Do you have a patient or client who seems lonely? How would you broach this sensitive topic? How do you normally assess this? Are there other things you could do to assess loneliness in your work?

How can you support a patient or client to increase their social participation? How do you find out what resources are available in your area? What barriers might there be to participation? Is there a way to overcome these barriers?

> **Key Points**
> - Up to 10 % of older people are thought to be severely lonely.
> - Loneliness can be conceptualised as a mismatch between the social relationships people desire and those that they actually have.
> - Loneliness increases the risk of depression and suicide in older people.
> - Interventions to increase social participation may reduce loneliness and depression.
> - A number of tools are available to measure loneliness and social participation.

References

1. Weeks DJ. A review of loneliness concepts, with particular reference to old age. Int J Geriatr Psychiatry. 1994;9(5):345–55.
2. Peplau LA, Perlman D. Perspectives on loneliness. In: Peplau LA, Perlman D, editors. Loneliness: a sourcebook of current theory, research and therapy. New York: Wiley; 1982. p. 1–18.
3. Cattan M, et al. Preventing social isolation and loneliness among older people: a systematic review of health promotion interventions. Ageing Soc. 2005;25(01):41–67.
4. Glass TA, Mendes De Leon C, Marottoli RA, Berkman LF. Population based study of social and productive activities as predictors of survival among elderly Americans. BMJ. 1999;319(7208):478–83.
5. Sirven N, Debrand T. Social participation and healthy ageing: an international comparison using SHARE data. Soc Sci Med. 2008;67(12):2017–26.

6. Chiao C, Weng L, Botticello A. Social participation reduces depressive symptoms among older adults: an 18-year longitudinal analysis in Taiwan. BMC Public Health. 2011;11:292.
7. Menec VH. The relation between everyday activities and successful aging: a 6-year longitudinal study. J Gerontol Ser B Psychol Sci Soc Sci. 2003;58(2):S74–82.
8. Berkman LF, Glass T, Brissette I, Seeman TE. From social integration to health: Durkheim in the new millennium. Soc Sci Med. 2000;51(6):843–57.
9. Thraen-Borowski KM, Trentham-Dietz A, Edwards DF, Koltyn KF, Colbert LH. Dose-response relationships between physical activity, social participation, and health-related quality of life in colorectal cancer survivors. J Cancer Surviv. 2013;7(3):369–78.
10. Levasseur M, Desrosiers J, Whiteneck G. Accomplishment level and satisfaction with social participation of older adults: association with quality of life and best correlates. Qual Life Res Int J Qual Life Asp Treat Care Rehab. 2010;19(5):665–75.
11. General Lifestyle Survey 2011, Table 3.3. ONS, 2013.
12. Victor CR, Bowling A. A longitudinal analysis of loneliness among older people in Great Britain. J Psychol. 2012;146(3):313–31.
13. Cacioppo JT, Hawkley LC. Perceived social isolation and cognition. Trends Cogn Sci. 2009;13:447–54.
14. De Jong Gierveld J, Van Tilburg T. The De Jong Gierveld short scales for emotional and social loneliness: tested on data from 7 countries in the UN generations and gender surveys. Eur J Ageing. 2010;7(2):121–30.
15. Brown GW, Harris T. Social origins of depression: a studyof psychological disorder in women. New York: Free Press; 1978.
16. Weeks DG, Michela JL, Peplau LA, Bragg ME. Relation between loneliness and depression: a structural equation analysis. J Pers Soc Psychol. 1980;39:1238–44.
17. Shaver PR, Brennan KA. Measures of depression and loneliness. In: Robinson JP, Shaver PR, Wrightsman LS, editors. Measures of personality and social psychological attitudes: measures of social psychological attitudes, vol. 1. San Diego: Academic; 1991. p. 195–289.
18. Cacioppo JT, et al. Loneliness as a specific risk factor for depressive symptoms: cross-sectional and longitudinal analyses. Psychol Aging. 2006;21(1):140.
19. O'Connell H, et al. Recent developments: suicide in older people. BMJ Br Med J. 2004;329(7471):895.
20. Wilson RS, Krueger KR, Arnold SE, et al. Loneliness and risk of Alzheimer disease. Arch Gen Psychiatry. 2007;64:234–40.
21. Hawkley LC, et al. Loneliness predicts increased blood pressure: 5-year cross-lagged analyses in middle-aged and older adults. Psychol Aging. 2010;25(1):132.
22. Burholt V, Scharf T. Poor health and loneliness in later life: the role of depressive symptoms, social resources, and rural environments. J Gerontol Ser B: Psychol Sci Soc Sci. gbt121. 2013;69(2):311–24.
23. Lyyra TM, Heikkinen RL. Perceived social support and mortality in older people. J Gerontol Ser B Psychol Sci Soc Sci. 2006;61(3):S147–52.
24. Luanaigh CÓ, Lawlor BA. Loneliness and the health of older people. Int J Geriatr Psychiatry. 2008;23(12):1213–21.
25. Marmot MG, et al. Fair society, healthy lives: strategic review of health inequalities in England post-2010. London: UCL; 2010.
26. Holt-Lunstad J, Smith TB, Layton JB. Social relationships and mortality risk: a meta-analytic review. PLoS Med. 2010;7(7):e1000316.
27. Hughes ME, Waite LJ, Hawkley LC, Cacioppo JT. A short scale for measuring loneliness in large surveys results from two population-based studies. Res Aging. 2004;26(6):655–72.
28. Russell D, Peplau LA, Ferguson ML. Developing a measure of loneliness. J Pers Assess. 1978;42(3):290–4.
29. Wilkie R, Peat G, Thomas E, Hooper H, Croft PR. The Keele assessment of participation: a new instrument to measure participation restriction in population studies. Combined qualitative and quantitative examination of its psychometric properties. Qual Life Res. 2005;4(8):1889–99.
30. Victor CR, Scambler S, Bowling A, Bond J. The prevalence of and risk factors for, loneliness in later life: a survey of older people in Great Britain. Ageing Soc. 2005;25:357–75.

31. Age UK. Loneliness in later life evidence review. London: Age UK; 2014.
32. Frost H, Haw S, Frank J. Promoting health and wellbeing in later life. Interventions in primary care and community settings. Edinburgh: MRC Scottish Collaboration for Public Health Research and Policy; 2010.
33. Dickens AP, Richards SH, Greaves CJ, Campbell JL. Interventions targeting social isolation in older people: a systematic review. BMC Public Health. 2011;11:647.
34. Tennstedt S, Howland J, Lachman M, Peterson E, Kasten L, Jette A. A randomized controlled trial of a group intervention to reduce fear of falling and associated activity restriction in older adults. J Gerontol B Psychol Sci Soc Sci. 1998;53:384–92.
35. Ciechanowski P, Wagner E, Schmaling K, Schwartz S, Williams B, Diehr P, et al. Community-integrated home-based depression treatment in adults. A randomized controlled trial. JAMA. 2004;291:1569–77.
36. McAuley E, Blissmer B, Marquez DX, Jerome GJ, Kramer AF, Katula J. Social relations, physical activity, and well-being in older adults. Prev Med. 2000;31:608–17.
37. Greaves CJ, Farbus L. Effects of creative and social activity on the health and well-being of socially isolated older people: outcomes from a multi-method observational study. J R Soc Promot Health. 2006;126(3):134–42.
38. Staricoff RL. Arts in health: the value of evaluation. J R Soc Promot Health. 2006;126:116–20.
39. Johnson V, Stanley J. Capturing the contribution of community arts to health and well-being. Int J Ment Health Promot. 2007;9:28–35.
40. Flood M. Exploring the relationships between creativity, depression, and successful aging. Act Adapt Aging. 2006;31:55–71.
41. Wikstrom BM. Social interaction associated with visual art discussions: a controlled intervention study. Aging Ment Health. 2002;6(1):82–7.
42. Everitt A, Hamilton R. Arts, health and community. Durham: Centre for Arts and Humanities in Health and Medicine; 2003.
43. Angus J. A review of evaluation in community-based art for health activity in the UK. London: Health Development Agency; 2002.
44. Resnik L, Plow MA. Measuring participation as defined by the international classification of functioning, disability and health: an evaluation of existing measures. Arch Phys Med Rehabil. 2009;90(5):856–66.
45. Noonan VK, Kopec JA, Noreau L, Singer J, Dvorak MF. A review of participation instruments based on the international classification of functioning, disability and health. Disabil Rehabil. 2009;31(23):1883–901.
46. Magasi S, Post MW. A comparative review of contemporary participation measures' psychometric properties and content coverage. Arch Phys Med Rehabil. 2010;91(9 Suppl):S17–28.
47. Wilkie R, Jordan JL, Muller S, Nicholls E, Healey EL, Van der Windt DA. Measures of social function and participation in musculoskeletal populations: impact on Participation and Autonomy (IPA), Keele Assessment of Participation (KAP), Participation Measure for Post-Acute Care (PM-PAC), Participation Objective, Participation Subjective (POPS), Rating of Perceived Participation (ROPP), and The Participation Scale. Arthritis Care Res. 2011;63(S11):S325–36.
48. Cardol M, de Haan RJ, de Jong BA, van den Bos GA, de Groot IJ. Psychometric properties of the impact on participation and autonomy questionnaire. Arch Phys Med Rehabil. 2001;82(2):210–6.
49. Gandek B, Sinclair SJ, Jette AM, Ware Jr JE. Development and initial psychometric evaluation of the participation measure for post-acute care (PM-PAC). Am J Phys Med Rehabil. 2007;86(1):57–71.
50. Brown, et al. Participation objective, participation subjective: a measure of participation combining outsider and insider perspectives. J Head Trauma Rehabil. 2004;19:459–81.
51. Sandström M, Lundin-Olsson L. Development and evaluation of a new questionnaire for rating perceived participation. Clin Rehabil. 2007;21(9):833–45.
52. Brakel WH, Anderson AM, Mutatkar RK, Bakirtzief Z, Nicholls PG, Raju MS, Das-Pattanayak RK. The participation scale: measuring a key concept in public health. Disabil Rehabil. 2006;28:193–203.

Link Between Anxiety and Depression and Pain and Sleep Disruption

John McBeth

7.1 Introduction

Musculoskeletal pain is one of the most common complaints in adults aged 50 years and over with 66 % reporting pain in the past 4 weeks. Up to 90 % of all pain complaints in older people relate to the musculoskeletal system [1], and chronic musculoskeletal pain accounts for more than 12 % of all consultations to primary care in people aged over 50 years [2]. Pain is often attributed to osteoarthritis and allied disorders of the musculoskeletal system. However, it has become clear that chronic pain may not necessarily represent disease of the joints: pain is not necessarily associated with advanced radiographic changes in joints in which the symptoms are located [3] and the genetic factors that predispose to developing pain are independent of the genetic factors that predispose to developing osteoarthritis [4]. Pain is the main cause of disability in later life [5]. With population ageing, the contribution of pain to long-term disability will increase relative to that of other chronic diseases in the next 20 years [6]. This chapter highlights how common pain is in older people and the relationship between pain, depression and anxiety; describes selected mechanisms that may explain those associations; and briefly discusses the primary care management of pain in older people.

J. McBeth, MA, PhD
Centre for Musculoskeletal Research, Arthritis Research UK Centre for Epidemiology, The University of Manchester, Manchester, UK
e-mail: john.mcbeth@manchester.ac.uk

© Springer International Publishing Switzerland 2016
C.A. Chew-Graham, M. Ray (eds.), *Mental Health and Older People: A Guide for Primary Care Practitioners*, DOI 10.1007/978-3-319-29492-6_7

7.2 How Common Is Pain?

Despite difficulties in classification and variation in the populations under study, it is clear that a high proportion of the general population reports pain [7]. The most common sites of pain reported by older people and for which they seek health care are the shoulder, knee and back [8]. However, it is common for persons to have chronic pain at multiple sites often referred to as chronic widespread pain [9]. The prevalence of pain *tends* (there are a few exceptions) to follow a clear pattern: increasing with age up until about the seventh decade at which point the prevalence plateaus or in some cases, for example, chronic widespread pain [9] decreases [10]. This is interesting since one would hypothesise that as age increases, the opportunity to 'accumulate' pain would also increase via associated degeneration of the musculoskeletal system, changes in pain processing pathways and other processes. However, whilst the prevalence of pain plateaus, the impact of that pain continues to increase. For example, Thomas and colleagues found that the prevalence of pain that interferes with daily life continues to increase with age, from 32 % in women aged 50–59 years to 50 % in those aged ≥80 years [1] (Fig. 7.1). The prevalence of pain appears to be increasing over time with increased rates of between two- and fourfold over 40 years [11] and is expected to continue rising with increases in life expectancy and ageing populations [12].

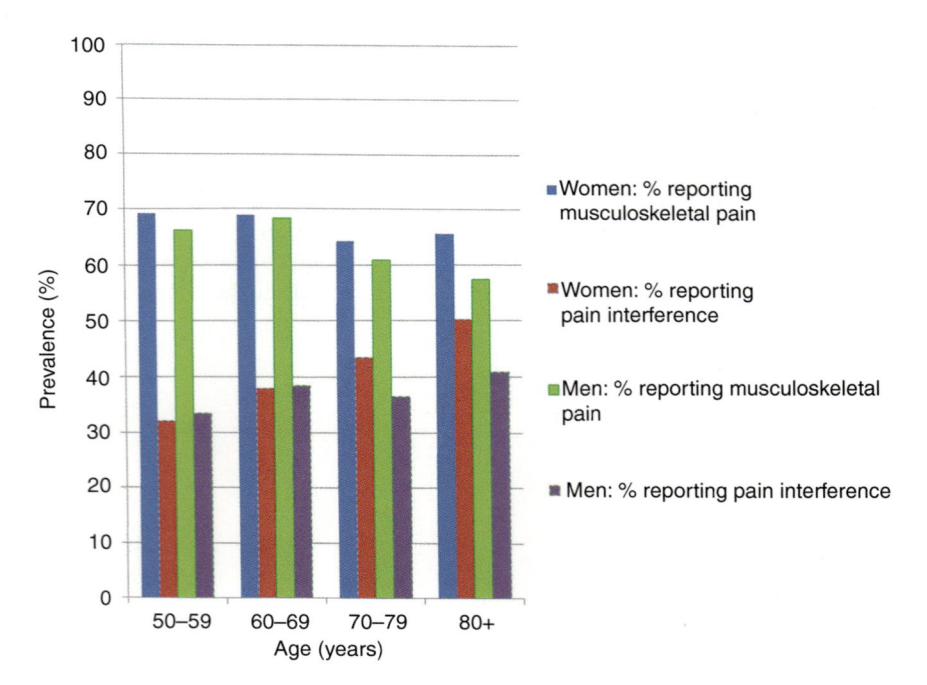

Fig. 7.1 The prevalence of pain and pain with interference separately by age and sex (Data from Thomas et al. [1])

7.3 The Relationship Between Depression, Anxiety and Pain

Up to 23 % of primary care patients seeking health care for pain have a major depressive disorder [13], and up to 50 % of patients with depression have pain [14]. Patients with co-morbid pain and depression had significantly lower quality of life [14] (Fig. 7.2) and higher rates of panic disorders, anxiety disorders and alcohol abuse than patients with either disorder alone [13]. As pain becomes more extensive, the likelihood of having co-morbid depression and anxiety increases: there was a linear relationship between an increasing number of pain sites and worsening psychological health [15] and probable major depressive disorder [14]; 13 % of persons with chronic widespread pain had *probable* depression compared to 2 % in those who were pain-free [16], and a study of US veterans found that when compared to patients without major depressive disorder, those with the disorder were almost twice as likely to have a diagnosis of one or more painful conditions in their medical records [17]. In a community-based study of 85,088 participants from 17 European countries [18], the relationship between pain and the prevalence of anxiety disorders (generalised anxiety disorder, panic disorder, post-traumatic stress disorder and social phobias) was examined. Compared to persons without pain, those with pain at a single site and those with pain in two or more sites were, respectively, two and four times more likely to have an anxiety disorder [18].

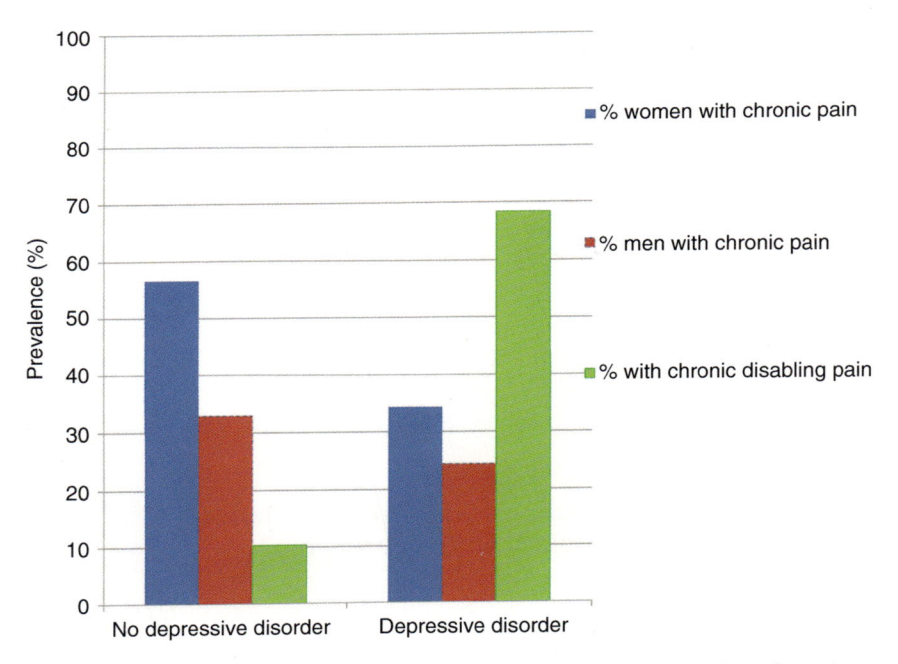

Fig. 7.2 The prevalence of pain stratified by major depressive disorder (Data from Arnow et al. [13])

Whilst the direction of association between pain and depression and anxiety has until recently been unclear, the weight of evidence suggests that the relationship is bidirectional. That is, deterioration in either pain or mood can lead to a paralleled worsening in their counterpart. Depression predicted the onset of low back pain in a large prospective cohort study ($N=4501$ adults aged 18–75 years) [19], the onset of knee pain independently of underlying osteoarthritis [20] and higher pain intensity scores and a worsening of pain in patients with knee pain [21, 22]. Depression is strongly associated with widespread pain disorders. In a study of post road traffic accident pain, depression predicted the development over a 12-month period of widespread pain in participants with localised neck and back pain [23] although that relationship is equivocal [24]. Forseth and colleagues [25] found that depression predicted the development of fibromyalgia, a disorder characterised by chronic widespread pain in the presence of multiple other somatic symptoms, in women with back pain. Among people with widespread pain, depression predicted symptom persistence over 12 months [26]. Pain catastrophising (the propensity to amplify the perception of a pain stimulus that is related to helplessness, active rumination and excessive magnification of cognitions and feelings towards the painful situation [27]) was associated with a significant increased risk of developing neck, shoulder, upper back, elbow, wrist/hand, lower back, hip, knee and ankle and foot pain [28, 29].

Conversely pain predicts the onset and course of depression and anxiety. Lower extremity pain predicted the onset of mild depressive symptoms, and the association was mediated by higher levels of fatigue and disability [30]. In the Netherlands Study of Depression and Anxiety, 614 participants with no previous history of depression or anxiety and no depression or anxiety when they entered the study were followed up over 4 years [31]. Participants reporting neck, back, head, orofacial and joint pain at baseline had between a two- and fourfold increased risk of incident depressive and anxiety disorders. The risk of incident depression and anxiety increased with the number of pain sites reported and that relationship was independent of subclinical depressive and/or anxiety symptoms that may have been present at baseline. Data from the same study showed that over 2 years a higher number of pain sites, having joint pain, pain duration of 90 days or more and daily use of pain medications predicted the persistence of anxiety and depression among those who were symptomatic at baseline [32]. Anxiety has also been associated with the persistence of chronic widespread pain. In a community-based prospective study, individuals whose chronic widespread pain persisted at 15-month follow-up had higher levels of anxiety at baseline [26].

7.4 What Are the Mechanisms of the Association Between Depression, Anxiety and Pain?

The factors and mechanisms linking psychological disorders such as depression with physical disorders such as pain are multifaceted. There are biological, behavioural, cognitive and social mechanisms by which pain may increase the risk of developing anxiety and depression and, conversely, by which the presence of anxiety and depression may increase the likelihood of experiencing pain. A detailed review is beyond the scope of this chapter. However, a brief discussion of selected mechanisms is presented below.

7.4.1 Pain Expectations and Modulation

The experience of pain can be influenced by a number of psychological factors, including attention and beliefs or expectations [33]. Pain expectancies (i.e. beliefs and predictions about future events or outcomes related to pain) were associated with higher levels of anxiety and depression and catastrophising in patients with fibromyalgia [34]. Within the nervous system, a modulatory system of ascending and descending pathways regulates the amount of pain perceived. The descending system receives input from the limbic system and can be affected by an individual's psychological state (interactions between anxiety, depression, attention and other factors), which may subsequently modulate the intensity of pain experienced [35].

7.4.2 Fear Avoidance

The fear-avoidance model of pain perception first proposed by Vlaeyen and Linton [36] proposes that in the event of a painful injury, the appraisal of whether that injury is threatening determines how the injury is interpreted and dealt with (see Fig. 7.3). If a painful injury is perceived as non-threatening, no fear will be associated with the injury leading to the continuation of daily activities (confrontation)

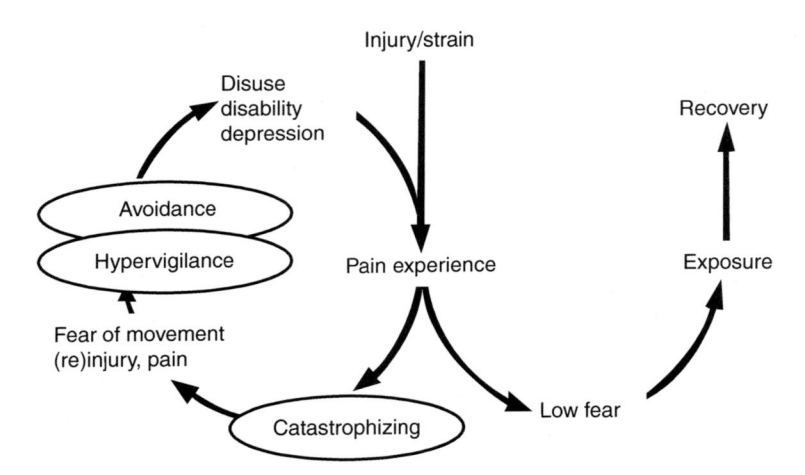

Fig. 7.3 The fear-avoidance model of pain and depression and anxiety (From Vlaeyen and Linton [36] with permission)

and rapid recovery [36]. If an injury is perceived as threatening, it can lead to the development of pain-related fear and hypervigilance to the painful sensation, as well as generating avoidance behaviours such as disability and disuse; this creates a negative feedback loop that could theoretically drive acute pain from an injury to develop into chronic pain, anxiety and depression [36]. A major limitation of the fear-avoidance model is that whilst it proposes a basis for the onset and persistence of chronic pain and associated mood disorders, it does not identify which factors in the 'threatening loop' should be targeted by interventions to reduce the risk of these negative outcomes [37].

7.4.3 The Physiological Response to Stress

Stress can be viewed as an adaptive response, involving physiological, psychological and behavioural changes aimed at maintaining stability (homeostasis). The *stress response* involves a cascade of autonomic, endocrine and immune system responses [38] aimed at achieving homeostasis. Failure to adapt to stress can lead to allostatic load marked by dysregulation of stress axes including the hypothalamic-pituitary-adrenal axis [39] and consequent insufficient or excessive secretion of stress products such as cortisol. Variations in cortisol levels were associated with pain in fibromyalgia patients [40], reporting chronic widespread pain [41] and predicted incident chronic widespread pain [42]. Depleted levels of associated stress products such as serotonin and norepinephrine were associated with higher levels of pain and the development of anxiety and depression [43–46].

7.4.4 Sleep Disruption

Pain and sleep problems are very clearly linked. Sleep problems are common in pain patients, with up to 90 % of patients with chronic pain reporting problems [47] including short sleep duration with frequent awakenings and periodic limb movements [48]. There is evidence that sleep problems can exacerbate pain [49, 50], whilst restorative sleep has been associated with the resolution of pain [26]. There is some evidence to suggest that sleep problems in patients with pain are associated with an increased likelihood of developing depression and anxiety. It is well established that independent of pain sleep problems are a risk factor for developing depression (e.g. [51, 52]) as well as predicting depression in those with pain [53]. In a prospective study, persons with pain who subsequently developed sleep problems were three times more likely to develop depression when compared to those who did not develop sleep problems [53]. Among those with pain, developing new depression was associated with an increased risk of subsequent sleep problems, although that association was weaker than the strength of the relationship between sleep and the onset of depression [54]. Two recent reviews reported evidence of bidirectional relationships between sleep and pain and depression and sleep problems [55, 56].

7.5 Primary Care Management of Pain, Depression and Anxiety in Older People

7.5.1 Case

Miriam is 76 years old and lives with her extended family. Her husband died from a heart attack 5 years ago. Since then, her sons say she has been 'depressed and sad'. She constantly complains of pain in her knees, back and shoulders. The GP has done lots of blood tests and X-rays, but told her that she has 'arthritis' and needs to take her painkillers regularly. Miriam says that everything would be alright if she could sleep: she often gets up in the night, 'because everything aches' and sits looking out of the window for an hour. She then feels tired when she has to get up to pray and tends to have a doze in the afternoon, even though the practice nurse has told her 'that is the worst thing to do'.

Older people with pain, like Miriam, are usually offered pharmacological treatment [57, 58] despite limited evidence of efficacy [59], significant increased risk of gastrointestinal bleeding with non-steroidal anti-inflammatory drug use and the increased risk of adverse side effects and drug interactions related to polypharmacy [60]. A systematic review of older people with arthritis pain and co-morbid depression demonstrated the short-term effectiveness of cognitive behavioural therapy, integrated depression care management and exercise therapy on depression symptoms [61]. However the long-term effectiveness of those interventions was not known. Referrals to non-pharmacological interventions such as cognitive behavioural therapy and exercise among patients with low back pain decrease with age [58]. This is perhaps unsurprising; older patients express a preference for pharmacological interventions for pain [62]; there is limited evidence of non-pharmacological treatment efficacy in older people, limited evidence to guide treatment decisions and a lack of availability of non-pharmacological interventions [57]. The GP could ask Miriam whether she would be interested in attending a pain management service (if one is available in the area).

The key to supporting Miriam and her family is listening to her concerns and getting her to prioritise her problems. The GP and/or practice nurse can offer advise about 'sleep hygiene' – avoiding stimulants like caffeine, ensuring activity during the day, keeping to the same bedtime and not getting up, even if awoken, rather using relaxation exercises to try to go back to sleep. If depression and anxiety are predominant, then the GP should offer referral for a 'talking treatment', explaining that this could help mood and sleep, which might impact positively on her perception of pain [63]. She could be offered referral to an activity or walking scheme (again, however, this will depend on whether such as service is commissioned locally), as walking regularly may improve mood and pain and ensure that she is tired by bedtime.

In working-age adults, self-management programmes reduce pain impact with recipients demonstrating increased active pain coping and self-efficacy for managing pain, decreased negative cognitive responses to pain [64–66] and increased physical activity [67]. Self-management programmes for older people with pain cover techniques to deal with frustration, fatigue, isolation and poor sleep; exercise for maintaining and improving strength, flexibility and endurance; use of medications; communicating effectively with family, friends and health professionals; nutrition; pacing activity and rest; and how to evaluate new treatments [64]. However as yet there is no evidence that these programmes decrease the impact of pain, including on depression and anxiety, on older people [68] and large high-quality randomised trials are required to test intervention clinical and cost-effectiveness.

> **Key Points**
> - Over 60 % adults over 50 years complain of pain in the previous 4 weeks, most commonly linked with the musculoskeletal system.
> - Depression and pain are interlinked – a quarter of people seeking help for depression will have pain, and 50 % of people with depression have pain.
> - Similarly, pain, anxiety and depression are linked with sleep disruption.
> - Treatment options offered are usually pharmacological, often leading to a combination of medication or polypharmacy.
> - There is limited evidence for the effectiveness of CBT-based interventions and pain management programmes for older people with depression, sleep disturbance and pain.

7.6 Suggested Activities

- What advice would you give to Miriam and her family if she were one of your clients/patients?
- How do you assess severity of pain in older people?
- If you are a prescriber, consider auditing your prescribing of analgesics, benzodiazepines and 'z' drugs to older people.
- What services are available in your locality for older people with pain?

References

1. Thomas E, Peat G, Harris L, Wilkie R, Croft PR. The prevalence of pain and pain interference in a general population of older adults: cross-sectional findings from the North Staffordshire Osteoarthritis Project (NorStOP). Pain. 2004;110(1–2):361–8.
2. Jordan KP, Kadam UT, Hayward R, Porcheret M, Young C, Croft P. Annual consultation prevalence of regional musculoskeletal problems in primary care: an observational study. BMC Musculoskelet Disord. 2010;11:144.
3. Neogi T, Felson D, Niu J, Nevitt M, Lewis CE, Aliabadi P, Sack B, Torner J, Bradley L, Zhang Y. Association between radiographic features of knee osteoarthritis and pain: results from two cohort studies. BMJ. 2009;339:b2844.
4. Williams FM, Spector TD, MacGregor AJ. Pain reporting at different body sites is explained by a single underlying genetic factor. Rheumatology (Oxford). 2010;49(9):1753–5.
5. World Health Organization. WHO technical report series: 919. Geneva. 2003.

6. Jagger C, Matthews R, Matthews F, Robinson T, Robine JM, Brayne C, Medical Research Council Cognitive Function and Ageing Study Investigators. The burden of diseases on disability-free life expectancy in later life. J Gerontol A Biol Sci Med Sci. 2007;62(4): 408–14.
7. McBeth J, Jones K. Epidemiology of chronic musculoskeletal pain. Best Pract Res Clin Rheumatol. 2007;21(3):403–25.
8. Abdulla A, Adams N, Bone M, Elliott AM, Gaffin J, Jones D, Knaggs R, Martin D, Sampson L, Schofield P, British Geriatric Society. Guidance on the management of pain in older people. Age Ageing. 2013;42 Suppl 1:i1–57.
9. Wolfe F, Clauw DJ, Fitzcharles MA, Goldenberg DL, Katz RS, Mease P, Russell AS, Russell IJ, Winfield JB, Yunus MB. The American College of Rheumatology preliminary diagnostic criteria for fibromyalgia and measurement of symptom severity. Arthritis Care Res (Hoboken). 2010;62(5):600–10.
10. Macfarlane GJ, Jones GT, McBeth J. Epidemiology of pain. In: McMahon SB, Klotzenburg M, editors. Wall and Melzack's textbook of pain. 5th ed. Philadelphia: Churchill Livingstone; 2006. p. 1199–214. Chapter 76.
11. Harkness EF, Macfarlane GJ, Silman AJ, McBeth J. Is musculoskeletal pain more common now than 40 years ago?: Two population-based cross-sectional studies. Rheumatology (Oxford). 2005;44(7):890–5.
12. Suka M, Yoshida K. The national burden of musculoskeletal pain in Japan: projections to the year 2055. Clin J Pain. 2009;25(4):313–9.
13. Arnow BA, Hunkeler EM, Blasey CM, Lee J, Constantino MJ, Fireman B, Kraemer HC, Dea R, Robinson R, Hayward C. Comorbid depression, chronic pain, and disability in primary care. Psychosom Med. 2006;68(2):262–8.
14. Nicholl BI, Mackay D, Cullen B, Martin DJ, Ul-Haq Z, Mair FS, Evans J, McIntosh AM, Gallagher J, Roberts B, Deary IJ, Pell JP, Smith DJ. Chronic multisite pain in major depression and bipolar disorder: cross-sectional study of 149,611 participants in UK Biobank. BMC Psychiatry. 2014;14(1):350.
15. Kamaleri Y, Natvig B, Ihlebaek CM, Benth JS, Bruusgaard D. Number of pain sites is associated with demographic, lifestyle, and health-related factors in the general population. Eur J Pain. 2008;12(6):742–8.
16. Aggarwal VR, McBeth J, Zakrzewska JM, Lunt M, Macfarlane GJ. The epidemiology of chronic syndromes that are frequently unexplained: do they have common associated factors? Int J Epidemiol. 2006;35(2):468–76.
17. Birgenheir DG, Ilgen MA, Bohnert AS, Abraham KM, Bowersox NW, Austin K, Kilbourne AM. Pain conditions among veterans with schizophrenia or bipolar disorder. Gen Hosp Psychiatry. 2013;35(5):480–4.
18. Gureje O, Von Korff M, Kola L, Demyttenaere K, He Y, Posada-Villa J, Lepine JP, Angermeyer MC, Levinson D, de Girolamo G, Iwata N, Karam A, Guimaraes Borges GL, de Graaf R, Browne MO, Stein DJ, Haro JM, Bromet EJ, Kessler RC, Alonso J. The relation between multiple pains and mental disorders: results from the World Mental Health Surveys. Pain. 2008;135(1–2):82–91.
19. Croft PR, Papageorgiou AC, Ferry S, Thomas E, Jayson MI, Silman AJ. Psychologic distress and low back pain. Evidence from a prospective study in the general population. Spine (Phila Pa 1976). 1995;20(24):2731–7.
20. Schiphof D, Kerkhof HJ, Damen J, de Klerk BM, Hofman A, Koes BW, van Meurs JB, Bierma-Zeinstra SM. Factors for pain in patients with different grades of knee osteoarthritis. Arthritis Care Res (Hoboken). 2013;65(5):695–702.
21. Phyomaung PP, Dubowitz J, Cicuttini FM, Fernando S, Wluka AE, Raaijmaakers P, Wang Y, Urquhart DM. Are depression, anxiety and poor mental health risk factors for knee pain? A systematic review. BMC Musculoskelet Disord. 2014;15:10.
22. Riddle DL, Kong X, Fitzgerald GK. Psychological health impact on 2-year changes in pain and function in persons with knee pain: data from the osteoarthritis initiative. Osteoarthritis Cartilage. 2011;19(9):1095–101.

23. Holm LW, Carroll LJ, Cassidy JD, Skillgate E, Ahlbom A. Widespread pain following whiplash-associated disorders: incidence, course, and risk factors. J Rheumatol. 2007;34(1):193–200.
24. Kindler LL, Jones KD, Perrin N, Bennett RM. Risk factors predicting the development of widespread pain from chronic back or neck pain. J Pain. 2010;11(12):1320–8.
25. Forseth KO, Husby G, Gran JT, Førre O. Prognostic factors for the development of fibromyalgia in women with self-reported musculoskeletal pain. A prospective study. J Rheumatol. 1999;26(11):2458–67.
26. Davies KA, Macfarlane GJ, Nicholl BI, Dickens C, Morriss R, Ray D, McBeth J. Restorative sleep predicts the resolution of chronic widespread pain: results from the EPIFUND study. Rheumatology (Oxford). 2008;47(12):1809–13.
27. Leung L. Pain catastrophizing: an updated review. Indian J Psychol Med. 2012;34(3):204–17.
28. Severeijns R, Vlaeyen JW, van den Hout MA, Picavet HS. Pain catastrophizing and consequences of musculoskeletal pain: a prospective study in the Dutch community. J Pain. 2005;6(2):125–32.
29. Picavet HS, Vlaeyen JW, Schouten JS. Pain catastrophizing and kinesiophobia: predictors of chronic low back pain. Am J Epidemiol. 2002;156(11):1028–34.
30. Hawker GA, Gignac MA, Badley E, Davis AM, French MR, Li Y, Perruccio AV, Power JD, Sale J, Lou W. A longitudinal study to explain the pain-depression link in older adults with osteoarthritis. Arthritis Care Res (Hoboken). 2011;63(10):1382–90.
31. Gerrits MM, van Marwijk HW, van Oppen P, van der Horst H, Penninx BW. Longitudinal association between pain, and depression and anxiety over four years. J Psychosom Res. 2015;78(1):64–70.
32. Gerrits MM, Vogelzangs N, van Oppen P, van Marwijk HW, van der Horst H, Penninx BW. Impact of pain on the course of depressive and anxiety disorders. Pain. 2012;153(2):429–36.
33. Atlas LY, Wager TD. How expectations shape pain. Neurosci Lett. 2012;520(2):140–8.
34. Brown CA, El-Deredy W, Jones AK. When the brain expects pain: common neural responses to pain anticipation are related to clinical pain and distress in fibromyalgia and osteoarthritis. Eur J Neurosci. 2014;39(4):663–72.
35. Brooks J, Tracey I. From nociception to pain perception: imaging the spinal and supraspinal pathways. J Anat. 2005;207(1):19–33.
36. Vlaeyen JW, Linton SJ. Fear-avoidance and its consequences in chronic musculoskeletal pain: a state of the art. Pain. 2000;85(3):317–32.
37. Leeuw M, Goossens ME, Linton SJ, Crombez G, Boersma K, Vlaeyen JW. The fear-avoidance model of musculoskeletal pain: current state of scientific evidence. J Behav Med. 2007;30(1):77–94.
38. Smith SM, Vale WW. The role of the hypothalamic-pituitary-adrenal axis in neuroendocrine responses to stress. Dialogues Clin Neurosci. 2006;8(4):383–95.
39. McEwen BS. Brain on stress: how the social environment gets under the skin. Proc Natl Acad Sci U S A. 2012;109 Suppl 2:17180–5.
40. McLean SA, Williams DA, Harris RE, Kop WJ, Groner KH, Ambrose K, Lyden AK, Gracely RH, Crofford LJ, Geisser ME, Sen A, Biswas P, Clauw DJ. Momentary relationship between cortisol secretion and symptoms in patients with fibromyalgia. Arthritis Rheum. 2005;52(11):3660–9.
41. McBeth J, Chiu YH, Silman AJ, Ray D, Morriss R, Dickens C, Gupta A, Macfarlane GJ. Hypothalamic-pituitary-adrenal stress axis function and the relationship with chronic widespread pain and its antecedents. Arthritis Res Ther. 2005;7(5):R992–1000.
42. McBeth J, Silman AJ, Gupta A, Chiu YH, Ray D, Morriss R, Dickens C, King Y, Macfarlane GJ. Moderation of psychosocial risk factors through dysfunction of the hypothalamic-pituitary-adrenal stress axis in the onset of chronic widespread musculoskeletal pain: findings of a population-based prospective cohort study. Arthritis Rheum. 2007;56(1):360–71.
43. Clauw DJ. Fibromyalgia: a clinical review. JAMA. 2014;311(15):1547–55.
44. Goddard AW, Ball SG, Martinez J, Robinson MJ, Yang CR, Russell JM, Shekhar A. Current perspectives of the roles of the central norepinephrine system in anxiety and depression. Depress Anxiety. 2010;27(4):339–50.

45. Popa D, Léna C, Alexandre C, Adrien J. Lasting syndrome of depression produced by reduction in serotonin uptake during postnatal development: evidence from sleep, stress, and behavior. J Neurosci. 2008;28(14):3546–54.
46. Ebner K, Singewald N. The role of substance P in stress and anxiety responses. Amino Acids. 2006;31(3):251–72.
47. Smith MT, Haythornthwaite JA. How do sleep disturbance and chronic pain inter-relate? Insights from the longitudinal and cognitive-behavioral clinical trials literature. Sleep Med Rev. 2004;8(2):119–32.
48. Choy EH. The role of sleep in pain and fibromyalgia. Nat Rev Rheumatol. 2015. doi:10.1038/nrrheum.2015.56. Epub ahead of print.
49. Morphy H, Dunn KM, Lewis M, Boardman HF, Croft PR. Epidemiology of insomnia: a longitudinal study in a UK population. Sleep. 2007;30:274–80.
50. Smith MT, Quartana PJ, Okonkwo RM, Nasir A. Mechanisms by which sleep disturbance contributes to osteoarthritis pain: a conceptual model. Curr Pain Headache Rep. 2009;13: 447–54.
51. Lustberg L, Reynolds CF. Depression and insomnia: questions of cause and effect. Sleep Med Rev. 2000;4:253–62.
52. Riemann D, Berger M, Voderholzer U. Sleep and depression – results from psychobiological studies: an overview. Biol Psychol. 2001;57:67–103.
53. Campbell P, Tang N, McBeth J, Lewis M, Main CJ, Croft PR, Morphy H, Dunn KM. The role of sleep problems in the development of depression in those with persistent pain: a prospective cohort study. Sleep. 2013;36(11):1693–8. doi:10.5665/sleep.3130.
54. Kelly GA, Blake C, Power CK, O'Keeffe D, Fullen BM. The association between chronic low back pain and sleep: a systematic review. Clin J Pain. 2011;27:169–81.
55. Staner L. Comorbidity of insomnia and depression. Sleep Med Rev. 2010;14:35–46.
56. Park J, Hughes AK. Nonpharmacological approaches to the management of chronic pain in community-dwelling older adults: a review of empirical evidence. J Am Geriatr Soc. 2012;60(3):555–68.
57. Macfarlane GJ, Beasley M, Jones EA, Prescott GJ, Docking R, Keeley P, McBeth J, Jones GT, MUSICIAN Study Team. The prevalence and management of low back pain across adulthood: results from a population-based cross-sectional study (the MUSICIAN study). Pain. 2012;153(1):27–32.
58. Reid MC, Bennett DA, Chen WG, Eldadah BA, Farrar JT, Ferrell B, Gallagher RM, Hanlon JT, Herr K, Horn SD, Inturrisi CE, Lemtouni S, Lin YW, Michaud K, Morrison RS, Neogi T, Porter LL, Solomon DH, Von Korff M, Weiss K, Witter J, Zacharoff KL. Improving the pharmacologic management of pain in older adults: identifying the research gaps and methods to address them. Pain Med. 2011;12(9):1336–57.
59. Decker SA. Behavioral indicators of postoperative pain in older adults with delirium. Clin Nurs Res. 2009;18(4):336–47.
60. Yohannes AM, Caton S. Management of depression in older people with osteoarthritis: a systematic review. Aging Ment Health. 2010;14(6):637–51.
61. Knauer SR, Freburger JK, Carey TS. Chronic low back pain among older adults: a population-based perspective. J Aging Health. 2010;22(8):1213–34.
62. Strauss VY, Carter P, Ong BN, Bedson J, Jordan KP, Jinks C, Arthritis Research UK Research Users' Group. Public priorities for joint pain research: results from a general population survey. Rheumatology (Oxford). 2012;51(11):2075–82.
63. McBeth J, Wilkie R, Bedson J, Chew-Graham CA, Lacey R. Sleep disturbance and chronic widespread pain. Curr Rheumatol Rep. 2015;17(1):1–10.
64. LeFort SM, Gray-Donald K, Rowat KM, Jeans ME. Randomized controlled trial of a community-based psychoeducation program for the self-management of chronic pain. Pain. 1998;74(2–3):297–306.
65. Lorig K, González VM, Laurent DD, Morgan L, Laris BA. Arthritis self-management program variations: three studies. Arthritis Care Res. 1998;11(6):448–54.

66. Moore JE, Von Korff M, Cherkin D, Saunders K, Lorig K. A randomized trial of a cognitive-behavioral program for enhancing back pain self care in a primary care setting. Pain. 2000;88(2):145–53.
67. Miles CL, Pincus T, Carnes D, Homer KE, Taylor SJ, Bremner SA, Rahman A, Underwood M. Can we identify how programmes aimed at promoting self-management in musculoskeletal pain work and who benefits? A systematic review of sub-group analysis within RCTs. Eur J Pain. 2011;15(8):775.e1–11.
68. Ersek M, Turner JA, Cain KC, Kemp CA. Results of a randomized controlled trial to examine the efficacy of a chronic pain self-management group for older adults [ISRCTN11899548]. Pain. 2008;138(1):29–40.

The Management of Depression and Anxiety in Older People: Evidence-Based Psychological Interventions, Stepped Care and Collaborative Care

8

Simon Gilbody

This chapter considers the main psychological approaches to the management of anxiety and depression in older people. It explores the challenges clinicians face when choosing the best treatment option and also the best way in which care can be organised and delivered in primary care.

The management of depression and anxiety amongst older people follows the same principles as the management of these disorders for working age adults. However, there may be cases where there is a need to adapt treatment to accommodate the presence of physical health problems, sensory impairments, physical frailty or cognitive impairment. This chapter covers the main approaches that are available or could feasibly be offered in primary care, with a specific focus on the most common evidence-supported psychological approaches (especially cognitive behaviour therapy) and innovative frameworks for delivering care for people with depression/anxiety such as stepped care or collaborative care.

8.1 Psychological Approaches to the Management of Depression and Anxiety

A number of psychological approaches can be used in the management of depression and anxiety, and each of these can be used in the treatment of depression amongst older people [1, 2]. Psychological treatments tend to focus on unhelpful ways of thinking or changes in behaviour which occur when someone is depressed or anxious. One of the most commonly used approaches is cognitive behaviour

S. Gilbody
Mental Health and Addictions Research Group, Department of Health Science,
University of York, York, UK
e-mail: simon.gilbody@york.ac.uk

therapy, but there are a number of alternative or complementary approaches which can also be offered and which might be more suited for use amongst older adults.

NICE produced two useful guidelines on the management of depression. The first guideline CG90 [3] relates to the management of depression amongst adults (including older adults) and the second relates to the management of depression amongst people with physical health problems (CG91) [4]. This latter guideline is especially important since a significant proportion of older people will also have coexisting long-term health problems. In relation to anxiety, there is a helpful guideline which summarises the evidential basis of psychological approaches to generalised anxiety disorder [5] and social anxiety [6].

This chapter will outline the main psychological approaches, first for depression and then for anxiety. Special consideration will be given to the adaptation and application of these therapies with regard to older adults.

8.2 Cognitive Behavioural Therapy (CBT) for Depression

Cognitive behavioural therapy (CBT) for depression is generally accepted to have been developed by Aaron T. Beck during the 1950s and became more readily available in the late 1970s when treatment manuals were developed [7, 8]. Beck first observed that people with depression have particular styles of thinking and reasoning which are based on their core beliefs [7]. Depressed people tend to hold negative views of themselves, the world and the future ('the Beckian cognitive triad'). People with depression also make logical errors of reasoning (cognitive distortions) by, for example, overgeneralising, magnifying negatives, minimising positives and catastrophising [9]. The process of CBT encourages people with depression to become aware of these characteristic thinking patterns and to re-evaluate their thinking. In relation to behaviours, CBT recognises that people with depression tend to withdraw from aversive situations and to reduce their levels of activity. This approach requires people to practice recognising and challenging their thoughts and developing new behaviours (by undertaking homework tasks) [10]. By changing patterns of thinking (cognitions) and behaviour, CBT leads to improvements in mood.

Typically CBT is given over 12–20 weekly sessions and requires the person to undertake homework tasks in between sessions [8, 11]. Early in the treatment, the person comes to recognise their unhelpful ways of thinking and acting. Some early improvements are often achieved by introducing new activities or re-engaging with activities which have been lost as depression has developed (by a technique known as 'activity scheduling'). Towards the middle of a course of therapy, the person challenges these patterns of thinking and puts new skills into practice. People undertaking CBT typically have to keep records of thoughts and behaviours (using daily diaries) and to devise 'behavioural experiments' whereby they make negative and positive predictions about what might happen in certain situations based on these predictions. This allows the validity of unhelpful and depressive assumptions to be tested in the 'real world'. Towards the end of therapy, the person develops a plan about how to 'stay well' based on what they have learned and about what to do when if they were to become depressed again (a relapse prevention plan).

8.2.1 What Is the Evidence Base for CBT for Depression?

A large number of high-quality studies have now been conducted which show that CBT is effective in treating depression symptoms and in improving function and quality of life (see Cuijpers and colleagues for a recent overview [12]). The effectiveness of CBT is likely to be comparable to that of antidepressants, and there is no reason why antidepressants and CBT cannot be used in combination with antidepressants. In fact there is some evidence that CBT and antidepressants in combination are more effective than either of these two approaches when offered alone [13]. CBT has been shown to reduce the rate of relapse for people with depression. When reviewing the evidence to support the use of CBT, NICE concluded that *'cognitive behavioural therapies have the largest evidence base. Within this group of studies the largest data set is that which compares individual CBT with antidepressant medication and which shows broad equivalence of effect across the range of severity. The clinical effectiveness data also clearly points to a clear advantage of combination treatment over antidepressants alone'*.

8.2.2 What Is the Evidence Base for CBT for Older People with Depression?

Though the evidence base for CBT is strong, most trials have been conducted amongst working age adults, and there are relatively few trials which have looked at the effectiveness of CBT in older adults. Trials in older adults have been summarised in a systematic review by Gould and colleagues [14]. They found that there is good evidence that CBT is effective in this group, but the evidence that CBT is superior to any other form of psychological treatment (including counselling and supportive therapies) is weak. They conclude that more research is needed before firm conclusions can be drawn in assuming that the effects of CBT are as strong as that observed in working age adults. Gould and colleagues also demonstrated that there is insufficient evidence from older populations to show that CBT is as effective as antidepressants, and it follows that CBT should be offered alongside antidepressant medication when this is indicated rather than as an alternative.

8.3 Behavioural Activation (BA) for Depression

Behavioural activation (BA) is an alternative to CBT which is now growing in popularity and in terms of the breadth of research evidence [15]. This approach for depression evolved from learning theory which proposes that depressive behaviours are learned through the consequences of those behaviours. In behavioural therapies, depression is seen as the result of a low rate of positive reinforcement in everyday life, and depression is maintained through negative reinforcement. People with depression typically use avoidance to minimise negative emotions and situations which they anticipate might be unpleasant [16]. Behavioural therapies focus on behavioural activation aimed at encouraging the patient to develop more rewarding and task-focused behaviours as well as moving away from patterns of negative reinforcement. In recent years, there has been renewed interest in behavioural activation (see, e.g. [17, 18]), as it is now known as a therapy in its own right although it has always been part of cognitive behavioural treatments of depression [19]. At the practical level, behavioural treatments also show some variability, but the monitoring and scheduling of activities are common components in all treatment protocols used in randomised studies of the approach [20].

8.3.1 What Is the Evidence Base for BA for Depression?

There is a very substantial body of evidence drawn from randomised controlled trials which demonstrates unequivocally that BA is an effective treatment for depression. A useful overview of the effectiveness is presented by Ekers and colleagues [21, 22]. In their systematic review, the benefit of BA is at least as large as that for CBT, and in head-to-head trials of CBT versus BA, they are generally found to be equivalent. Though there are fewer trials of BA versus antidepressants than is the case for CBT versus antidepressants, there is still convincing evidence that BA is at least as effective as drug-based treatments. An advantage that is claimed for BA is that it is easier to teach people to deliver this treatment and that patients prefer the simplicity of behavioural approach which does not require more complex cognitive diaries [16].

8.3.2 What Is the Evidence Base for BA for Older People with Depression?

As is the case for CBT, there are relatively few trials of BA for older people compared to the evidential basis of BA in working age adults [22]. In a systematic review by Samad and colleagues [23], four trials were found which provided supportive evidence that BA was superior to usual care and was as effective as CBT. Taken together with the substantial evidence base in working age adults, there is convincing evidence that BA can be assumed to be effective for this age group.

8.4 Psychological Approaches to the Management of Anxiety Disorders in Older People

Anxiety disorders are also common in older people. 'Anxiety' covers the terms generalised anxiety disorder (GAD), panic disorder and phobic anxiety disorders. GAD is a common disorder, of which the central feature is excessive worry about a number of different events associated with heightened tension. Anxiety and depression often co-exist (or overlap) in older people and may also be co-morbid with physical conditions (leading to poorer outcomes in those conditions). Typically an older person with anxiety might worry excessively (ruminate) and experience physical symptoms of overarousal such as a racing heart, overbreathing and gastrointestinal disturbance. Where anxiety is related to specific situations, then avoidance can emerge as a means of managing distressing anxiety symptoms. Older people commonly suffer with intense anxiety on leaving the house (agoraphobia) which can make them housebound or dependent on others to leave the house. Problems commonly arise when they are prevented from shopping or visiting the doctors. For these reasons, people with situational anxieties including agoraphobia often fail to present to their GP. The mainstay of treatment for anxiety disorders is through the use of psychological approaches. As with depression, the mainstay of treatment for anxiety disorders focuses on unhelpful cognitions relating to anxiety-provoking situations and the meaning of somatic anxiety symptoms or the association between aversive stimuli and anxiety responses which is best understood in behavioural terms. Short-term relief from anxiety is achieved by avoidance of aversive situations, and this in turn maintains an anxiety disorder. Effective psychological approaches seek to challenge unhelpful cognitions and to use a process of exposure to aversive stimuli or situations to reduce the severity of anxiety response over time. This takes time and requires people with anxiety to do something which initially makes them more anxious and is counter to most people's long-established form of coping.

There is abundant research evidence drawn from randomised controlled trials to show that cognitive and behavioural approaches are highly effective treatments for anxiety disorders, including generalised anxiety disorder, specific phobias, panic disorder and social anxiety (see Hoffman and colleagues [24] for a review of evidence in this area). As is the case with depression, the evidential basis to support the use of CBT and behavioural approaches to anxiety disorders is smaller, but trials suggest that such strategies are effective in older people (see Hendriks and colleagues [25] for a review of the effectiveness of psychological treatments in older people). However, very few older people are offered these effective forms of treatment.

8.5 Collaborative Care and Stepped Care Frameworks for Depression and Anxiety

Most older people with depression and/or anxiety are managed entirely by the GP within a primary care setting. Only a small proportion of people will be referred for treatment to secondary or specialist care services. Within primary care, there may be poor co-ordination of care for people with depression which results in suboptimal outcomes. Medications are not taken as they are intended, and psychological therapies are not offered or are not in line with evidence. The volume of anxiety and depression in primary care means that it is not feasible to refer all patients to secondary care services, and a response has been to re-engineer or redesign primary care services for people with depression or anxiety to ensure better co-ordination (see Bower and Gilbody for a review [26]). The NICE guidelines (3, 4 and 5) suggest that a 'stepped care' model is utilised, so that patients receive a brief, low-intensity intervention initially but are 'stepped up' to receive higher-intensity psychological input where their symptoms are not improving or 'stepped down' when their symptoms are resolving. This stepped care approach is illustrated diagrammatically in Figs. 8.1 and 8.2.

Collaborative care (CC) is an innovative model of care with a good evidence base for the management of depression. Collaborative care generally involves the case manager actively co-ordinates the care of a person with depression. The case manager delivers an intervention directly to the patient, offering 'person-centred' care (so, a flexible intervention),and working in collaboration with the GP to ensure evidence-supported drug treatments and psychological therapies are offered in an optimal manner. In trials of CC, the intervention has been delivered over the telephone, and case managers are often skilled in the delivery of lower-intensity psychological treatments such as BA over the telephone. A central feature of collaborative care is symptom-tracking whereby standard measures of depression or anxiety severity are used in each session to judge progress and to recognise deterioration. When symptoms do not improve, the person with depression or anxiety can be referred to their GP for a review of their medication or stepped up to receive higher-intensity psychological input.

Stepped care model for depression

Focus of the intervention	Nature of the intervention
STEP 4: Serve and complex[1] depression; risk to life; serve self-neglect	Medication, high-intensity psychological interventions, electroconvulsive therapy, crisis service, combined treatments, multiprofessional and inpatient care
STEP 3: Presistent subthreshold depressive symptoms or mild to moderate depression with inadequate responce and serve depression	Medication, high-intensity psychological interventions, combined treatments, collaborative care[2] and refferal for further assessment and interventions
STEP 2: Presistent subthreshold depressive symptoms; mild to moderate depression	Low-intensity psychosocial interventions, psychological interventions, medication and referral for further assessment and interventions
STEP 1: All konown and suspected presentations of deperssion	Assessment, support, psychoeducation, active monitoring and referral for further assessment and interventions.

Fig. 8.1 Stepped care model for depression (From NICE guidelines [CG90] https://www.nice.org.uk/guidance/cg90/chapter/1-Guidance)

Stepped care model for GAD

Focus of the intervention	Nature of the intervention
STEP 4: Complex treatment-refractory GAD and very marked functional impairment, such as self-neglect or a high risk of self-harm	Highly specialist tratment, such as complex drug and/or psychological traetment regimens; input form multi-agency teams, crisis services, day hospitals or inpatient care
STEP 3: GAD with an inadequate response to step 2 interventions or marked functional impairment	Choice of a high-intensity psychological intervention (CBT/applied relaxation) or a drug treatment
STEP 2: Diagnosed GAD that has not improved after education and active monitoring in primary care	Low-intensity psychological interventions: individual non-facilitated self-help*, individual guided self-help and psychoeducational groups
STEP 1: All known and suspected presentations of GAD	Identification and assessment; education about GAD and treatment options; active monitoring

Fig. 8.2 Stepped care model for generalised anxiety disorder (From NICE guidelines [CG113] https://www.nice.org.uk/guidance/CG113/chapter/1-Guidance)

There is a substantial evidence base to support the use of collaborative care. Over sixty trials of this model of care were included in a Cochrane review by Archer and colleagues (see [27]), and the effectiveness of collaborative care has been demonstrated in the short and longer term. Collaborative care has been shown to improve both depression and quality of life. For older people, there are large-scale trials of this model of care. For example, the IMPACT trial included over 1,800 participants and showed collaborative care to be effective in older people in the USA [28] with effects still apparent 2 years following the input of a case manager [29]. This has led to calls for collaborative care to be more widely implemented for older people in primary care [30].

8.6 Are There Any Special Considerations When Using Psychological Therapy for Older People?

The seminal texts by Beck and colleagues make no reference to psychological approaches being suitable or unsuitable for older people [7, 8, 31]. Older people are not readily offered psychological therapy, and there are sometimes age-based assumptions that evidence-supported approaches such as CBT or BA cannot be as readily used for amongst older people. There are important differences between older and younger people in terms of the cause, presentation and course of depression. One of the most important differences is the coexistence of depression alongside physical health problems and physical decline. An additional factor is the onset of cognitive problems and the importance of social isolation and bereavement in depression for older people. It is clear therefore that some consideration of the role of age in the delivery of CBT needs to be made. This was clearly articulated by Koder and colleagues in relation to CBT [32]: '[T]*he debate is not whether cognitive therapy is applicable to the elderly … but rather how to modify existing cognitive therapy programmes so that they incorporate differences in thinking styles in elderly people, and age-related adjustment*'. This general ethos is one which should guide the delivery of all psychological approaches amongst older people.

In a helpful review of the application of psychological approaches for older people, Evans highlights a number of modifications which need to be made to the delivery and content of therapy [33]. In terms of the delivery of therapy, chronological age alone is not a helpful marker for deciding whether modifications are necessary, and part of the process of assessment for therapy requires some consideration of each of a range of factors highlighted in Table 8.1. A robust cognitive assessment (using an instrument such as the MMSE) and some assessment of sensory difficulties enables adaptations to these factors to be incorporated into the delivery of CBT. Evans also highlights that the content of therapy may be different for older people in order to reflect the common experiences of bereavement, social isolation and physical impairment.

In terms of the content of therapy, Evans [33] also highlights that there are certain age-related themes and factors that may emerge more frequently and thus require a modified focus. By way of example, older people and society at large often holds negative views of ageing, and there is a belief that depression and physical decline

Table 8.1 Procedural modifications to psychological therapy for older people

Tackling cognitive changes
Repeat and summarise information
Present information in multiple modalities
Use folders and notebooks
Consider offering memory training
Tackling sensory impairment
Help to correct it where possible
Prepare written materials in bold print
Use tape recorders
Physical health
Agree realistic goals
Tackle dysfunctional beliefs that limit activity
Input from a 'medicine for the elderly' team
Therapy setting and format
Be flexible
Adapted from Evans [33] with permission

are inevitable. These factors may impact on core beliefs and unhelpful assumptions that emerge in the form of negative automatic thoughts and unhelpful depressive overgeneralisations. Family dynamics may also be more complex with potential for tensions and disagreements in the context of intergenerational relationships. A central tenet of CBT and BA is the importance of increasing a depressed person's repertoire of activities and reintroducing positively re-enforcing behaviours. A barrier to this might be the presence of physical impairments or frailty. When addressing physical impairment, there needs to be careful balance between remaining attentive to any physical limitations a person may have and awareness that individuals may have excessively negative appraisals of their own limitations. Realistic goals need to be agreed when planning behavioural experiments which acknowledge that patients can be severely limited by physical problems. It also requires that more time be spent examining dysfunctional thoughts and assumptions that may be preventing them from making the most of ongoing activities. Increasing activity levels and the reintroduction of positively reinforcing behaviours are at the centre of behavioural activation. For people with reduced physical capacity or increased frailty, this can be seen to be a barrier to 'doing more', and it is important to make use of techniques such as 'activity substitution' and 'functional equivalence'.

Pasterfield and colleagues [34] provide a useful overview of some of the adaptations that can be made to behavioural activation in order for it to be used to the greatest benefit for older people. Behavioural activation pays particular attention to the function that the behaviour holds for an individual and that reinforcement is determined functionally [35]. An important consequence of this view is the concept of 'functional equivalence'. A specific form of behaviour may have served a particular function for a person; however, that behaviour may no longer be possible due to physical health problems. In this situation, an aim of treatment may be to identify a functionally equivalent behaviour that is different in focus and therefore still possible despite physical changes. This concept may be particularly beneficial in the treatment of older people who, for example, may reduce previously enjoyed activities due to physical limitations [36]. If an older person with depression is unable to undertake a previously rewarding activity, they should ask the person why they enjoyed doing it, what else it offered them over and above just doing the activity and what made them keep on doing it and use this information to come up with alternative activities with the participant.

Depression is associated with cognitive impairment in older people [37], and studies have found that some people with early-stage cognitive impairment report feelings of inadequacy and low self-esteem [38]. This could have a potential impact on treatment because problems associated with short-term memory and the recall of information may lead to difficulties in the learning of new material [39]. Proponents of behavioural approaches to depression have argued that they are simpler to deliver than other more complex psychological interventions such as CBT [16, 40], and this may be an advantage of this approach in older people compared to cognitively based treatments. The simplicity of behavioural activation may be particularly beneficial for older adults who may be experiencing cognitive difficulties [41]. Additional reasons to consider behavioural activation as a suitable treatment for older adults include that it conceptualises the onset of depression as being associated with situational factors and changes in a person's environment [42]. Depressive behaviours are seen as being linked to the individual's attempts to cope with these shifts, which are often characterised by a lack of positive reinforcement opportunities [17]. This may be particularly relevant for the treatment of depressive symptoms in older adults who can experience life events such as financial difficulties, bereavement and physical illness, as well as changes in social roles and living situations [43].

8.7 Case Studies

8.7.1 Case Study 1 Treating Anxiety and Depression with CBT: Peter C

Peter, 80, lives with his 78-year-old wife in a terraced house. Peter has chronic obstructive pulmonrary disease (COPD) and is finding that he is increasingly breathless on very minor exertion. He avoids activity and develops pains in his chest. He thinks he might cause himself to have a heart attack. He rarely leaves the house in case when this happens whilst he cannot summon help. Scrutiny of his medical records shows that he has called the ambulance on three occasions in the past few months. On each occasion, he has been taken to A&E where his breathing has settled and he has had normal tests (thus, excluding a heart attack).

When he was asked about his previous leisure activities, he mentioned that he used to play crown green bowls, and he and his wife played in matches and met with people. They no longer do this, and they rarely leave the house together.

When asked about his drinking, he noticed that alcohol temporarily made him feel happier and reduced the degree to which he ruminated about his difficulties. He felt less anxious when he drank, and he noticed that his breathlessness was less prominent.

In previous chapters, we recognised that Peter's problems are suggestive of an anxiety disorder, which is very common amongst people with COPD. Depression is also common in people with COPD, so anxiety and depression may be co-morbid in a patient like Peter. People with anxiety may use alcohol to manage their anxiety, and the clinician should always explore alcohol use.

A psychological approach to Peter's problems would readily identify a number of psychological problems which might be tackled with psychological approaches such as CBT and BA.

A cognitive understanding of anxiety would readily reveal that as part of his COPD, Peter experiences worsening of breathlessness and also develops chest pains. He seeks reassurance and has on many occasions summoned the help of his wife and has called 999 resulting in admission to A&E. He misinterprets the pains in his chest as indicative of an imminent heart attack, but when admitted to A&E, there has never been evidence of this (his tests are always normal). Peter catastrophises and misinterprets his physical symptoms. He has a belief that he will die and seeks reassurance in order to minimise his subjective distress. He is avoidant of situations which might provoke this situation, particularly exercise. As a consequence, he does less and his physical fitness is reducing more quickly than it ought to. He previously was physically active and was an accomplished bowls player. His increasing lack of physical fitness means that he is now unable to get up the stairs which further limits his activity around the house. By recognising the misinterpretation of physical symptoms and engaging in behavioural experiments, he was able to begin to walk longer distances and exert himself, even if this made him breathless. His confidence improved, and in time he was able to start using the stairs again and was able to contemplate leaving the house.

It was decided that it was unrealistic to begin playing bowls again, but a functional analysis as part of BA identified that bowls fulfilled an important role in his life. It meant that he got out of the house with his wife and met old friends with a shared interest. Since he stopped playing bowls, a range of positively re-enforcing and mood-enhancing activities have ceased, and this contributes to his depression. By putting in place some functionally equivalent strategies, Peter was able to start attending social gatherings at the local bowls club, and in time he took up a less physically demanding but important role at the club. He and his wife took on the joint role of treasurer. His mood improved over time, and he came to look forward to twice weekly meetings at the bowls club. Peter reconnected with old friends, and he met them outside of club meetings by visiting their homes and receiving guests at his own home.

Peter developed some mastery of anxiety and some improvements in mood. He found less need for a drink at night-time, and in time his mood further improved as he reduced his alcohol intake to within recommended limits.

8.7.2 Case Study 2 Diabetes and Depression: Afzal K

Mr K is 75 years old and lives with his eldest son, who works as an accountant, daughter-in-law and their four children. His wife died suddenly 2 years ago following a subarachnoid haemorrhage. He stopped working in the family shop following his bereavement and gave the business to his second son. He has had diabetes since the age of 50 and tries hard to watch his diet; he usually takes his medication regularly but struggles to know what to do during Ramadan. His son has just been told he, too, has diabetes, and now the family meals are more focused on ensuring that all the family eat plenty of fruit and vegetables. Mr K rarely attends his general practice, except when he is told to make an appointment for an annual review with the practice nurse.

Mr K tries to speak to his grandchildren, who are teenagers, but they all seem so busy, so he spends a lot of time on his own. He goes to the Mosque but, otherwise, rarely leaves the house. Sometimes he wishes he didn't wake up in the morning but feels guilty about this.

In previous chapters, we have recognised that Mr K is likely to have a depressive illness, which is quite common amongst people with diabetes. He had also experienced a number of significant life events including the loss of his wife and the loss of role in managing his shop. A psychological approach using CBT or BA is especially helpful in this case. A cognitive understanding of Mr K's depression would first examine his core beliefs. Mr K feels very guilty about having diabetes and thinks that something he did as a younger man might have caused him to become diabetic. He feels a burden on his family and has experienced a change in role. He has experienced a transition from being the head of the family who had built up the family business and provided for the family. His role had changed to being someone who could no longer manage the business and was financially dependent on the labours of his son. When asked about his views of himself, he felt a failure in many aspects of his life. Looking to the future, his view was that he would forever be a burden on his family and that it was inevitable that he would develop severe complications of diabetes irrespective of what he did. He was hopeless and had contemplated suicide in order to relive his family of the burden of caring for him. He worried about his diabetes and thought this prevented him engaging in new activities. He displayed a typical cognitive triad described earlier with a negative view of himself, his environment and the future. When asked about the future of his family and the business, he felt that bad things would always happen and the business would fail and the family would be separated. He demonstrated an overgeneralisation, assuming that if one bad thing happened, then things would always be bad for his family.

Mr K was encouraged to keep a diary to capture some examples of these thoughts, and he worked collaboratively with a therapist to challenge some of the underlying assumptions. In time Mr K came to recognise some of these thoughts and to challenge them for himself. In relation to his diabetes, he came to recognise that there was no inevitability to his physical deterioration and recognised that he could take greater control of the outcome of his diabetes by engaging in treatment and improving his diabetic control.

Using a behavioural activation approach, Mr K quickly realised that he avoided any reminder of his diabetes including making visits to the diabetic nurse. He recognised that he was doing much less and there was an absence of positively reinforcing activities including going to the Mosque, where he previously enjoyed social interaction and contemplating his faith. Functional equivalence and activity substitution helped him recognise that there were things which he could do at the Mosque whilst observing Ramadan and maintaining control over his diabetes. He found that diabetes was quite common amongst other members of the Mosque and there were certain accommodations for people of the Moslem faith with diabetes who have to observe Ramadan. His experience of therapy was improved through the recognition that there were specific adaptations that can be made for people of the Moslem faith [44]. He increased his activity levels and found some early gains and improvements in his mood. In turn this made him more positive and optimistic that he could make further changes in his life. His relationship with his son improved, and he began working in the shop on 1 or 2 days per week. His diabetic control improved after visiting the diabetic nurse, and this in turn made him take an active role in choosing his food, doing the weekly food shop and helping with the cooking.

8.8 Opportunities for Reflection

- How does CBT and BA help us understand depression and anxiety?
- What is the evidence that CBT is effective?
- What is the evidence that BA is effective?
- How would you access psychological therapy for your patients?
- Are there any adaptations which need to be made in order to help an older person engage with psychological therapy?
- Can psychological therapy be used alongside medication?
- What is collaborative care and how does this improve the outcomes of primary care for depression?

References

1. Scogin F, McElreath L. Efficacy of psychosocial treatments for geriatric depression: a quantitative review. J Consult Clin Psychol. 1994;62(1):69.
2. Lebowitz BD, et al. Diagnosis and treatment of depression in late life: consensus statement update. JAMA. 1997;278(14):1186–90.
3. National Institute for Health and Clinical Excellence. Depression in adults: the treatment and management of depression in adults (update – NICE clinical guideline 90). Manchester: National Institute for Health and Clinical Excellence; 2009.
4. National Institute for Clinical Excellence. The treatment and management of depression in adults with chronic physical health problems (partial update of CG23). London: NICE; 2009.
5. National Institute for Clinical Excellence. Generalised anxiety disorders, (with or without agoraphobia in adults) (CG113). London: NICE; 2011.
6. Pilling S, et al. Recognition, assessment and treatment of social anxiety disorder: summary of NICE guidance. BMJ. 2013;346:f2541.
7. Beck AT, et al. Cognitive therapy for depression. New York: Guilford Press; 1979.
8. Beck JS. Cognitive therapy: the basics and beyond. New York: Guilford Press; 1995.
9. Beck AT. Thinking and depression 1: Idiosyncratic content and cognitive distortions. Arch Gen Psychiatry. 1964;9:324–33.
10. Beck AT. Cognitive therapy: nature and relation to behavior therapy. Behav Ther. 1970;1(2):184–200.
11. Beck AT, Steer RA. The beck depression inventory manual. San Antonio: The Psychological Corporation, Harcourt Brace Janovich; 1987.
12. Cuijpers P, et al. A meta-analysis of cognitive-behavioural therapy for adult depression, alone and in comparison with other treatments. Can J Psychiatry Rev Can Psychiatr. 2013;58:376–85.
13. Cuijpers P, et al. Psychotherapy versus the combination of psychotherapy and pharmacotherapy in the treatment of depression: a meta-analysis. Depress Anxiety. 2009;26(3):279–88.
14. Gould RL, Coulson MC, Howard RJ. Cognitive behavioral therapy for depression in older people: a meta-analysis and meta-regression of randomized controlled trials. J Am Geriatr Soc. 2012;60(10):1817–30.
15. Veale D. Behavioural activation for depression. Adv Psychiatr Treat. 2008;14(1):29–36.
16. Ekers D, et al. Behavioural activation. In: Dryden W, editor. Cognitive behaviour therapies. London: SAGE Publications Ltd; 2012.
17. Jacobson NS, Martell CR, Dimidjian S. Behavioral activation treatment for depression: returning to contextual roots. Clin Psychol Sci Pract. 2001;8(3):255–70.
18. Hopko DR, et al. Contemporary behavioral activation treatments for depression: procedures, principles, and progress. Clin Psychol Rev. 2003;23(5):699–717.

19. Beck AT. The past and future of cognitive therapy. J Psychother Pract Res. 1997;6:276–84.
20. Kanter JW, et al. What is behavioral activation?: A review of the empirical literature. Clin Psychol Rev. 2010;30(6):608–20.
21. Ekers D, Richards D, Gilbody S. A meta-analysis of randomized trials of behavioural treatment of depression. Psychol Med. 2008;38(5):611–23.
22. Ekers D, et al. Behavioural activation for depression; an update of meta-analysis of effectiveness and sub group analysis. PLoS One. 2014;9(6):e100100.
23. Samad Z, Brealey S, Gilbody S. The effectiveness of behavioural therapy for the treatment of depression in older adults: a meta-analysis. Int J Geriatr Psychiatry. 2011;26(12):1211–20.
24. Hofmann SG, et al. The efficacy of cognitive behavioral therapy: a review of meta-analyses. Cogn Ther Res. 2012;36(5):427–40.
25. Hendriks G, et al. Cognitive behavioural therapy for late life anxiety disorders: a systematic review and meta-analysis. Acta Psychiatr Scand. 2008;117(6):403–11.
26. Bower P, Gilbody S. Managing common mental health disorders in primary care: conceptual models and evidence base. BMJ. 2005;330:839–42.
27. Archer J, et al. Collaborative care for depression and anxiety problems. Cochrane Database Syst Rev, 2012;(10):CD006525.
28. Unutzer J, et al. Collaborative care management of late-life depression in the primary care setting: a randomized controlled trial. JAMA. 2003;288:2836–45.
29. Hunkeler EM, et al. Long term outcomes from the IMPACT randomised trial for depressed elderly patients in primary care. BMJ. 2006;332(7536):259–63.
30. Chew-Graham CA, Burns A, Baldwin RC. Treating depression in later life: we need to implement the evidence that exists. BMJ. 2004;329:181–2 [Invited Editorial].
31. Beck AT. Cognitive therapy of the emotional disorders. New York: New Americal Library; 1976.
32. Koder DA, Brodaty H, Anstey KJ. Cognitive therapy for depression in the elderly. Int J Geriatr Psychiatry. 1996;11(2):97–107.
33. Evans C. Cognitive–behavioural therapy with older people. Adv Psychiatr Treat. 2007;13(2):111–8.
34. Pasterfield M, et al. Adapting manualized behavioural activation treatment for older adults with depression. Cogn Behav Ther. 2014;7:e5.
35. Martell CR, Addis MA, Jacobson NS. Depression in context: strategies for guided action. New York: Norton; 2001.
36. Yon A, Scogin F. Behavioral activation as a treatment for geriatric depression. Clin Gerontol. 2008;32(1):91–103.
37. Vinkers DJ, et al. Temporal relation between depression and cognitive impairment in old age: prospective population based study. BMJ. 2004;329(7471):881.
38. Clare L. Managing threats to self: awareness in early stage Alzheimer's disease. Soc Sci Med. 2003;57(6):1017–29.
39. Zeiss AM, Steffen A. Treatment issues with elderly clients. Cogn Behav Pract. 1997;3(2):371–89.
40. Ekers D, et al. Behavioural activation delivered by the non-specialist: phase II randomised controlled trial. Br J Psychiatry. 2011;198(1):66.
41. Porter JF, Spates CR, Smitham S. Behavioral activation group therapy in public mental health settings: a pilot investigation. Prof Psychol Res Pract. 2004;35(3):297.
42. Quijano LM, et al. Healthy IDEAS A depression intervention delivered by community-based case managers serving older adults. J Appl Gerontol. 2007;26(2):139–56.
43. Fiske A, Wetherell JL, Gatz M. Depression in older adults. Annu Rev Clin Psychol. 2009;5:363.
44. Mir G, et al. Adapted behavioural activation for the treatment of depression in Muslims. J Affect Disord. 2015;180:190–9.

Pharmacological Management of Anxiety and Depression in Older People

Philip Wilkinson and Sophie Behrman

9.1 Introduction: Pharmacological Treatments in Context

Depressive and anxiety disorders are commonly encountered in older patients in primary care. They may present with psychological or physical symptoms or a combination and may impact on the course and management of coexisting physical disorders. Depression and anxiety often coexist; up to a quarter of older people with anxiety disorders also meet criteria for major depression [1] and the presence of anxiety in depressed patients is associated with a greater risk of relapse [2]. Not surprisingly, therefore, their causes and treatments also overlap. Most anxiety disorders are diagnosed by the age of 40, but a few people will develop them after 65 years [3]; generalised anxiety and social phobia appear to be the more common disorders in older people. They typically run a cyclical course and are unlikely to remit completely, even with long-term treatment. Around two thirds of people with Alzheimer's disease experience anxiety symptoms and 5–6 % have diagnosable generalised anxiety disorder [4] so it is important to assess for cognitive impairment when deciding on management. Risk factors for anxiety in older people include female gender, multiple physical conditions, residing in a care home, and physical disability [3]. Anxiety is specifically linked to thyroid problems, respiratory and gastrointestinal disorders, and arthritis; anxiety disorders may also precede the onset of physical illness and worsen quality of life and disability [5].

Depression may also precede the onset of physical illness, such as Parkinson's disease [6]. Suffering with depression worsens the outcome of physical illness via reduced treatment adherence, increased disability, and higher mortality. Physical

---

P. Wilkinson, BM, BS, FRCPsych (✉) • S. Behrman, BA, BMBCh, MRCPsych
Department of Psychiatry, Warneford Hospital, Oxford, Oxfordshire, UK
e-mail: philip.wilkinson@psych.ox.ac.uk; sophie.behrman@psych.ox.ac.uk

symptoms influence the course of depression; ongoing pain is particularly linked to the recurrence of depression [7]. While in younger adults antidepressants are as efficacious in people with comorbid physical illnesses as those without [8], in older people specific neurobiological changes such as cerebral white matter disease are associated with a poorer response to antidepressant treatment [9, 10]. Poorer response is also predicted by advanced age, higher levels of stress, poorer social support, younger age at first episode, higher anxiety, and poorer sleep [11]. Compared with younger patients, older people may take longer to respond to antidepressant medication and as many as half may not achieve remission with their first treatment [12]. There is marked variation in rate and stability of recovery ranging from rapid sustained improvement to partial response or lack or response.

Older patients may be reluctant to take antidepressant medication due a lack of understanding of depression, fear of drug dependence, and negative experiences with medication [13]. Stigma against seeking help for psychological problems may also be a barrier. It is worthwhile, therefore, exploring a patient's attitude and backing up treatment with factsheets and active monitoring [14]. The prescriber should be aware of relevant guidelines in the treatment of depression and anxiety. However, it is important to recognise that the evidence base for drug treatment of anxiety and depression in older people is significantly smaller than in younger adults as drug trials typically exclude patients with complex physical illness and those taking multiple medications [15]. For instance, there is a paucity of randomised controlled trials in anxiety disorders in older people not responding to first line treatments [16]. In addition, guidelines may not easily map onto the management of patients with complex multimorbidity [17]. Potential adverse effects will need to be taken into the equation and weighed against the negative consequences for physical and psychological health of leaving anxiety or depression untreated. Non-pharmacological treatments should always be considered. The best results are obtained by a collaborative approach between primary care and a depression case manager using both psychological and pharmacological interventions [18, 19], if such a service is available.

9.2 Drugs Used in the Treatment of Anxiety and Depression

Antidepressants are the principal group of medications used in the treatment of anxiety and depression. Their main therapeutic mechanisms of action are enhancement of the activity of the neurotransmitters serotonin (5-HT) and noradrenaline (norepinephrine); antidepressants can be subdivided into those acting solely on one neurotransmitter (single action) and those acting on both (dual action). The first antidepressants to be developed also acted on other neurotransmitter systems, such as cholinergic pathways, causing undesirable side effects. The diversity of actions of antidepressant drugs allows prescribers to individualise treatment decisions and to avoid specific side effects [20]. Specialist prescribers may also institute

Table 9.1 Main classes of antidepressant

Class	Examples
Serotonin reuptake inhibitors (SSRIs)	Sertraline, citalopram
Tricyclic antidepressants (TCAs)	Amitriptyline, imipramine, lofepramine
Serotonin/noradrenaline reuptake inhibitors (SNRIs)	Venlafaxine, duloxetine
Noradrenergic and specific serotonergic antidepressants (NaSSAs)	Mirtazapine
Serotonin antagonist/serotonin reuptake inhibitors (SARIs)	Nefazodone
Noradrenaline/dopamine reuptake inhibitors (NDRIs)	Bupropion
Monoamine oxidase inhibitors (MAOIs)	Phenelzine, tranylcypromine

Data from Stahl [20]

combinations of drugs to enhance efficacy and reduce adverse effects. The main classes of antidepressants currently in use are listed in Table 9.1.

9.2.1 Serotonin Reuptake Inhibitors (SSRIs)

SSRIs are single-action antidepressants and currently are the first line in the pharmacological treatment of depression and anxiety in late life. The group includes citalopram (and its isomer escitalopram), sertraline, fluoxetine, and paroxetine. SSRIs have a lower rate of cardiac conduction abnormalities in overdose than older antidepressants and a low propensity to cause seizures. However, frequent side effects include nausea, vomiting, dry mouth, insomnia, weight gain, and sexual dysfunction. Therefore they may not be suitable in patients with insomnia and agitation. SSRIs may also worsen parkinsonism. Naturalistic studies indicate that treatment of older adults with SSRIs is not associated with increased risk of completed or attempted suicide, in contrast with their use in adolescents. In fact, treatment reduces risk of suicide by over 50 % [21].

9.2.2 Tricyclic Antidepressants

These dual-action drugs were amongst the earliest antidepressants. The group includes amitriptyline, nortriptyline, dothiepin, clomipramine, and imipramine. As well as the desired action on serotonin and noradrenaline receptors, they also act at other receptors (acetylcholine, adrenergic, and histamine) giving rise to dry mouth, constipation, tachycardia, cognitive impairment, postural hypotension, and sedation. Nortriptyline has been well evaluated in older people with well-established efficacy and tricyclics retain a place in the treatment of depression and anxiety under specialist supervision.

9.2.3 Other Classes of Antidepressant

Venlafaxine and duloxetine are dual-action serotonin/noradrenaline reuptake inhibitors (SNRIs) that also have an inhibiting effect on the neurotransmitter dopamine. Some flexibility is offered by the use of venlafaxine which, at lower doses, functions as a single-action SSRI. SNRIs may be more beneficial than SSRIs in treatment-resistant depression [22]. Mirtazapine and nefazodone are dual-action antidepressants that have additional properties of postsynaptic serotonin antagonism which can reduce adverse effects such as sexual dysfunction and nausea associated with serotonin reuptake inhibition. They also antagonise alpha-adrenergic receptors causing adverse effects of postural hypotension and dizziness. Mirtazapine also has some histamine blocking effect, causing sedation and weight gain. Monoamine oxidase inhibitors were the original antidepressant class. Now generally avoided due to dietary restrictions and interactions, they still have a place in the treatment of atypical and treatment-resistant depression under specialist supervision.

9.2.4 Lithium

Lithium (as its carbonate or citrate salt) is a well-established and effective mood-stabilising treatment in the management of bipolar disorder, including the treatment of bipolar depression. Lithium can also be used in the augmentation of antidepressant treatment in patients with unipolar depression who have failed to respond to antidepressant treatment alone. From the limited number of studies of different augmentation strategies in older people, lithium has the strongest evidence of efficacy [23] and it also reduces suicide risk [24]. Prescribing with diuretics (particularly thiazides) and non-steroidal anti-inflammatory drugs should usually be avoided, but, otherwise, lithium can generally be used safely in older patients taking other drugs for comorbid medical conditions. Monitoring of serum levels, renal function, thyroid function, and weight is essential and particular care is necessary in patients with chronic renal impairment. Therefore, lithium should usually be initiated and monitored by a specialist.

9.2.5 Antipsychotics

Antipsychotic drugs are primarily used in the treatment of schizophrenia, other psychoses, and bipolar disorder. Their main action is through the blockade of dopaminergic pathways. Newer ("atypical") antipsychotics also interact with serotonin receptors and have a role in the specialist management of depressive illness to augment the effects of antidepressants [25] although extrapyramidal and metabolic side effects may limit their use in certain patients. There are only limited data to support the use of antipsychotics in the treatment of anxiety disorders [26], so given the risk of adverse effects in older people, their use should be limited to more severe or treatment-refractory cases, under specialist supervision. Antipsychotic use in people with dementia is associated with increased risk of stroke and death [27] and so should be limited to specialist prescribing.

9.2.6 Benzodiazepines

Benzodiazepines, such as lorazepam and diazepam, act by enhancing the effect of the inhibitory neurotransmitter gamma-aminobutyric acid (GABA). Although of benefit in the short-term management of severe anxiety, their side effects of sedation, falls and cognitive impairment, and the potential for dependence mean that long-term use is best avoided. However, under specialist supervision, they might be used in disabling anxiety that is refractory to a range of pharmacological and psychological interventions [28].

9.2.7 Buspirone

Buspirone is a partial serotonin agonist with some dopaminergic action that acts to reduce anxiety. It has the advantage over benzodiazepines of not suppressing breathing and lacks dependence risk. However its benefits in the long-term management of generalised anxiety are not clear and it appears to be ineffective in patients who have been dependent on benzodiazepines [29].

9.2.8 Pregabalin

Pregabalin is an anticonvulsant drug that decreases the release of glutamate and noradrenaline; unlike benzodiazepines, it does not act on GABA receptors. Although less commonly used than antidepressant drugs, it appears to be of benefit in the treatment of generalised anxiety disorder and social anxiety and may also relieve depressive symptoms. As it is excreted unmetabolised, it may be more suitable than other drugs for patients with hepatic impairment [28].

9.3 Pharmacological Considerations in Treating Older Patients

9.3.1 Drug Interactions

Knowledge of the interaction potential of antidepressants helps clinicians to predict and avoid certain drug combinations, making prescribing safer [30]. This applies particularly to older patients who often take a range of medications and in whom reduced serum albumin levels may give rise to interactions with other plasma-bound drugs such as warfarin. The hepatic cytochrome p450 enzymes are involved in the metabolism of a large proportion of psychotropic drugs which also can lead to the inhibition of warfarin metabolism in patients taking antidepressants. Therefore, patients taking warfarin who are starting antidepressant treatment will require closer anticoagulant monitoring. Sertraline and citalopram are the SSRIs least likely to interact with warfarin. SSRIs can also increase levels of tricyclic antidepressants so this combination should only

Table 9.2 Important drug interactions in older patients taking antidepressants

Drugs causing interaction	Effect of interaction
Antipsychotic drugs Loop and thiazide diuretics Antiepileptic drugs Antiparkinsonian drugs	Hyponatraemia
Anticoagulants Non-steroidal anti-inflammatory drugs	Increased bleeding
Erythromycin Tamoxifen Quinine Antiarrhythmic drugs	Impaired cardiac conduction
Other classes of antidepressant with serotonergic action	Serotonin syndrome

be used under specialist supervision. See Table 9.2 for a summary of important drug interactions.

9.3.2 Hyponatraemia

The prevalence of hyponatraemia in older people treated with antidepressants as a probable consequence of treatment is around 9 %. Mechanisms include syndrome of inappropriate antidiuretic hormone secretion (SIADH) and nephrogenic syndrome of inappropriate antidiuresis [31]. Although most often associated with SSRI treatment, hyponatraemia can occur with all classes of antidepressant. While routine monitoring of serum sodium in patients taking antidepressants is not recommended, the prescriber should consider monitoring in the presence of certain risk factors and potential interactions (see Tables 9.2 and 9.3) and when symptoms of confusion and fatigue are present. Management of hyponatraemia involves reviewing the indication for the antidepressant, review of other medications, fluid restriction, and possible trial of different classes of antidepressant. Left undetected, severe hyponatraemia can lead to seizures, permanent neurological damage, and death so discussion with a general physician is advised when serum sodium is lower than 125 mmol/l.

9.3.3 Risk of Bleeding

In patients taking SSRIs, a decrease in platelet serotonin release is thought to lead to reduced platelet aggregation, increasing the risk of gastrointestinal bleeding. Therefore, the prescriber should consider the addition of a proton pump inhibitor when an SSRI is prescribed with other medications that increase risk of gastric bleeding (non-steroidal anti-inflammatory drugs and anticoagulants) [32] and in patients drinking large amounts of alcohol. Concern has been expressed about the possibility of an increased risk of haemorrhagic stroke in people taking SSRIs, but,

Table 9.3 Risk factors for hyponatraemia in patients taking antidepressants

Previous hyponatraemia
Low weight
Psychosis
Heart failure
Severe renal impairment
Diabetes mellitus
Hypertension
Chronic obstructive pulmonary disease

based on current evidence, there is no reason to restrict their use in depressed older people with cerebrovascular risk factors or post-stroke depression [33].

9.3.4 Cardiac Effects

Antidepressants are associated with changes in cardiac conduction, with prolongation of the PR, QRS, and QT intervals. At clinical doses, these changes are most likely to occur with tricyclics; most SSRIs do not appear to be associated with an increased risk of adverse events in people with cardiac disease [34]. However, the SSRI citalopram and its isomer escitalopram are associated with significant risk of QT prolongation at higher clinical doses so that maximum daily doses of 20 mg and 10 mg, respectively, are recommended (www.hma.eu). Risk of QT prolongation is increased by prescribing with certain other drugs, including erythromycin, tamoxifen, and quinine. It should be remembered that treatment of depression may actually improve the prognosis of cardiovascular disease by reducing mortality associated with depression or through effects on platelet function and modification of arrhythmias [35].

9.3.5 Other Adverse Effects of Antidepressants

SSRIs can induce or worsen movement disorders such as tremor, dyskinesia, dystonia, and parkinsonism, so monitoring for side effects is recommended in patients with these problems. Sertraline may be the least likely to cause movement disorders [33]. Sexual side effects of SSRIs include delayed or absent orgasm; this may respond to a change to an alternative antidepressant such as mirtazapine. Older antidepressants (tricyclics and monoamine oxidase inhibitors) may worsen glycaemic control in patients with diabetes, while SSRIs and SNRIs appear to have no effect; mirtazapine is not known to affect glycaemic control but can produce weight gain. Although it has been suggested that serotonergic antidepressants can accelerate osteoporosis, there is no sound evidence for this [36]. Serotonin syndrome is a rare complication of treatment with serotonergic drugs manifesting as mental state changes, autonomic instability, and neuromuscular abnormalities; those at greater risk are patients taking more than one serotonergic drug [37].

9.3.6 Antidepressant Discontinuation Syndromes

Although antidepressants are not addictive, patients should be aware that abrupt cessation of treatment can produce unpleasant symptoms that may be similar to those of their anxiety or depression, such as irritability, nausea, and neuromotor changes. Apart from fluoxetine, which has a long half-life, antidepressants should be tapered and withdrawn over a 1-month period. On rare occasions, it may be appropriate to stop antidepressants suddenly (e.g. after a cardiac arrhythmia with a tricyclic antidepressant); on such occasions it would be prudent to seek specialist advice.

9.4 Making Prescribing Decisions for Depression in Older People

As in all clinical situations, the decision on whether or not to prescribe depends on a weighing-up of the potential pros and cons of treatment. Ideally, this should be a collaborative process with the clinician, the patient, and his/her relatives or friends. For some, a good assessment will itself be therapeutic, giving an opportunity for the clinician and patient to come to a shared understanding of the biological, psychological, and social factors impacting on the patient's condition. For mild depression, the patient may benefit from self-help strategies and addressing some of the stressors in their life. If the patient is found to have moderate depression, i.e. impacting on day-to-day functioning, they may have a view as to whether to pursue psychological or pharmacological therapy which may be based on some assumptions which might be helpful to explore. For example, some are wary to take antidepressants, believing that they are addictive; if this view is dispelled, it might persuade a patient to try antidepressants. Alternatively, a patient with a very medical view of depression may be encouraged to take a more psychological stance on considering his/her illness and may gain further insight and improve further than would have been possible with medication alone. In certain situations, following assessment, the primary care physician may recommend referral to a specialist service (see Table 9.4).

Evidence with younger adults indicates that 50 % of those in a depressive episode will respond to an antidepressant, compared to 30 % of those taking a placebo [38]. As with younger adults, antidepressant drugs are more likely to be of benefit if an older person's depression is of at least moderate severity [39]. The NICE clinical practice guideline for depression [14] advocates a stepwise approach to treatment, with active monitoring and psychological therapies being first-line treatments. Antidepressants are reserved for episodes of moderate or greater severity and for patients who have had a less intense low mood for 2 years or more (dysthymia) and those who have had previous episodes of severe depression. If antidepressants are started, NICE recommends an SSRI as first line, with a gastroprotective agent for older patients and/or those taking NSAIDs or aspirin. A Cochrane systematic review supports this approach, finding that SSRIs and tricyclics have similar efficacy in

Table 9.4 Indications for referral to a specialist older people's mental health service

Suspected bipolar affective disorder
Presence of delusions and hallucinations (psychotic depression)
Concurrent significant alcohol or substance abuse
Failure of anxiety or depression to respond to two different classes of antidepressant
Possibility of dementia
Significant risks (suicidality, self-neglect, risk to others)

older people but with SSRIs being better tolerated [40]. Sertraline and escitalopram are the better tolerated SSRIs [41].

Contrary to widely held beliefs, the beneficial effect of antidepressants is most pronounced in the first week of use, with continuing improvement seen for the first 6 weeks of treatment [42]. Guidelines suggest increasing the chosen antidepressant to recommended therapeutic dose and monitoring for 4 weeks to see if it is effective [38]. Subtherapeutic dosing has previously been found to be a significant cause of non-response in older people [43]. This may reflect low expectations on behalf of the prescriber or patient or fear of the harm; however, with newer antidepressants there is no reason to avoid recommended doses. When a first-line antidepressant trial has failed, subsequent prescribing choices are guided by the findings of the "STAR-D" study [44]. In this, with citalopram as first-line treatment, 30 % of participants achieved remission. After a switch to bupropion, venlafaxine, or sertraline, or augmenting with bupropion or buspirone about a further 25 % more remitted. In further treatment stages of change of drug class or augmentation, smaller proportions each time achieved remission. The NICE Depression Guideline [14] recommends that if there is an inadequate response or intolerable side effects with a first-line SSRI, treatment be changed to another SSRI or another better tolerated newer generation antidepressant such as mirtazapine. As a third-line strategy, a switch to a different class that is usually less well tolerated is indicated (e.g. venlafaxine, a tricyclic, or a MAOI). At all steps of the guideline, it is recommended that psychological therapies as an adjunct be considered. If some benefit is seen, but the patient is struggling with side effects, it may be appropriate to provide reassurance and to continue the drug (perhaps reducing the dose or offering non-pharmacological strategies to manage the side effect), as many side effects dissipate over time. If side effects persist or are intolerable, a second medication may be added to help, such as mirtazapine for sexual dysfunction. While first- and second-line treatments may be initiated in primary care, it would be usual for further interventions to be introduced under specialist supervision.

As well as switching between antidepressants, a specialist in secondary care may also suggest augmenting antidepressants with other drugs, particularly if some initial benefit has been seen. Agents used to augment antidepressants include lithium, mirtazapine, and atypical antipsychotics, including aripiprazole, olanzapine, quetiapine, and risperidone. Before starting lithium, a baseline ECG is recommended in patients with cardiovascular disease. Once stabilised, lithium levels are monitored

12 h post dose every 3 months, and renal function, thyroid function, and calcium monitored every 6 months. If a patient develops dehydration or altered renal function, more frequent monitoring is advised. Patients who have failed to respond to multiple courses of different antidepressants may be seen as being "treatment resistant" and some of the more complex strategies outlined above can be adopted. Before labelling a patient as "treatment resistant", however, it is prudent to review the diagnosis and to look at drug interactions, poor compliance, and comorbid substance abuse.

Depression is typically a recurrent disorder. Of those with one episode of major depression, 50–80 % will go on to have a second episode, and of those who have had two episodes, 80–90 % will have a third [35]. Risk factors for recurrence include being female, having a longer and more complex episode of depression, comorbid physical illness, recurrent dysthymia, psychosocial stressors, and poor social support. Guidelines for younger adults recommend continuing the antidepressant(s) at full therapeutic dose for 6–9 months from full remission of a first episode of depression in order to reduce the risk of relapse [14, 38]. In patients with recurrent depression, continuing antidepressants reduces the risk of relapse by two thirds [45] and NICE recommends continuing antidepressants for at least 2 years [14], but, again, this is based on studies with younger adults. A Cochrane review of continuation and maintenance studies of antidepressant treatment in older people did not find evidence of benefit based on a small number of trials [46]. The risks and benefits of continuing antidepressants must always be weighed up on an individual basis to allow the patient and doctor to make a decision about ongoing treatment. In the absence of contraindications, the prescriber is likely to base the decision on the available guidelines for younger adults and to consider long-term treatment when depression is severe or highly recurrent. A pathway for prescribing decisions is shown in Fig. 9.1.

St John's wort (*Hypericum perforatum*) is a commonly used herbal antidepressant that is available without prescription. The active ingredient and mechanism of action are unclear but they possibly involve inhibition of breakdown and reuptake of monoamines and action on serotonin receptors. St John's wort is generally well tolerated and has been found to be effective for mild to moderate depression and dysthymia [47]. However, the product is poorly regulated, the therapeutic dose is unknown, and it may interact with a number of other medications. Patients taking it may omit to mention it to their doctor assuming that, as a herbal medicine, it will be harmless. NICE does not recommend the use of St John's wort in the management of depression [14].

9.5 Case 1: Mr A, Initial Presentation of Depression

Mr A, a 70-year-old man, presents to his general practitioner (Dr X) with a month-long history of low mood, poor sleep, poor appetite, lack of motivation, and reduced enjoyment of his usual activities. He has no prior history of mental disorder and no physical illnesses.

9 Pharmacological Management of Anxiety and Depression in Older People

Initial assessment
- confirm diagnosis
- discuss with patient (and family) self-help strategies, active monitoring, and psychological therapies
- refer to specialist if indicated (see Table 9.4)

↓

If medication appropriate, discuss with patient different options (see Tables 9.2 and 9.3), taking into account.
- past response
- likely therapeutic response
- adverse effects and interactions
- time to respond
- likelihood/risks of discontinuation reactions

↓

- Start antidepressant (SSRI first line or mirtazapine if sedation required)
- Titrate dose (increase 1–2 weekly)
- Monitor carefully first 2–4 weeks (risk of side effects)
- Assess efficacy

↓

No effect
Assess weekly for further 1–2 weeks, increase dose if tolerated

Good effect. Continue for 6-9 months at treatment does for single episode, longer for recurrent depression. Withdraw antidepressants gradually and warn about discontinuation symptoms.

Partial effect/poorly tolerated
Adjust dose
Weigh up risks/benefits of switching antidepressant

Intolerable/inadequate effect
Switch to a different antidepressant (may wish to try a different class) and reasess

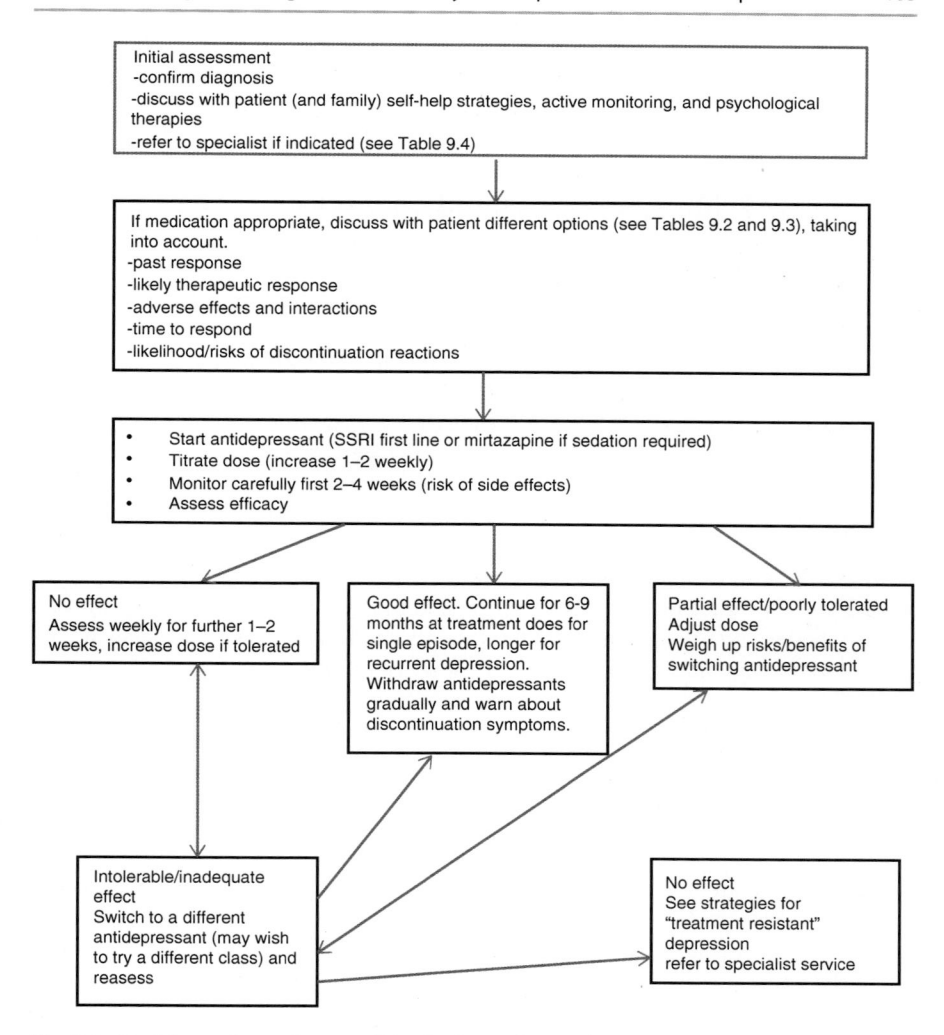

No effect
See strategies for "treatment resistant" depression
refer to specialist service

Fig. 9.1 Decision pathway for prescribing in depression

This would seem to be a depressive episode. A biopsychosocial assessment should confirm the diagnosis and identify precipitating and maintaining factors and risks.

Dr X completes a full assessment and diagnoses a moderate depressive episode with no major risks and no significant functional impairment. Dr X outlines treatment options, gives some written information about depression and sleep hygiene, and asks Mr A to make a follow-up appointment. Mr A returns the following week and is keen to be referred for psychological therapy but not sure about medication as he has heard it is addictive and would prefer to try a natural option like St John's wort. Dr X discusses the pros and cons of medication and St John's wort and addresses some of Mr A's misunderstandings. Mr A decides to try psychological therapy alone (an online course while waiting for an assessment with the psychological therapy service). Dr X supports the decision and advises Mr A to return for a follow-up appointment in 2 weeks or sooner if necessary.

9.6 Case 2: Mr A, Starting an Antidepressant

Mr A returns to Dr X after a month as he feels no better and would like to consider starting an antidepressant. Dr X discusses the pros and cons of different medications. Although Mr A has difficulty getting to sleep, this has improved slightly with exercise and Mr A does not like the idea of taking mirtazapine due to the risks of daytime sedation and weight gain. They agree on a trial of sertraline, starting at 50 mg. Dr X discovers that Mr A occasionally takes ibuprofen for joint pain and advises him about the risk of gastrointestinal bleeding with both NSAIDs and SSRIs. Mr A agrees to try different analgesic options if required, rather than start a proton pump inhibitor as a gastroprotective agent. Dr X advises Mr A of possible side effects of sertraline and asks him to return in a week's time.

On return a week later, Mr A feels slightly better. He has had some symptoms of nausea and diarrhoea but these seem to be settling. One week later, Mr A still feels slightly better and asks to increase the dose of sertraline to see if this leads to any further improvement. Dr X increases the dose to 100 mg and asks Mr A to return again for a further appointment. Mr A feels a great deal better on 100 mg and decides to stay on this dose while continuing psychological treatment.

9.7 Case 3: Mr A, Stopping an Antidepressant

Mr A returns to Dr X after 5 months of treatment and asks about stopping the sertraline as he does not feel he needs it any longer. Dr X discusses the pros and cons of stopping the medication and the potential risk of relapse with Mr A. Mr A decides to continue for another couple of months until he has finished his course of psychological treatment before stopping the medication. The sertraline is reduced to 50 mg daily for 1 month and then discontinued.

NICE guidelines recommends continuing antidepressants for 6 months from remission of a first episode of depression [14] *although at present there is a lack of evidence specific to older people* [45].

9.8 Case 4: Mr A, Recurrence of Depression

Nine months later, Mr A returns with another episode of depression and feels worse than he did previously. He restarts sertraline and finds he needs a higher dose this time (150 mg). After 6 weeks of treatment, he feels much better and would like to reduce the dose and eventually stop the sertraline again. Dr X and Mr A discuss the increased risk of relapse; now Mr A has had two episodes of depression. Dr X informs Mr A of the guidelines which recommend continuing it for 2 years for relapse prevention. Mr A decides to continue at 150 mg.

9.9 Case 5: Mrs B, a Patient Who Does Not Respond to Treatment

Mrs B presents with a first episode of moderate depression aged 75. She is not keen to try any psychological therapy and so starts a course of sertraline increasing the dose to 100 mg over 2 weeks. She does not notice any improvement in her symptoms and asks Dr X if she can try something else. Dr X discusses the pros and cons of different options with her, suggesting trying either mirtazapine or a different SSRI. Mrs B decides to try mirtazapine as she has been having trouble sleeping.

9.10 Case 6: Mrs B, No Response to a Change of Antidepressant

After 4 weeks, Mrs B has still not noticed any improvement in her symptoms. Dr X explores her problems further and discovers that she is using significant alcohol in order to help her sleep. He discusses the possibility of alcohol being a maintaining factor of her problems and suggests ways of cutting down her intake, offering specialist support and advice on sleep hygiene. Dr X explores again Mrs B's reticence towards psychological therapies but she remains unwilling to consider this as an option.

Mrs B manages to cut down her alcohol intake, but her depressive symptoms get worse, despite good compliance with mirtazapine 45 mg nightly. Dr X is concerned that Mrs B has been having more suicidal thoughts and is neglecting her self-care and refers her to the older adult community mental health team (CMHT). She sees a psychiatrist who adds venlafaxine to her mirtazapine and a community psychiatric nurse assesses Mrs B at home to support her through her recovery.

9.11 Case 7: Mr C, Depression After a Stroke

Dr X sees Mr C 2 weeks after his return from hospital following a large ischaemic cerebrovascular event. Mr C is receiving intensive support from the community physiotherapists but is not making as much progress as they would like as he lacks motivation to complete the rehabilitation exercises. The physiotherapist has discussed the case with Dr X as he is concerned Mr C may be depressed.

It is estimated that 40 % of patients who survive a stroke suffer from depression and that this slows down rehabilitation [48]. There is also some evidence that, regardless of depressive symptoms, antidepressants may enhance recovery of motor skills in the rehabilitation process [49]. Although theoretically there is potential for SSRIs to worsen haemorrhagic stroke, in practice this does not seem to be the case and the benefits of antidepressants (including SSRIs) outweigh the risks for both haemorrhagic and ischaemic stroke[48], with there currently being evidence for citalopram, fluoxetine, and nortriptyline [35].

Mr C starts a course of fluoxetine (with omeprazole as he is already taking clopidogrel after his stroke) and finds his mood and motivation improve, with subsequent benefits for his recovery and rehabilitation.

9.12 Case 8: Mrs D, Depression After Previous Deliberate Overdoses

Mrs D has a history of recurrent depression with previous suicide attempts by overdose. She consults Dr X about starting antidepressants. She cannot recall what treatments have helped previously and her old records are not available. She currently has no specific plans to take an overdose but explains that previous overdoses have been impulsive and often after drinking alcohol.

Dr X considers the pros and cons of different medication options with Mrs D. Tricyclic antidepressants and venlafaxine are least safe in overdose so are best avoided. There would be a risk of oversedation if Mrs D were to take an overdose of mirtazapine, particularly if combined with alcohol. SSRIs would be the safest option but Mrs D will still need careful monitoring and possible referral to the CMHT. It is agreed that her neighbour will look after her stocks of medication.

9.13 Case 9: Mrs E, Hyponatraemia and Confusion with an SSRI

Mrs E is aged 85 and living in a nursing home. She has a history of heart failure following a myocardial infarction and a degree of renal impairment and takes (amongst other medications) bendroflumethiazide and omeprazole. She was started on fluoxetine by a colleague 2 weeks ago and the nursing home call Dr X as she appears muddled and lethargic. Dr X completes a full assessment and requests serum electrolytes. Mrs E is found to have a serum sodium of 127 mmol/L (normal range 135–145 mmol/L), which is the likely cause of her confusion and lethargy.

See Table 9.3 *for risk factors for developing hyponatraemia. When sodium is greater than 125 mmol/l, the patient can be monitored daily and the team may consider withdrawing the likely causal agent. If sodium drops below 125 mmol/l, it is prudent to seek specialist medical advice and to stop the SSRI. Fluid restriction alone may correct the sodium. It is possible to repeat a trial of an SSRI or to use a less serotonergic antidepressant, such as lofepramine* [35].

Dr X slowly withdraws the fluoxetine and monitors her sodium, but three days later it has dropped to 124 mmol/L. Mrs E is treated in a general hospital and returns to the nursing home. Dr X weighs up the pros and cons of further antidepressant treatment with Mrs E and her key nurse and they decide to avoid further antidepressants for the time being.

9.14 Case 10: Mr F, Sexual Dysfunction with an SSRI

Mr F presents to Dr X requesting to stop the fluoxetine he started a month ago. Dr X explores this further with him, and, although he reports some improvement in his depression, he has been suffering from erectile dysfunction and sees that this might be a side effect of the medication. Dr X discusses this further and Mr F recognises that the erectile dysfunction may also be linked to the depression, given that some of his difficulties occurred before starting fluoxetine. Dr X excludes other contributory factors to the erectile dysfunction, such as substance misuse, side effects of other medications, and diabetes. Dr X reassures Mr F that sexual dysfunction side effects of SSRIs are reversible and discusses different options with Mr F. Options include continuing on the same dose of fluoxetine and monitoring, trying a reduced dose, switching to or adding a different antidepressant with likely lower risk (e.g. mirtazapine), or considering adding sildenafil as an adjunct. Mr F decides to switch to mirtazapine which helps both his erectile dysfunction and his mood.

Bupropion is thought to be the antidepressant with the least likelihood of sexual dysfunction side effects, but it is currently not licensed for use as an antidepressant in the UK [35].

9.15 Case 11: Mrs G, Psychotic Depression

Mrs G's daughter asks Dr X to urgently assess her mother as she has rapidly lost weight. Dr X finds no physical cause for her weight loss. Mrs G has not been eating and explains to Dr X that her "insides have rotted away" and that she is somehow culpable for her granddaughter's recent miscarriage. Dr X explores this further and diagnoses Mrs G with a psychotic depression. Due to the severity of her illness, Dr X discusses her case with the CMHT who arrange an urgent assessment. Mrs G is supported in her home with daily visits from a care agency and frequent contact from the CMHT. She is started on olanzapine, an antipsychotic, and sertraline. Dr X continues to work closely with the mental health team and to manage her physical health, with regular reviews and blood tests as she begins to eat again. Over time, Mrs G's psychotic symptoms diminish and she is able to look after herself without the support of carers.

9.16 Case 12: Mr H, Depression with a Background of Bipolar Affective Disorder

Mr H presents to Dr X with a moderate depressive episode. He is known to have bipolar affective disorder with numerous previous admissions to hospital with mania. His last admission was 5 years ago, and he has been taking lithium since, but stopped it a year ago, with the support of the CMHT, as he was beginning to develop renal failure. Dr X discusses the case with the CMHT as there would be a risk of Mr

H developing another manic episode if he started antidepressant treatment. The CMHT psychiatrist assesses Mr H and discusses the pros and cons of different treatment options with him, including the possibility of trying quetiapine (an antipsychotic with an antidepressant action) or restarting lithium. Mr H agrees to try quetiapine and his depressive symptoms improve without any manic relapse.

9.17 Making Prescribing Decisions for Anxiety in Older People

Anxiety disorders are highly prevalent in older people although sufferers may be unlikely to seek help. Anxiety symptoms are associated with increased disability and mortality, increased burden on health service, and decreased cognitive and functional abilities [15]. As already described, anxiety often coexists with depression and chronic physical health conditions which may blind the clinician to identifying the anxiety disorder and offering appropriate treatment. Different types of anxiety disorder also often coexist – for example, a patient with generalised anxiety may also have a specific phobia. When considering more than one diagnosis, it is advisable to perform a thorough assessment of all symptoms in order to gain an understanding of the patient's experience, to treat the predominant disorder and then reassess the effect on other symptoms, and offer further treatment if necessary.

The largest evidence base in the management of anxiety disorders is for psychological interventions, particularly cognitive behavioural therapy (CBT) [50]; pharmacological therapy is reserved for patients who experience functional impairment or do not respond to psychological therapy. For treatment-refractory anxiety, the combination of pharmacotherapy and psychological therapy can be considered but there is little evidence to guide decisions [16]. Benzodiazepines are only recommended for short-term use in generalised anxiety disorder and extra caution should be taken when prescribing in the elderly due to risk of sedation and falls. Table 9.5 summarises current prescribing guidance. Patients whose anxiety does not respond to an SSRI are likely to be referred to a specialist for advice on further management.

9.18 Case 13: Mrs I, Generalised Anxiety Disorder

Mrs I presents to Dr X following an admission to hospital. She is highly anxious about falling and so has not felt able to leave the house since her discharge 2 months ago. She is frequently seeking reassurance from her daughter who asks if she can be started on benzodiazepines. Dr X assesses Mrs I and finds that she has numerous physical and psychological symptoms of anxiety and specific worries about falling consistent with generalised anxiety disorder. Dr X discusses different treatment options with Mrs I and her daughter and explains the risks of increased falls and dependence with benzodiazepines. Mrs I is too anxious to leave the house to attend

Table 9.5 Prescribing decisions for anxiety disorders

Anxiety disorder	Acute management	Long-term first-line management	Other drug treatments	Comments
Generalised anxiety disorder	Benzodiazepines (short-term use only – weeks)	Start with sertraline and then try another SSRI or venlafaxine. Use low starting dose and increase gradually. If lack of response, try pregabalin	Buspirone, beta blockers for somatic symptoms (with caution due to cardiovascular effects)	Continue treatment for a year. May prevent development of depression
Panic disorder	Benzodiazepines not recommended by NICE	SSRIs – as above	Imipramine or clomipramine if no improvement after 12 weeks (with caution due to cardiovascular effects)	Assess for comorbid depression and/or substance abuse
Post-traumatic stress disorder	Nil	SSRIs (paroxetine or sertraline) and then venlafaxine	Other antidepressants	Continue for 12 months
Obsessive compulsive disorder	Nil	SSRIs, clomipramine. May take up to 12 weeks to respond	Augment with antipsychotics or mirtazapine	May need higher dose of antidepressants than dose for depression. May take longer to remit. Continue for 12 months
Social phobia	Occasional short-acting benzodiazepines	SSRIs and then venlafaxine. Consider MAOIs (phenelzine, moclobemide)	Buspirone as adjunct to SSRIs, propranolol for performance anxiety (with caution due to cardiovascular effects)	Treat for at least 6 months

Data from National Institute for Health and Clinical Excellence [50] and Baldwin et al. [28]

a psychological therapy group and there is a waiting list for individual CBT at home. Mrs I and Dr X agree that she should start sertraline while waiting for the individual CBT. Mrs I responds well to sertraline and bibliotherapy about anxiety and the CBT model. After a month of treatment, she is able to leave the house and attends the group CBT with good effect.

9.19 Case 14: Mr J, Mixed Anxiety and Depression

Mr J presents 6 months after the death of his wife with symptoms of low mood and anxiety. After careful assessment Dr X diagnoses Mr J with a moderate depressive episode with prominent anxiety symptoms. Dr X and Mr J agree to initiate treatment with antidepressants and CBT. Mr J responds well to antidepressants and both his depressive and anxiety symptoms resolve.

9.20 Case 15: Mrs K, Anxiety in Chronic Disease

Mrs K frequently attends Dr X's practice with symptoms of breathlessness. Mrs K has a history of chronic obstructive pulmonary disease (COPD) with frequent exacerbations. Dr X diagnoses features of generalised anxiety disorder as well as poorly controlled COPD. Mrs K is not keen on taking medication and Dr X sees from old notes that many of her infective exacerbations of COPD have been complicated by her poor compliance with antibiotics and steroid regimes. Dr X refers Mrs K to the practice nurse for education about her COPD and intensive support in enabling her to manage her own symptoms. Mrs K's compliance with inhalers improves, her peak flow improves, and she has fewer exacerbations of her COPD, which improves her breathlessness and anxiety symptoms.

9.21 Suggested Topics for Clinical Audit in Primary Care

- Rates of follow-up appointments within 2 weeks of initiating antidepressant treatment
- Rates of 6-month review of antidepressant treatment with decision on whether to continue
- Identification of drug combinations associated with important interactions (SSRIs with NSAIDs or anticoagulants; lithium with diuretics)
- Monitoring of renal and thyroid function and lithium levels in patients taking lithium

9.22 Appendix 9.1: Suggested Reading for Patients

Age UK website, including printable factsheets on depression: www.ageuk.org.uk/health-wellbeing/conditions-illnesses/depression/

Mind website, including factsheets on depression and anxiety: www.mind.org.uk/information-support/types-of-mental-health-problems/depression
NHS Choices website: www.nhs.uk/conditions

9.22.1 Appendix 9.2: Recommended Reading for Prescribers

Cleare A, Pariante C, Young AH, et al. Evidence-based guidelines for treating depressive disorders with antidepressants: a revision of the 2008 British Association for Psychopharmacology guidelines. J Psychopharmacol 2015;29(5): 459–525.

Baldwin DS, Anderson IM, Nutt DJ, et al. Evidence-based pharmacological treatment of anxiety disorders, post-traumatic stress disorder and obsessive-compulsive disorder: A revision of the 2005 guidelines from the British Association for Psychopharmacology. J Psychopharmacol (Oxf). 2014;28(5):403–39.

Taylor D, Paton C, Kapur S. The Maudsley prescribing guidelines in psychiatry. 11th edn. Chichester: Wiley-Blackwell; 2012.

Stahl S. The prescriber's guide: antidepressants. New York: Cambridge University Press; 2006.

References

1. Cairney J, Corna L, Veldhuizen S, et al. Comorbid depression and anxiety in later life: patterns of association, subjective well-being, and impairment. Am J Geriatr Psychiatry. 2008;16(3): 201–8.
2. Andreescu C, Lenze E, Mulsant BH, et al. High worry severity is associated with poorer acute and maintenance efficacy of antidepressants in late-life depression. Depress Anxiety. 2009; 26(3):266–72.
3. Wolitzky-Taylor KB, Castriotta N, et al. Anxiety disorders in older adults: a comprehensive review. Depress Anxiety. 2010;27(2):190–211.
4. Ferretti L, McCurry S, Logsdon R, et al. Anxiety and Alzheimer's disease. J Geriatr Psychiatry Neurol. 2001;14(1):52–8.
5. Sareen J, Jacobi F, Cox BJ, et al. Disability and poor quality of life associated with comorbid anxiety disorders and physical conditions. Arch Intern Med. 2006;166(19):2109–16.
6. de la Riva P, Smith K, Xie S, Weintraub D. Course of psychiatric symptoms and global cognition in early Parkinson disease. Neurology. 2014. doi:10.1212/WNL.0000000000000801.
7. Gerrits M, van Oppen P, Leone S, et al. Pain, not chronic disease, is associated with the recurrence of depressive and anxiety disorders. BMC Psychiatry. 2014;14:187.
8. Rayner L, Price A, Evans A, et al. Antidepressants for depression in physically ill people. Cochrane Database Syst Rev. 2010;3.
9. Alexopoulos G, Murphy C, Gunning-Dixon F, et al. Microstructural white matter abnormalities and remission of geriatric depression. Am J Psychiatry. 2008;165:238–44.
10. Sheline Y, Pieper C, Barch D, et al. Support for the vascular depression hypothesis in late-life depression: results of a two-site, prospective, antidepressant treatment trial. Arch Gen Psychiatry. 2010;67:277–85.
11. Dew MA, Reynolds III CF, Houck P, et al. Temporal profiles of the course of depression during treatment. Arch Gen Psychiatry. 1997;54:1016–24.
12. Roose SP, Schatzberg A. The efficacy of antidepressants in the treatment of late-life depression. J Clin Psychopharmacol. 2005;25(4 Suppl 1):S1–7.

13. Fawzi W, Abdel Mohsen MY, Hashem AH, et al. Beliefs about medications predict adherence to antidepressants in older adults. Int Psychogeriatr. 2012;24(01):159–69.
14. National Institute for Health and Clinical Excellence. The treatment and management of depression in adults (updated version). National Clinical Practice Guideline 90. 2010.
15. Gonçalves DC, Byrne GJ. Interventions for generalized anxiety disorder in older adults: systematic review and meta-analysis. J Anxiety Disord. 2012;26(1):1–11.
16. Barton S, Karner C, Salih F, et al. Clinical effectiveness of interventions for treatment-resistant anxiety in older people: a systematic review. Health Technol Assess Rep. 2014;18(50).
17. Greenlagh T, et al. Evidence based medicine: a movement in crisis? BMJ. 2014;348:18–21.
18. Hunkeler E, Katon W, Tang L, et al. Long term outcomes from the IMPACT randomised trial for depressed elderly patients in primary care. Br Med J. 2006;332:259–62.
19. Richards DA, Hill JJ, Gask L, et al. Clinical effectiveness of collaborative care for depression in UK primary care (CADET): cluster randomised controlled trial. BMJ. 2013;347:f4913.
20. Stahl S. Selecting an antidepressant by using mechanism of action to enhance efficacy and avoid side-effects. J Clin Psychiatry. 1998;59(18):23–9.
21. Barbui C, Esposito E, Cipriani A. Selective serotonin reuptake inhibitors and risk of suicide: a systematic review of observational studies. Can Med Assoc J. 2009;3:291–7.
22. Mazeh D, Shahal B, Aviv A, et al. A randomized single-blind comparison of venlafaxine with paroxetine in elderly patients suffering from resistant depression. Int Clin Psychopharmacol. 2007;22:371–5.
23. Cooper C, Katona C, Lyketsos K, et al. A systematic review of treatments for refractory depression in older people. Am J Psychiatry. 2011;168(7):681–8.
24. Cipriani A, Hawton K, Stockton S, Geddes J. Lithium in the prevention of suicide in mood disorders: updated systematic review and meta-analysis. BMJ. 2013;346:3646.
25. Sheffrin M, Driscoll H, Lenze EJ, et al. Pilot study of augmentation with aripiprazole for incomplete response in late-life depression: getting to remission. J Clin Psychiatry. 2009;70:208–13.
26. Depping A, Komossa K, Kissling W, Leucht S. Second-generation antipsychotics for anxiety disorders. Cochrane Database Syst Rev. 2010;(12):CD008120.
27. Banerjee S. The use of antipsychotic medication for people with dementia: time for action. London: Department of Health; 2009.
28. Baldwin DS, Anderson IM, Nutt DJ, et al. Evidence-based pharmacological treatment of anxiety disorders, post-traumatic stress disorder and obsessive-compulsive disorder: a revision of the 2005 guidelines from the British Association for Psychopharmacology. J Psychopharmacol (Oxf). 2014;28(5):403–39.
29. Chessick C, Allen M, Thase M. Azapirones for generalized anxiety disorder. Cochrane Database Syst. Rev. 2006;(3):CD006115.
30. Spina E, Trifirò G, Caraci F. Clinically significant drug interactions with newer antidepressants. CNS Drugs. 2012;26(1):39–67.
31. Mannesse C, Jansen P, van Marum RP, et al. Characteristics, prevalence, risk factors, and underlying mechanism of hyponatraemia in elderly patients treated with antidepressants: a cross-sectional study. Maturitas. 2013;76:357–63.
32. de Abajo F. Effects of selective serotonin reuptake inhibitors on platelet function: mechanisms, clinical outcomes and implications for use in elderly patients. Drugs Aging. 2011;28(5):345–67.
33. Chemali Z, Chahine LM, Fricchione G. The use of selective serotonin reuptake inhibitors in elderly patients. Harv Rev Psychiatry. 2009;17(4):242–53.
34. Lespérance F, Frasure-Smith N, Koszycki D, et al. Effects of citalopram and interpersonal psychotherapy on depression in patients with coronary artery disease: the Canadian Cardiac Randomized Evaluation of Antidepressant and Psychotherapy Efficacy (CREATE) trial. JAMA. 2007;297:367–79.
35. Taylor D, Paton C, Kapur S. The Maudsley prescribing guidelines in psychiatry. 11th ed. Chichester: Wiley-Blackwell; 2012.
36. Gebara MA, Shea MLO, Lipsey KL, et al. Depression, antidepressants, and bone health in older adults: a systematic review. J Am Geriatr Soc. 2014;62(8):1434–41.

37. Buckley N, Dawson A, Ibister G. Serotonin syndrome. BMJ. 2014;348:33–5.
38. Cleare A, Pariante C, Young AH, et al. Evidence-based guidelines for treating depressive disorders with antidepressants: a revision of the 2008 British Association for Psychopharmacology guidelines. J Psychopharmacol 2015;29(5):459–525.
39. Nelson J, Delucchi K, Schneider L. Moderators of outcome in late-life depression: a patient-level meta-analysis. Am J Psychiatry. 2013;170:651–9.
40. Mottram P, Wilson K, Strobl J. Antidepressants for depressed elderly. Cochrane Database Syst Rev. 2006;(1):CD003491.
41. Cipriani A, Furukawa TA, Salanti G, et al. Comparative efficacy and acceptability of 12 new-generation antidepressants: a multiple-treatments meta-analysis. Lancet. 2009;373(9665):746–58.
42. Taylor MJ, et al. Early onset of selective serotonin reuptake inhibitor antidepressant action: systematic review and meta-analysis. Arch Gen Psychiatry. 2006;63:1217–23.
43. Heeren TJ, Derksen P, van Heycop Ten Ham BF, van Gent PP. Treatment, outcome and predictors of response in elderly depressed in-patients. B J Psychiatry. 1997;170:436–40.
44. Gaynes BD, Warden D, Trivedi MH, et al. What did the STAR*D teach us? Results from a large-scale, practical, clinical trial for patients with depression. Psychiatr Serv. 2009;60(11):1439–45.
45. Geddes JR, Carney SM, Davies C, et al. Relapse prevention with antidepressant drug treatment in depressive disorders: a systematic review. Lancet. 2003;361:653–61.
46. Wilkinson P, Izmeth Z. Continuation and maintenance treatments for depression in older people (review). Cochrane Database Syst Rev. 2012;(11):CD006727. doi:10.1002/14651858.CD006727,pub2.
47. Linde K, Berner M, Egger M, Mulrow C. St John's wort for depression: meta-analysis of randomised controlled trials. Br J Psychiatry. 2005;186:99–107.
48. Sarkstein SE, Mizrahi R, Power BD. Antidepressant therapy in post-stroke depression. Expert Opin Pharmacother. 2008;9(8):1291–8.
49. Chollet D, Tardy J, Albucher J-F, Berard E, et al. Fluoxetine for motor recovery after acute ischaemic stroke (FLAME): a randomised placebo-controlled trial. Lancet Neurol. 2011;10:123–30.
50. National Institute for Health and Clinical Excellence. Generalised anxiety disorder and panic disorder (with or without agoraphobia) in adults. Management in primary, secondary and community care. National Clinical Practice Guideline 113. www.niceorguk. 2011.

Depression and Anxiety: Admission and Discharge

10

Alan Thomas

10.1 Introduction

Depression is more common in older people with long-term physical conditions (see Chap. 5). As expected this is particularly true in people with brain diseases: 20–40 % of people with Parkinson's disease, [1] 25–50 % with dementia [2] and about a third of people after stroke [3]. Anxiety is also common in older adults, though consistently reported as less so than in younger adults. A problem with prevalence figures is the variety of anxiety disorders and their different definitions, but overall anxiety disorders occur in about 5 % of people over 65 during a 12-month period, compared with about three times this prevalence in younger adults [4]. The development of anxiety in an older person with no previous history of anxiety should be taken to suggest the real problem is depression with anxiety [5], and anxiety is a predictor of poor outcome [6].

Anxiety may increase the risk of hospital admission, and the presence of both anxiety and depression can lead to difficulties for discharge back home and in the immediate post-discharge period.

The impact of anxiety and depression on hospital admission and discharge will be considered in the following cases.

10.2 Case Study 1

Mrs H is a 74-year-old woman living alone in a deprived urban area. She had apparently enjoyed good physical and mental health although seemed to have been a little too dependent on her husband and their three children. She had never worked

---

A. Thomas, MRCPsych, PhD
Institute of Neuroscience, Newcastle University, Newcastle upon Tyne, UK
e-mail: alan.thomas@ncl.ac.uk

© Springer International Publishing Switzerland 2016
C.A. Chew-Graham, M. Ray (eds.), *Mental Health and Older People:
A Guide for Primary Care Practitioners*, DOI 10.1007/978-3-319-29492-6_10

outside the home and had only a limited social network, all of whom were joint friends with her husband. When her husband died suddenly of a stroke when she was 72, she was bereft. Her children rallied round to support her, and all initially seemed well. However, after 6 months or so, she began ringing the out-of-hours service frequently and making appointments at her GP practice weekly or more often. Her concerns were about vague physical symptoms, such as headache, dizziness, palpitations and pain, which were always difficult to localize, and she appeared increasingly tense. Physical assessment and blood tests were normal, and on questioning by her GP, she admitted to worrying about how she would cope and when anxious to experiencing tingling in her limbs and palpitations.

Paracetamol and other analgesics did not help her vague pain symptoms, and she declined referral to the primary care mental health team (PCMHT), or third sector agencies (Anxiety UK), [7] to help with her anxiety symptoms. She became increasingly withdrawn, and her children became concerned about her weight loss and requested a home visit. The GP found her very low in mood, complaining of headache and vague pain and possibly having lost weight. She said she could not sleep, and there were again no features on examination suggesting a physical cause of her symptoms. Mrs H denied any thoughts of harming herself, but admitted that she sometimes wished she was dead. This GP suggested that she might take an antidepressant but she declined.

That evening Mrs H called an ambulance and was taken to A&E, where she became distressed, crying and saying she was going to die, pleading for someone to help her. After several hours, having been refused assessment as 'too old' by the local crisis team, she was assessed by the on-call junior psychiatrist who admitted her.

On the ward, she did not exhibit any significant depressive symptoms, but the nurses found her very dependent, frequently asking for help to do ordinary tasks such as dressing. If left alone for much time, she sought out staff, often in a flustered state complaining of feeling worried about her health and that she was a terrible burden on her family. She often caught one of the ward doctors to plead for a physical assessment, though these and investigations never identified any physical health concerns. Discussion with her children during visits gradually revealed that Mrs H had not only always wanted her husband to do everything but that she had 'always been a worrier' and 'complained about her health all the time'.

A case conference was held, and her social worker reported Mrs H to be well known as a frequent caller over the last couple of years who had had undergone assessments but then declined the services offered. At the case conference, it was agreed with Mrs H and her family that she return home to have a home assessment by a social worker, to have weekly input from the community mental health nurse, and a follow up by a consultant psychiatrist in 6 weeks. However, some concern was expressed about how agreeable Mrs H really was to this as she had seemed to enjoy being on the ward and was unsettled by the prospect of discharge. The day before her discharge she cut herself on the left forearm, pleading that she could not cope, but it appeared with no intention of significantly harming herself.

Somatic symptoms in older people may be manifestations of an affective illness, although exclusion of underlying physical causes should be more carefully considered than in younger adults, so it is important that physical examination and investigations, including indicated blood tests, are conducted.

The presence of anxiety and depression increases use of services including GP attendance [8] ('frequent attenders') and admission [9].

The use of case-finding questions for anxiety (see Chap. 5) is key to the identification of anxiety in patients who attend frequently, particularly with a range of physical symptoms. The clinician should also be aware of the increased use of alcohol in people with anxiety. Key informant information can be useful, as in case 1 where it became apparent that anxiety and 'dependent' traits were longstanding features of Mrs H. Such features may only surface when the social circumstances alter, in this case, the loss of her husband on whom she had depended. Assessment of risk is just as important in patients where anxiety symptoms appear to predominate (see Chap. 5) as in depression. Residual anxiety symptoms are a problematic feature in late-life depression and frequently refractory to standard drug treatments.

Admission of people with anxiety to hospital can exacerbate their problems, and intensive home-based support would have been more appropriate, in the above case, including the clinical team encouraging Mrs H to have a social work assessment and support through community-based services. This can be facilitated through an integrated care approach [10].

10.3 Case Study 2

Mr Patel is an 82-year-old man who lives with his extended family in the suburbs of a large city. He has asthma and diabetes, treated hypertension and was recently told that he has 'something wrong with his kidneys', but he is normally mobile and active. One evening, his family took to A&E following an episode of chest pain. They were keen to take him home, but the doctor told him that he might have had a heart attack, so he was admitted to the Coronary Care Unit, although he only stayed there one night and is now on a ward surrounded by 'old people'. He is now very worried about his heart, but no one has confirmed whether he had a heart attack, and no one has explained why all his tablets have been changed. He cannot sleep because of all the noise in the ward at night. He pleads with his family to take him home and is discharged after two further days in hospital.

Following discharge, his sons become increasingly concerned that their father is withdrawn and quiet; he used to be such a pleasure to be with but is now irritable if anyone speaks to him. He has started to take his meals into his own room and declines to go out on family visits. The family is upset that no one from Mr Patel's practice have visited since he was discharged, and the social care package that was promised lasted only a week, because they were told that there were sufficient family members in the house to support Mr Patel to get dressed and take his tablets. They began to agree when Mr Patel said that 'no one cares' and were concerned that he was not taking his tablets properly.

Depression is two to three times more common in a range of cardiovascular diseases including cardiac disease, coronary artery disease, stroke, angina, congestive heart failure, or following a heart attack [11]. Prevalence estimates vary between around 20 % and 50 % depending on the conditions studied and the assessment approach used, but the two- to threefold increase compared with controls is consistent across studies. Anxiety problems are also common in cardiovascular disease [12, 13]. Outcomes from cardiovascular care are poorer for patients with co-morbid mental health problems, even after taking severity of cardiovascular disease and patient age into account. Cardiovascular patients with depression experience 50 % more acute exacerbations per year [12] and have higher mortality rates [14]. People with diabetes who also have co-morbid mental health problems are at increased risk of poorer health outcomes and premature mortality [14].

Given the significant impact on prognosis, it is unsurprising that co-morbid mental health problems also substantially increase patients' use of health services for their physical problems. Increased service use translates into substantial additional costs. Not only does depression increase the risk of hospital admission, but it can also cause delayed discharge, so highlighting the role of hospital clinicians in detecting depression in in-patients under their care. Case 2 illustrates the need for social care professionals not to assume that because a person is living with an extended family, they would not benefit from input. Again, the role of the primary care team in case-finding for depression in patients [15] recently discharged from hospital for their physical health problems is vital. If depression is detected in patients with physical health problems, collaborative care arrangements between primary care and mental health specialists can improve outcomes with no or limited additional net costs [16].

10.4 Suggestive Activities

Do you have any patients or clients who are 'frequent attenders' or make what you feel are unnecessary demands on your service? How could you manage them better?

A person who has had a recent hospital admission is at risk of depression: what systems do you have in place to identify this?

> **Key Points**
> - Somatic symptoms in older people may be manifestations of an affective illness, although exclusion of physical causes needs to be more carefully considered than in younger adults.
> - The first presentation with anxiety-related symptoms in an older person may suggest a depressive illness.
> - Residual anxiety symptoms are a problematic feature in depression in older people and frequently refractory to standard drug treatments.

- Admission of people with anxiety disorders to hospital can exacerbate their problems.
- Hospital admission can precipitate depression in older people.
- Collaborative care arrangements between primary care and mental health specialists can improve outcomes with no or limited additional net costs.
- Innovative forms of liaison psychiatry demonstrate that providing better support for co-morbid mental health needs can reduce physical health care costs in acute hospitals.
- Practitioners should be aware of the risk of depression in patients as an inpatient and then after discharge.

References

1. Lieberman A. Depression in Parkinson's disease – a review. Acta Neurol Scand. 2006;113(1): 1–8.
2. Ballard C, Bannister C, Solis M, Oyebode FWilcock G. The prevalence, associations and symptoms of depression amongst dementia sufferers. J Affect Disord. 1996;36(3–4):135–44.
3. Gaete JM, Bogousslavsky J. Post-stroke depression. Expert Rev Neurother. 2008;8(1):75–92.
4. Byrne G. Anxiety disorders in older people. In: Dening T, Thomas AJ, editors. Oxford textbook of Old Age psychiatry. Oxford: Oxford University Press; 2013. p. 589–602.
5. Thomas AJ. Depression in older people. In: Dening T, Thomas AJ, editors. Oxford textbook of old age psychiatry. Oxford: Oxford University Press; 2013. p. 545–69.
6. Azar AR, Chopra MP, Cho LY, Coakley E, Rudolph JL. Remission in major depression: results from a geriatric primary care population. Int J Geriatr Psychiatry. 2011;26(1):48–55.
7. https://www.anxietyuk.org.uk.
8. Neal RD, Heywood PL, Morley S. 'I always seem to be there' – a qualitative study of frequent attenders. Br J Gen Pract. 2000;50:716–23.
9. Morriss et al. BMC family practice. 2012; 13:39 http://www.biomedcentral.com/1471-2296/13/39.
10. https://www.gov.uk/enabling-integrated-care-in-the-nhs.
11. Fenton WS, Stover ES. Mood disorders: cardiovascular and diabetes comorbidity. Curr Opin Psychiatry. 2006;19(4):421–7.
12. Goodwin RD, Davidson KW, Keyes K. Mental disorders and cardiovascular disease among adults in the United States. J Psychiatr Res. 2009;43(3):239–46.
13. Whooley MD, de Jonge P, Vittinghoff E, Otte C, Moos R, Carney RM, Ali S, Dowray S, Na B, Feldman MD, Schiller NB, Browner WS. Depressive symptoms, health behaviors, and risk of cardiovascular events in patients with coronary heart disease. JAMA. 2008;300(20):2379–88.
14. Katon WJ. Clinical and health services relationships between major depression, depressive symptoms, and general medical illness. Biol Psychiatry. 2003;54(3):216–26.
15. Meader N, Mitchell AJ, Chew-Graham C, Goldberg D, Rizzo M, Bird V, et al. Case identification of depression in patients with chronic physical health problems: a diagnostic accuracy meta-analysis of 113 studies. Br J Gen Pract. 2011;61(593):e808–20.
16. Katon WJ, Lin EHB, Von Korff M, Ciechanowski P, Ludman EJ, Young B, et al. Collaborative care for patients with depression and chronic illnesses. N Engl J Med. 2010;363(27): 2611–20.

Depression and Anxiety: The Role of the Third Sector

11

Christopher Dowrick and Susan Martin

11.1 Introduction

The *third sector* refers to those organisations and groups which make a non-governmental and not-for-profit contribution to civic society. It is also known as the voluntary or community sector or the civic or societal sector [1]. It includes charities and co-operatives, social enterprises and self-help groups. The third sector has an expanding role in those western societies, including England, whose governments are seeking to reduce direct statutory involvement in the running of public services [2].

One way of understanding the role of the third sector is to consider it as positioned in the middle of a continuum or pyramid of care, stretching from self-help at one end to specialist care at the other (see Fig. 11.1).

Third-sector organisations such as charities, self-help groups and faith communities can play a substantial role in addressing those mental health problems, such as anxiety and depression, which are commonly experienced by older people. However many primary care professionals, including general practitioners, are unaware that such potentially rich resources and support may be available nearby. This chapter is designed to give primary care professionals some new perspectives and ideas on how the third sector can provide much needed help and support in the identification and management of common mental health problems in older people.

In this chapter, we describe four ways in which the third sector may be involved in helping to reduce symptoms of depression and anxiety amongst older people. These are befriending, increasing physical activity, guided self-help and

---

C. Dowrick, BA, MSc, MD, FRCGP (✉)
Department of Psychological Sciences, University of Liverpool, Liverpool, UK
e-mail: cfd@liv.ac.uk

S. Martin, BA, MSc, PhD
Netherton Feelgood Factory, Liverpool, UK
e-mail: hilbilsue@gmail.com

Fig. 11.1 Third sector and pyramid of care

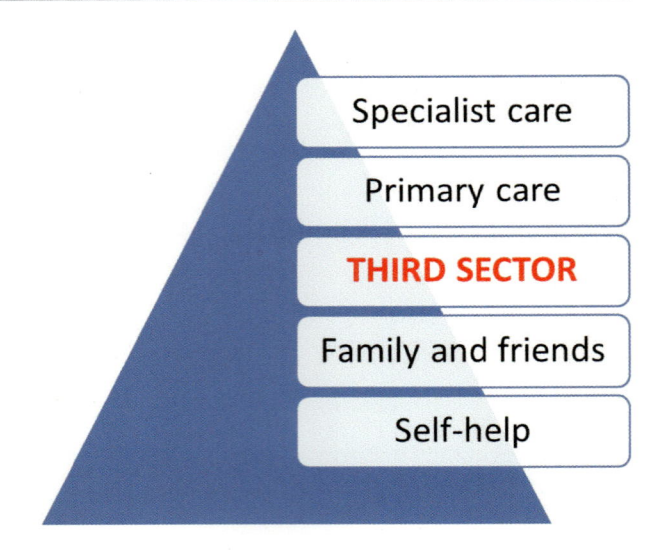

- Specialist care
- Primary care
- **THIRD SECTOR**
- Family and friends
- Self-help

collaboration between community groups and health-care providers. The first three are examples of how the third sector can deliver services to the benefit of older primary care patients with mental health problems. The fourth offers insights into how community groups and primary care teams can work together to improve services for older patients.

This is by no means an exhaustive list: there are many other examples we could have chosen, for example, debt or bereavement counselling, arts-based activities such as reading or singing groups and the act of volunteering itself. We have focused on these four because they are examples of third-sector activities that are supported by evidence of benefit for older people with symptoms of anxiety and depression.

We then provide a case study of one successful third-sector intervention, a guided self-help initiative for older people, and include the perspective of a service user.

Finally we offer readers the opportunity to reflect on their own practice.

11.2 Befriending

Befriending is an emotional support intervention commonly offered by the voluntary sector. It is usefully defined as 'a relationship between two or more individuals which is initiated, supported and monitored by an agency that has defined one or more parties as likely to benefit. Ideally the relationship is non-judgemental, mutual, and purposeful, and there is a commitment over time' [3]. In the UK, for example, more than 500 charitable and voluntary sector organisations currently offer befriending services [3].

Befriending can be helpful in reducing depressive symptoms and emotional distress amongst older people, particularly those who are isolated and lonely.

Mead and colleagues conducted a systematic review of randomised trials of interventions focused on providing emotional support to individuals in the community. Their aim was to examine the clinical and cost-effectiveness of befriending for individuals in the community, with a focus on the impact on depressive symptoms and emotional distress. They found 24 suitable trials, of which five were focused on older people. Compared with usual care or no treatment, they found that befriending has a modest but significant effect on depressive symptoms and emotional distress, both in the short term and the long term [4].

A good example of a befriending service is *Reclaiming Joy*, a mental health peer support programme for low-income older adults in Kansas, USA. In this programme, an older adult volunteer is paired with another older adult with mental health problems who is in need of peer support. Volunteers receive training on the strengths-based approach, mental health and ageing, goal setting and attainment, community resources and safety. The pairs meet once a week for 10 weeks. Participants establish and work towards goals that they feel will improve their mental health and wellbeing. In a pilot study of this service, 32 participants completing the intervention were assessed. There was statistically significant improvement for symptoms of depression, although not for symptoms of anxiety. Quality-of-life indicators for health and functioning improved for participants with symptoms of both depression and anxiety [5].

Telephone friendship support has been suggested as an alternative and perhaps more cost-effective method of providing befriending services. A study in Sheffield, UK, tested a service for people aged 75 and older where 6 weeks of short one-to-one telephone calls were followed by 12 weeks of group telephone calls with up to six participants, led by a trained volunteer facilitator. Although it was feasible to find suitable study participants, it proved more challenging to identify sufficient volunteer facilitators to run the service. The study leaders suggest that, to be a success, a programme like this would need to recruit volunteers from more than one city and might also need dedicated management of the volunteers [6].

11.3 Increasing Physical Activity

Physical exercise, especially when linked to social and communal activities, is beneficial for the mental health of older people. Third-sector organisations can be effective in providing opportunities for older people to experience these benefits.

This is the case when physical exercise is considered generally. Older people living in two low-income housing estates in San Francisco were encouraged to increase their physical activity by taking part in existing community-based physical activity classes and programmes of their choice. Participants were encouraged to adopt activities tailored to their preferences, physical abilities, health status, income and resources for transport. Those who adopted and maintained a new physical activity over 6 months experienced greater improvements in anxiety, depression and overall psychological wellbeing relative than those who did not [7].

It is also the case for physical activity tailored specifically to the needs and interests of older people. We note here the evidence for the beneficial effects of two types of activity supported by third-sector organisations: gardening or green gyms and the 'Men's Sheds' movement.

The cultivation of a garden plot can contribute to good mental health. In a seminal qualitative study on this subject, Milligan and colleagues note the importance of the wider landscape and the domestic garden in the lives of older people and illustrate the sense of achievement, satisfaction and aesthetic pleasure that older people can gain from their gardening activity. They propose that communal gardening on allotment sites 'creates inclusionary spaces in which older people benefit from gardening activity in a mutually supportive environment that combats social isolation and contributes to the development of their social networks' [8]. Evidence is accumulating in support of these propositions, including statistically significant improvement in measures of mental health and self-esteem [9]. The awareness of being away from one's usual setting and fascination with the processes and achievements of gardening are important components of its therapeutic effects on older people with depression [10].

The Men's Sheds movement is a rapidly developing intervention for older men, which has spread from Australia to several parts of the Anglophone world including the UK and Ireland [11]. Men's Sheds provide a communal space for older men to voluntarily engage in practical activities, particularly woodwork. It is estimated that across Australia there are more than 550 Men's Sheds with approximately 50,000 older men, attending on a regular basis. There is expanding evidence to indicate positive effects of Men's Sheds on the mental health of older men [12]. The consistency and frequency of such reports suggests that older men find benefits to their mental health from participating in social and physical activities in Sheds, due primarily to a greater sense of belonging and purpose in their lives:

> Men experience a range of very positive benefits as a result of participating. They feel better about themselves, are happier at home, have a strong sense of belonging and enjoyment and greatly appreciate the opportunity to be accepted by, and give back to, the community through what they make and do. [13]

11.4 Guided Self-Help

Third-sector organisations have an important role to play in the provision of low-intensity psychological interventions, which are of particular benefit to people with mild to moderate symptoms of anxiety and depression [14]. The role of third-sector organisations is expanding in countries such as England, where there is currently a policy imperative to allow any qualified provider to tender for previously statutory services [2]. It is also valuable in situations where long waiting lists cause delays for face-to-face treatment and for those people who prefer not to seek health service help. This is of particular importance to older people, who may be less likely to see primary care as an appropriate place to present or discuss mental health problems [15].

Cognitive behavioural therapy (CBT) can be effectively implemented by third-sector self-help clinics. *Beating the Blues* is a computerised CBT package which has been shown to reduce symptoms of depression and anxiety. In England, a third-sector organisation led by service users set up a self-help clinic to guide people through this package. They received over 500 referrals during their initial evaluation period. They found good evidence of recovery in half of those who met case criteria for anxiety or depression and had completed at least two sessions of CCBT [16].

In Scotland the charity Action on Depression is offering a life skills community course to people with symptoms of low mood. This is an eight-session community-based cognitive behaviour therapy group intervention called *Living Life to the Full*. It can also be taken up online if people prefer. Participants are recruited from the community through newspaper adverts and via the charity's website. This intervention is currently being evaluated by a randomised controlled trial [17].

The Netherton Feelgood Factory is a community-led healthy living centre based in Merseyside, England. Amongst its activities, it offers the *Positive Thoughts Course*, a group psycho-education programme which combines CBT and social network approaches. This programme is based on the Coping with Depression course, which has been shown to be effective in reducing symptoms of depression in community settings [18, 19]. One of the Positive Thoughts Courses is designed specifically for older people. We described this course in more detail later in this chapter, in our case study.

11.5 Collaboration Between Community Groups and Health-Care Providers

The previous examples have all been of services provided by third-sector organisations, which are likely to be of benefit to older primary care patients with mental health problems. In this section, we describe innovative ventures in which primary care or mental health-care teams have worked together with voluntary community organisations to achieve more accessible and acceptable services for older people.

11.5.1 The Amalthea Project

It is well recognised that, due in part to time constraints and lack of local knowledge, general practitioners and other primary care health professionals are often unable to refer patients with mental health problems to voluntary services that might be able to help them. In Bristol, England, the *Amalthea Project* was commissioned by general practitioners who wanted improved access to the numerous voluntary organisations with a potentially useful role in the management of psychosocial problems. This NHS-funded project was set up to collect information about the voluntary sector. Referral facilitators were employed to assess patients and recommend appropriate voluntary organisations. The project aimed to improve patients' quality of life and to decrease time spent by health-care professionals dealing with psychosocial problems. In a randomised controlled trial, patients referred to the Amalthea Project made greater use of more than 25 voluntary sector services (including local social groups for the elderly, bereavement charities, the University of the Third Age and the Royal British Legion) than those who received usual care. They showed significantly greater improvements in anxiety, other emotional feelings and quality of life, although no differences were detected in depression or perceived social support [20].

11.5.2 Beat the Blues

It is important to ensure that services meet the needs of the people they are supposed to help. Community organisations can provide crucial intelligence in ensuring that this actually happens. Older African Americans, for example, are at high risk for depression due to high levels of chronic illness, disability and socioeconomic distress. However they often do not access existing primary care or mental health services because they do not see them as likely to meet their needs. In Baltimore, USA, a collaboration between a senior centre and a local mental health resource has resulted in the creation of a new programme called Beat the Blues (different from the Beating the Blues CCBT package we noted in the previous section), designed specifically to meet the mental health needs of older African Americans. Licensed senior centre social workers trained in Beat the Blues meet with participants at home for up to ten sessions over 4 months. They assess care needs and make referrals and linkages with other community resources. They also provide depression education, instruct in stress reduction techniques and use behavioural activation to identify goals and steps to achieve them. They are currently conducting a trial to test whether Beat the Blues reduces depressive symptoms and improve quality of life in more than 200 African Americans aged 55 and over [21].

11.5.3 The AMP Programme

A potentially powerful example of involving third-sector organisations in the planning and delivery of high-quality services for older people with common mental health problems is the *AMP Programme* from north-west England [22].

The AMP Programme created a multilevel intervention model designed to increase equity of access to high-quality mental health services in primary care. The model involved intervening simultaneously at three levels: community engagement, primary care training and tailored psychosocial interventions (see Fig. 11.2).

This model is based on the assumption that intervening at three levels would be mutually reinforcing and thus more effective than intervening at one or two levels. We describe here how the model was deployed to meet the mental health needs of older people living in an area of high social deprivation.

The community engagement element involved gathering information about existing local resources, identifying a community champion and setting up a consultative group to identify key issues and set an agenda for action. The consultative group was based in a resource centre for older people and brought together, for the first time, representatives of local third-sector organisations (including faith groups,

Fig. 11.2 The AMP intervention model

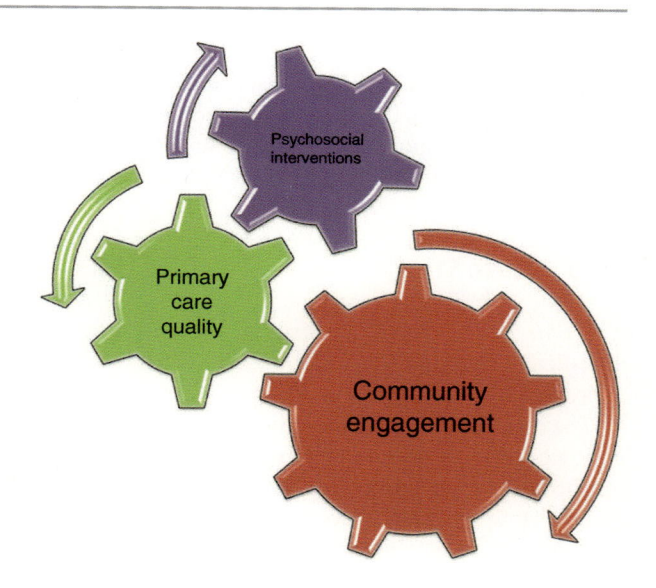

education providers and older people's advocacy groups) and primary care teams and also representatives of the police, housing associations, employment, health commissioners and local politicians. Its main activities were disseminating information about locally availably services for older people and strategic involvement with citywide mental health policy. These activities provided opportunities to increase cooperation between third-sector organisations, develop links between these organisations and primary care and raise the profile of the mental health needs of older people across the city.

The primary care element consisted of an interactive training package: a training component, advice on practice organisational features that may impede or promote access by underserved groups and raising awareness of relevant third-sector organisations and resources. It was particularly effective in practices where a senior member of the team acted as an advocate or champion of the interactive training package.

The psychosocial or 'wellbeing' interventions were based on cognitive-behavioural principles, with an emphasis on social participation. They were modified to suit the needs of older people following consultation with local focus groups. There were positive effects on depression and wellbeing for those older people who received the interventions, compared with those who received usual care [23].

A health commissioner was enthusiastic about the benefits of the integrated AMP model:

> I think about the whole thing . . . so the AMP is improving access to mental health and primary care and then you have got the well-being facilitators and – really exciting and well done – for the bit that says in our, you know, here are the facilities, here are the local things that we have in our local community, which for us in a practical world is really helpful. Really helpful for GPs, really good to say, listen here's – you know – here's what you've got.

Community engagement led to an increase in referrals to the AMP psychosocial interventions. The quality of mental health care for older people within primary care was enhanced by the information-gathering element of the community engagement strategy, enabling more active linkage with community-based resources, and by the offer of access to the AMP psychosocial interventions [22].

11.6 Case Study

The *Elderly Positive Thoughts Course* is a group psycho-education programme, specifically designed for older people, which combines CBT and social network approaches.

The course takes a cognitive-behavioural approach, based on the assumption that how we think and feel affects what we do [24]. But what we have forgotten, or maybe never even worked out, is how we really feel. How many times when we are asked "How are you?" Do we say, "Fine thanks", without even thinking for a moment how we actually feel? Or do we say, "Oh, I've been so busy", which completely bypasses the question of feeling? Each week, every participant gets the opportunity to say how they feel in a safe, accepting environment. We do not "fix" feelings, but acknowledge their validity and explain the importance and value they have in our lives. It is important that each participant understands from the start that this is not a therapy where they just talk but that they will be required to learn and practise new techniques that will make them feel more positive about their lives. In practice we have found this is a plus for most people who can see no value in "just talking about my problems over and over again".

The basic structure and content of each session is a combination of feedback, discussion, relaxation and homework. It is acceptable that the style and manner of presentation may vary. Every week there is homework and one component is always a mood chart, a daily record of how we feel on a score of 1–10. This keeps the theme of feelings high on the agenda. Each session lasts approximately 2 h. This includes a tea break which further encourages social support amongst the group. The lecture notes for the instructor are intended to be the basis of the group discussion with the more detailed information being given to the participants in the form of a handout. This means that during the group there is little reading to be done. This bypasses problems with sight and reading skills.

The course covers different themes, for example, how our activities affect our mood, finding out the things we can do to make ourselves feel better and some ways to help us change our thoughts. Themes are developed in the course, both from the taught material and also from the contributions of course members. People are encouraged to bring in material and ideas that have helped them. These are discussed in the course and then there is appropriate homework. The discussions and the social support these generate are important in helping people find their own solutions.

During the course, we hope that participants will come to realise a number of things. Firstly, many other people have similar problems. They will realise that there are a number of ways of dealing with any given set of circumstances. They are likely to have both given and taken advice over the time of the course. Practical suggestions will have been made to everyone on how they can lift their mood. Everyone's feelings will have been acknowledged, accepted and thus validated. A lot of this information would have come from within the group.

The course provides many alternative ways of looking at our lives. Some problems do not have easy solutions. Instead we need to learn to live with them or, better still, bypass them. There are sessions on good eating habits, rewarding yourself, letting others help you and having fun.

If participants can take even one change on board, they feel more in charge of their own lives. This heralds the belief that the future can improve and that they are people with the skills to improve it.

11.6.1 Service User Perspectives

We recently asked participants 'What do you find helpful about coming to the Positive Thoughts Course?'

They describe the course as an important source of social support: "We have a good laugh.... Tea and biscuits and a natter". It is also part of their routine: "It's regular, it happens every month". The anticipation of its occurrence is something good, a positive fixed point in an often difficult life.

It provides a safe and open space for reflection: "I can have a good moan in a neutral atmosphere – with people who usually take my side!" "There's space for everyone to speak.... You can talk about anything". People's views are taken seriously: "We aren't spoke to like we were kids". And there is opportunity speak differently: "Sometimes I can say things I can't say at home".

It leads to new ways of thinking and dealing with life: "You get lots of advice from others". "It helps you think and find other solutions". "The course makes me feel better".

11.7   Conclusions

The third sector is an important source of support for GPs and their older patients who are experiencing common mental health problems. However its potential contribution all too often goes unrecognised and underutilised.

We have provided evidence of four ways in which third-sector, voluntary, community organisations can provide tangible benefits in this field. We see these simply as examples, and there are many others that could have been presented.

GPs and other primary care health professionals are hard-pressed to deliver the quality of care to which we aspire and which we consider our patients need and deserve. It is timely – perhaps even essential – for us to have the courage and imagination to expand beyond our habitual range of contacts. We need to identify and make productive links with those many third-sector organisations that are undoubtedly flourishing within easy reach of our surgeries and clinics.

11.8 Opportunity for Reflection

Here are three questions to help you to think about your engagement with local third-sector, voluntary, community groups and organisations

- What third-sector resources are you aware of locally, which could help you with the common mental health problems experienced by your older patients?
- How many of these resources have you visited or invited to meet you?
- How can you find out about other relevant local third-sector resources?

References

1. Frumkin P. On being nonprofit: a conceptual and policy primer. Cambridge, MA: Harvard University Press; 2005.
2. https://www.gov.uk/government/collections/civil-society-update-series. Accessed 1 Jul 2014.
3. Dean J, Goodlad R. Supporting community participation; the role and impact of befriending. Pavilion: Pavilion Publishing & Joseph Rowntree Foundation; 1998.
4. Mead N, Lester H, Chew-Graham C, Gask L, Bower P. Effects of befriending on depressive symptoms and distress: systematic review and meta-analysis. Br J Psychiatry. 2010;196:96–101.
5. Chapin RK, Sergeant JF, Landry S, Leedahl SN, Rachlin R, Koenig T, Graham A. Reclaiming joy: pilot evaluation of a mental health peer support program for older adults who receive Medicaid. Gerontologist. 2013;53:345–52.
6. Mountain GA, Hind D, Gossage-Worrall R, Walters SJ, Duncan R, Newbould L, Rex S, Jones C, Bowling A, Cattan M, Cairns A, Cooper C, Edwards RT, Goyder EC. 'Putting Life in Years' (PLINY) telephone friendship groups research study: pilot randomised controlled trial. Trials. 2014;15:141.
7. Stewart AL, Mills KM, Sepsis PG, King AC, McLellan BY, Roitz K, Ritter PL. Evaluation of CHAMPS, a physical activity promotion program for older adults. Ann Behav Med. 1997;19:353–61.
8. Milligan C, Gatrell A, Bingley A. "Cultivating health": therapeutic landscapes and older people in northern England. Soc Sci Med. 2004;58:1781–93.
9. Pretty J, Peacock J, Hine R, Sellens M, South N, Griffin M. Green exercise in the UK countryside: effects on health and psychological well-being, and implications for policy and planning. J Environ Plann Manag. 2007;50:211–31.
10. Gonzalez MT, Hartig T, Patil GG, Martinsen EW, Kirkevold M. Therapeutic horticulture in clinical depression: a prospective study of active components. J Adv Nurs. 2010;66:2002–13.
11. Wilson NJ, Cordier R. A narrative review of Men's Sheds literature: reducing social isolation and promoting men's health and well-being. Health Soc Care Community. 2013;21:451–63.
12. Milligan C, Neary D, Hanratty B, Payne S, Dowrick C. Older men and social activity: a systematic review of Men's Sheds and other gendered interventions. Ageing and Soc. FirstView Article. 2016, pp 1–29; Published online: 2015.
13. Golding B, Brown M, Foley A, Harvey J, Gleeson L. Men's sheds in Australia: learning through community contexts. National Centre for Vocational Education Research (NCVER) Australia; 2007.
14. NICE. Depression in adults: the treatment and management of depression in adults [CG 90]. London: National Institute for Health and Clinical Excellence; 2009.
15. Kovandžić M, Chew-Graham C, Reeve J, Edwards S, Peters S, Edge D, Aseem S, Gask L, Dowrick C. Access to primary mental health care for hard-to-reach groups: from 'silent suffering' to 'making it work'. Soc Sci Med. 2011;72:763–72.

16. Cavanagh K, Seccombe N, Lidbetter N. The implementation of computerized cognitive behavioural therapies in a service user-led, third sector self help clinic. Behav Cogn Psychother. 2011;39:427–42.
17. McClay CA, Morrison J, McConnachie A, Williams C. A community-based group-guided self-help intervention for low mood and stress: study protocol for a randomized controlled trial. Trials. 2013;14:392.
18. Dowrick C, Dunn G, Ayuso-Mateos JL, Dalgard OS, Page H, Lehtinen V, Casey P, Wilkinson C, Vazquez-Barquero JL, Wilkinson G. Problem solving treatment and group psychoeducation for depression: multicentre randomised controlled trial. Outcomes of Depression International Network (ODIN) Group. BMJ. 2000;321:1450–4.
19. Dalgard OS. A randomized controlled trial of a psychoeducational group program for unipolar depression in adults in Norway. Clin Pract Epidemiol Ment Health. 2006;2:15.
20. Grant C, Goodenough T, Harvey I, Hine C. A randomised controlled trial and economic evaluation of a referrals facilitator between primary care and the voluntary sector. BMJ. 2000;320:419–23.
21. Gitlin LN, Harris LF, McCoy M, Chernett NL, Jutkowitz E, Pizzi LT, Beat the Blues Team. A community-integrated home based depression intervention for older African Americans: description of the Beat the Blues randomized trial and intervention costs. BMC Geriatr. 2012;12:4.
22. Dowrick C, Chew-Graham C, Lovell K, Lamb J, Aseem A, Beatty S, Bower P, Burroughs H, Clarke P, Edwards S, Gabbay M, Gravenhorst K, Hammond J, Hibbert D, Kovandžić M, Lloyd-Williams M, Waheed W, Gask L. Increasing equity of access to high quality mental health services in primary care: a mixed-methods study. Program Grants Appl Res. 2013;1(2):1–184.
23. Lovell K, Gask L, Bower P, Aseem S, Beatty S, Burroughs H, Chew-Graham C, Clarke C, Dowrick A, Edwards S, Gabbay M, Kovandzic M, Lamb M, Lloyd-Williams M, Waheed W, Dowrick C. Development and evaluation of a psychosocial intervention for hard to reach groups in primary care. BMC Psychiatry. 2014;14:217.
24. Martin S. Management of late life depression in primary care: case studies UK. In: Chew-Graham C, Baldwin R, Burns A, editors. Integrated management of depression in the elderly. Cambridge: Cambridge University Press; 2008. p. 43–5.

Creativity and the Arts for Older People Living with Depression

12

Mo Ray

12.1 Context/Introduction

The right to participate in cultural life and enjoy the arts is enshrined in Article 27 of the 1948, Universal Declaration of Human Rights [1]. In a contemporary context, there is an appreciation that the arts and creative activities can support the development and maintenance of good mental health across the life course. Policies in each of the devolved nations recognise the positive role of culture and the arts in the lives of its citizens and the part that it plays in supporting vibrant and creative communities. More recently, arts and creativity as non-pharmacological interventions in the treatment and management of mental health conditions has received considerable attention. The Department of Health and Arts Council England [2], for example, has highlighted that the arts have an important role to play in the delivery of health care, in promoting social wellbeing and in delivering demonstrable benefits across the life course against a wide range of health priorities. Arguably, older people have been at the vanguard of community arts and crafts through their leadership and participation in the many voluntary organisations, such as the Women's Institute (WI), which exist at least in part, to support and encourage such activities. However, the involvement of older people in participatory arts in the form of community projects or as interventions in the support, management and treatment of mental or physical health needs has traditionally been less visible [3].

This chapter begins by defining participatory arts and other kinds of arts activity. It briefly considers the role of the arts and creativity in the treatment of mental health conditions with a focus on depression in later life. The chapter then takes a broader perspective and reviews some of the evidence which illustrate the ways in

M. Ray, PhD
Gerontological Social Work and Programme, School of Social Science and Public Policy, Keele University, Keele, Staffordshire, UK
e-mail: m.g.ray@keele.ac.uk

which participatory arts support more generally the promotion of mental health and contribute to developments such as age-friendly cities and places.

12.2 Defining Terms

Taking part in the arts incorporates a diverse range of activities informed by different theoretical perspectives and with different ambitions in respect of their purpose, process, degrees of participation and outcomes. The Mental Health Foundation [4] identifies various forms of arts engagement which include audience participation, 'passive' engagement (e.g. listening to music), doing art and craft through personal hobbies, the arts as therapy and participatory arts. Arts as therapy (e.g. art therapy, music therapy, drama therapy) have been defined as expressive or creative therapy that introduces action to psychotherapy [5]. The British Association of Art Therapy defines its discipline as 'a form of psychotherapy that uses art media as its primary mode of expression and communication. Within this context, art is not used as a diagnostic tool but as a medium to address emotional issues which may be confusing and distressing [6].

Participatory arts are distinct from other forms of artistic endeavour as they are underpinned by a belief in the right to access culture and the arts, to create environments which give voice and the means of expression to people who often have less power or who are recognised as marginalised people [3]. Participatory art involves people in collaboration with professional artists representing diverse forms of expression, to develop artistic work, which reflects, represents or relates in some way, to participant experience [4].

Participatory art is defined as an emergent research field which is not yet in a position to provide scientific evaluation which can make confident comparisons between art forms or draw conclusions about impact from a number of studies [4, 7]. Nevertheless, there is a growing and often compelling body of literature which supports the view that older people benefit from arts engagement, suggesting positive impact on health and wellbeing and value in supporting the promotion of good mental health and in the management and treatment of a wide range of health contexts.

12.3 Arts and Creative Interventions with Older People with Depression

It is increasingly accepted that arts engagement with older people can impact positively on health, improve health outcomes, support people to cope with the challenges associated with poor health and provide a means of developing protective resources to combat the risk of mental ill health [8–11]. There is evidence to suggest that older people are more likely to prefer to participate in psychosocial interventions than to use medication to treat depression [4] and some of the evaluations of participatory arts projects appear to corroborate this view by presenting evidence of higher rates of participation amongst older people when compared with participation in more 'traditional' interventions [3, 7]. There is too the potential for arts-based interventions to offer opportunities to older people who, across the course of their lives, have experienced inequality of opportunity and who may, as a result, be at particular risk of poor mental health and with limited opportunities to access culture and the arts [7, 12].

Reminiscence with older people has had a lengthy and significant presence in practice with older people. Organisations such as 'Age Exchange' started by Pam Schweitzer MBE in 1983 developed ground-breaking participatory theatre linked with reminiscence practice with older people and across generations. Reminiscence has a significant place in therapeutic practice with older people with physical and mental health needs, including people living with depression. A number of studies have concluded that reminiscence can lead to constructive outcomes in the management and treatment of depression evidenced by improvement in symptoms of depression, an increase in wellbeing and growth in confidence [13–15]. Gibson [16], who has researched and written extensively on the use of reminiscence and life story work with older people, cautiously concluded that a combination of talking, reflection, life review and production of a tangible record can have constructive outcomes for older people with depression. At the time of writing, there has not been a systematic review utilising Cochrane standards to assess the impact of reminiscence as an intervention for older people with depression. The waters are further muddied by the potential to conflate different kinds of reminiscence – for example, reminiscence work, reminiscence therapy, life review, life history or life story work – and for reminiscence to become a 'casual' activity or form of distraction in collective settings which Organ [3] argues reduces reminiscence to an end in itself and another form of 'care'.

The potential health benefit of older people with mental health needs participating in musical activity has also received significant attention. Although there has been a growth of research reporting on the impact of participation in music, they are of variable quality evidenced by a variety of approaches in operationalising concepts, problematic sample sizes and research design weaknesses [17]. A study to systematically identify and critically appraise existing published research on singing, wellbeing and health [18] yielded analysis of 35 articles which, methodological weaknesses notwithstanding, evidenced benefit for older participants with long-standing psychological distress, including depression. Research focusing on the effects of community choir membership also suggests important benefits for people with long-term mental health needs [19, 20]. Case studies have provided a rich source of qualitative testimony from older participants highlighting improvement in the symptoms of depression and are perceived to give a range of other benefits such as increased social confidence, self-esteem, developing social networks and friendships [21]. The authors reason that 'people with mental health issues would not continue attending singing groups if they didn't derive substantial benefits from the experience'. Recently, a pilot randomised control trial compared group singing with usual activities amongst 258 participants aged 60 and over and followed participants up at 3 and 6 months [22]. Findings included a significant positive effect on alleviating loneliness and isolation and statistically significant improvement on ratings of anxiety and depression. Coulton et al. [22] conclude that community singing can have a significantly positive impact for older people living with mental health problems, including depression.

Similar observations about the quality of research in assessing impact of participatory arts are made for other art forms. A Cochrane review of dance movement therapy, for example [23], found that due to the low number of studies, combined with quality of evidence, it was not possible to draw any firm conclusions about the impact of the use of this art form. Moreover, it was not possible to compare dance with other treatments and interventions. Taking methodological weaknesses into consideration, a wealth of qualitative and case study evidence exists which supports the benefit of dance and movement for older people with impact upon physical strength, balance and confidence and emotional wellbeing [24]. In a review of exemplary arts practice, Organ [3] cites the Akademi group which offers dance with older women from a Bangladeshi community in London where opportunities for social participation are circumscribed by gender and cultural norms. Organ comments 'The very act of coming to the class is crossing borders of participation that they will have seldom transgressed' [3]. In posing the question 'is this a good thing?', she observes that attendance and participation exceeds groups such as physiotherapy and provides considerable emotional benefit to its members.

Arts on prescription schemes provide arts and creative activities for participants who are often experiencing mental health problems or the difficulties associated with social isolation and loneliness. The 'Good Times' participatory arts project with Dulwich Picture Gallery was based on GP practices connecting older people who were at risk of or experiencing mental health problems, including depression. Based on a retrospective qualitative evaluation of the project, Harper and Hamblin [7] commented that 'prescription for art' led to positive evaluations from professional and family carers who saw a reduction in depressive symptoms from individual older people who took part. Qualitative evaluations from older participants highlighted many social, emotional and psychological benefits to participation. Other projects such as the 'Arts in Mind' project (www.nottinghamshire.gov.uk/artsonprescriptioncasestudy.pdf) have demonstrated similar findings [25].

12.3.1 Social Prescribing and Participatory Arts: Art Lift

In recognition that 30 % of GP consultations are about mental health problems, the 'Art Lift' project was developed as a form of social prescribing for people with identified mental health needs or who were at risk of developing mental health needs. Participants took part in 10-week courses with a variety of artists representing different art forms took place over the period 2009/2011 and included 202 participants in the evaluation. Measures included the Warwick-Edinburgh Mental Well-being Scale (WEMWBS), artists' subjective ratings of participant engagement and the Index of Multiple Deprivation. Both the 7- and 14-item WEMWBS demonstrated statistically significant improvement [7-item ($t=-6.049$, d.f.$=83$, $P<0.001$, two tailed) and 14-item ($t=-6.961$, d.f$=83$, $P<0.001$, two tailed) scaled]. The evaluation reported high levels of participation in Art Life when compared to other types of referral to schemes such as exercise. The oldest members of the sample had the best participation and completion rates [26].

Overall, the study concluded that the project offered a relevant and effective intervention for people with mental health needs and who were at risk of developing mental health problems [26].

The researchers suggested further longitudinal research in order to assess longer-term impact on mental health. Further research examining cost-effectiveness against uptake, adherence and outcome would also be of benefit [26].

12.4 Participatory Arts, Ageing and Mental Health Promotion

The World Health Organisation [27] defines mental health as a 'state of well being in which the individual realises his or her own abilities, can cope with the normal stresses of life, can work productively and fruitfully, and is able to make a contribution to his/her community'. Thus good mental health has an intrinsic value as well as contributing to overall health, personal capital, wellbeing and functioning. It is recognised that older people may face particular barriers including isolation, disability and ageism which are of themselves debilitating but also act as barriers to participating in social and creative activities that protect and support good mental health and wellbeing. The value of arts in respect of ageing has tended to focus on health benefits derived from participation for those older people who are using health and social care services [3]. But the importance of all people across the life course having the right to access to art and culture and the general benefit to good mental and physical health, social capital and the sheer enjoyment of being creative must not be overlooked.

A systematic evidence review of participatory art projects for people aged 60 and over identified a number of benefits which, despite the limitations of evidence in this area, are argued to be sufficiently compelling to suggest significant impact on mental and physical wellbeing [4]. Specifically, benefits to the individual highlighted in the review were:

- Increased confidence and self-esteem
- Feelings of mastery and accomplishment
- Positive aspects to identity
- Counterbalancing challenges to wellbeing associated with experiences of loss and change
- Increased levels of daily activity

Research exploring various aspects of creativity and ageing has highlighted similar benefit for older citizens across many art forms and means of creative expression.

12.4.1 Participatory Arts Research Projects Funded by the New Dynamics of Ageing Research Programme

Example One

The 'Ages and Stages' project included as one of its research aims, addressing the relationship between older people's involvement in theatre and drama and continued social engagement in later life. The research project demonstrated impact for older participants in enhanced self-esteem and self-confidence through participation in theatre and drama and crucially challenged a stereotype that creativity declines with age [28].

Example Two

The 'Music for Life' research project aimed to explore the ways in which participation in creative music making could enhance the lives of older people and to explore the potential impact on wellbeing [29].

Results found that participants experienced enhanced wellbeing and quality of life as well as benefitting from acquiring new skills and enjoying social and community activities and the relationships that developed from those activities. In terms of perceived emotional health benefits, findings included improved mental health for participants experiencing mental health problems and emotional distress (e.g. associated with loss and bereavement) and that participation in music making may act as a protective factor against depression [29].

Example Three

The 'Look at Me' research project focused on visual representations of ageing women and included in its aims enabling women from different settings to create their own images of ageing supported by participatory visual methods. The research findings highlighted that the participatory process gave women a sense of solidarity and ownership of the process. Crucially the research challenged stereotypes of ageing women and impacted on participant wellbeing [30].

The importance of accessing culture and the arts as part of social participation is highlighted in the World Health Organisation's Age-Friendly Cities movement which aims to promote active ageing in cities and to optimise opportunities for health, participation and security [31]. Removing barriers to the social participation of older people in the life of the city is vital to the wellbeing of older citizens and to the development of the city [32].

12.4.2 Manchester, UK

Manchester was the first city in the UK to become a member of the WHO network of age-friendly cities after establishing a 'valuing older people' programme to improve services and opportunities for older residents in Manchester. Since 2007 a key activity has been to work with older citizens and cultural providers to make sure that Manchester's cultural offer is available to older people in the city and to address or remove the barriers that they may face [32].

A network of over 100 voluntary cultural champions act as ambassadors to:

- Inform older people's networks and communities within Manchester about the variety of cultural events taking place in the city throughout the year
- Encourage older people's networks to attend and try out a variety of cultural events taking place in the city throughout the year [32]

In partnership with a range of arts and cultural providers in the city, a comprehensive cultural offer is available to older citizens. For example:

Theatre and performance

- Developmental projects
- Intergenerational performance

Music

- Club nights
- Dance workshops
- Live music
- The development of the Golden Voices Choir
- Outreach work 'Musicians on Call'

Museums and galleries

- Arts led workshops
- Adult learning programmes
- Living history performance
- Outreach work [32]

12.5 Discussion

This chapter has briefly reviewed some of the many developments currently taking place in the field of participatory arts with older people. The potential for the arts to impact positively on alleviating the distress associated with mental health problems, emotional distress and isolation is clearly very significant. Taking a wider perspective, arts and culture has always had a vitally important role to play in promoting mental health across the life course and contributing to developing and sustaining vibrant and creative communities. And of course, enjoying the arts or immersing oneself in creative activity, however defined, is important in and of itself. Organ [3] argues that the joy, personal accomplishment, challenge and benefit that individual people derive from doing art or creative activity means that we must be critical of a direction of travel which places an emphasis on health outcomes as the main justification for arts activity. Examples such as the cultural offer in Manchester show how barriers to older peoples' participation in the arts may be reduced. Such developments add value and benefit to the lives of older citizens and contribute to the development of inclusive practice in supporting older people to participate in the city.

The place of participatory arts in ameliorating the experience of older people living with depression or other mental health problems remains an important element of participatory arts. In order to consider the kinds of arts intervention that work most effectively with particular populations, there is a need to continue to develop research which addresses some of the methodological challenges that have hitherto affected the confidence with which impact can be claimed. Nevertheless, qualitative evidence in the form of the voice of older people and their lived experience is and should remain a central part of evaluation. This is especially important as older people with the most complex needs are also most likely to experience significant marginalisation. This is important not only in order to properly involve older people but also ensure that the kinds of opportunities that are offered are acceptable and appropriate for those people and status as adults. As Organ comments, 'activities that are reminiscent of playschool, sing-alongs, waving parachutes, visiting clowns, making pictures out of pasta are not associated with a sense of agency in the world. For adults fearing a loss of dignity, uncertainty with strangers, lacking a sense of autonomy, child-like activities can feel very uncomfortable, patronising and plain weird. They can be awkward and uncomfortable reminders of our diminished status and threatened dignity' [3]. Participating in the arts and creativity should provide every opportunity to reaffirm and validate participants' status as adults regardless of the complexity of their needs.

12.6 Questions for Reflection

- How could social prescribing support the work of primary care in their practice with older people?
- How do projects such as participatory arts fit with the GP commitment to biopsychosocial care and support for individual patients and local communities?
- What role should primary care have in supporting wider developments in mental health promotion such as supporting the development of age-friendly communities?

Appendix 12.1 Useful Resources

ageofcreativity.co.uk
UK wide website for professionals and organisations working in the field of the arts and older people
www.baringfoundation.org.uk
Baring Foundation focusing on participatory arts and ageing
New Dynamics of Ageing Research http://www.newdynamics.group.shef.ac.uk
Research summaries funded by the New Dynamics of Research fund

Appendix 12.2 Further Reading

Clift S, Hancox G, Staricoff R, Whitmore C. Singing and health: a systematic mapping and review of non-clinical research, Canterbury, Sidney De Haan Research Centre for Arts and Health. http://www.canterbury.ac.uk/centres/sidney-de-haan-research/

Cutler D. Ageing artfully. London: Baring Foundation; 2011. Accessed via, http://baringfoundation.org.uk/wp-content/uploads/2009/08/AgeingArtfully.pdf.

Mental Health Foundation. Review of the impact of participatory arts in older people. London: Mental Health Foundation; 2011. Accessed via, www.mentalhealth.org.uk.

Organ D. After you are two: exemplary practice in participatory arts. London: Baring Foundation; 2013. Accessed via, http://baringfoundation.org.uk/wp-content/uploads/2013/09/AfterYAT.pdf.

References

1. United Nations. Universal declaration on human rights. 1948. http://www.un.org/Overview/uninbrief/hr.shtml
2. Department of Health/Arts Council for England. A prospectus for arts and health, London, DoH and ACE. 2007. Retrieved on 2nd June 2015. http://www.artscouncil.org.uk/media/uploads/documents/publications/phpYUAxLH.pdf
3. Organ D. After you are two: exemplary practice in participatory arts. London: Baring Foundation; 2013. Retrieved on: 2nd April 2015. http://baringfoundation.org.uk/wp-content/uploads/2013/09/AfterYAT.pdf.
4. Mental Health Foundation. Review of the impact of participatory arts in older people. London: Mental Health Foundation; 2011. Retrieved on: 15 May 2015www.mentalhealth.org.uk.
5. Malchiodi C. Expressive therapies. In: Malchiodi C, editor. Expressive therapies. New York: Guilford Press; 2005. p. 1–15.
6. British Association of Art Therapy (undated) What is art therapy? Retrieved on. 30 June 2015. http://www.baat.org/
7. Harper S, Hamblin K. 'This is living' good times: art for older people at Dulwich Picture Gallery. Oxford: Oxford Institute of Ageing/Dulwich Picture Gallery; 2010.
8. Batt-Raden KB, Tellnes G. Nature-culture-health activities as a method of rehabilitation: an evaluation of participants' health, quality of life and function. Int J Rehabil Res. 2005;28:175–80.

9. Greaves CJ, Farbus L. Effects of creative and social activity on the health and well being of socially isolated older people: outcomes from a multi method observational study. J R Soc Promot Health. 2006;126(3):134–42.
10. Crone DM, O'Connell EE, Tyson PJ, Clark-Stone F, Opheer S, James DVB. 'Art Lift' intervention to improve mental well-being: an observational study from UK general practice. Int J Ment Health. 2013;22:279–86. a partnership arts and health project.
11. Cutler D. Tackling loneliness in older age: the role of the arts. London: Baring Foundation/Campaign to end loneliness; 2012. Retrieved on 2 June 2015www.baringfoundation.org.uk.
12. Murray M. Scharf T, Maslin Protheroe S, Beech R, Ziegler F. Call me: promoting social engagement and participation amongst older people living in disadvantaged communities. Findings 18. University of Sheffield, NDA. 2013. Retrieved on: 2 June 2015. http://www.newdynamics.group.shef.ac.uk/assets/files/NDA%20Findings_18.pdf
13. Chiang KJ, Lu RB, Chu H, Chang YC, Chou KR. Evaluation of the effect of a life review group program on self-esteem and life satisfaction in the elderly. Int J Geriatr Psychiatry. 2008;23:7–14.
14. Preschl B, Maercker A, Wagner B, Forstmeier S, Ban RM, Alcan M, Castilla D, Botella C. Life-review therapy with computer supplements for depression in the elderly: a randomized control trial. Aging Ment Health. 2012;16(8):964–74.
15. Housden S. The use of reminiscence in the prevention and treatment of depression in older people living in care homes. Groupwork. 2009;19(2):28–45.
16. Gibson F. Reminiscence and life story work. 4th ed. London: Jessica Kingsley; 2011.
17. Skingley A, Bungay K. The silver song club: singing to promote the health of older people. Br J Community Nurs. 2010;15(3):135–40.
18. Clift S, Hancox G, Morrison I, Hess B, Stewart D, Kreutz G. Choral singing, wellbeing and health: findings from a cross-national survey. Canterbury: Canterbury Christ Church University; 2008. Retrieved on: 1 May 2015. http://www.canterbury.ac.uk/ centres/sidney-de-haan-research.
19. Clift S, Hancox G. The significance of choral singing for sustaining psychological wellbeing: findings from a survey of choristers in England, Australia and Germany. Music Health. 2010;3(1):79–96.
20. Skingley A, Clift SM, Coulton SP, Rodriguez J. The effectiveness and cost-effectiveness of a participative community singing programme as a health promotion initiative for older people: protocol for a randomised control trial. Public Health. 2011;11:142.
21. Morrison I, Clift S. Singing and mental health. Canterbury: Sidney de Haan Research Centre for Arts and Health; 2012. Retrieved on: 8 June 2015http://www.artsandhealth.ie/wp-content/uploads/2013/01/Singing-and-Mental-Health-PDF.pdf.
22. Coulton S, Clift S, Skingley A, Rodriguez J. Community singing and health in the older population: a randomised controlled trial. Br J Psychiatry. 2015;207:250.
23. Meekums B, Karkou V, Nelson E. Is dance movement an effective treatment for depression: a review of the evidence. 2015. Retrieved on: 10th May 2015 http://www.cochrane.org/CD009895/DEPRESSN_is-dance-movement-therapy-an-effective-treatment-for-depression-a-review-of-the-evidence
24. Keogh JWL, Kilding A, Pidgeon P, Ashley L, Gillis D. Physical benefits of dancing for healthy older adults: a review. J Aging Phys Act. 2009;17:479–500.
25. Arts in Mind (undated) Nottingam County Council. Retrieved on: 15 June 2015. http://www.nottinghamshire.gov.uk/enjoying/artsandculture/arts/
26. World Health Organisation. Mental health: new understanding, new hope. 2001. Retrieved on: 30 May 2015. http://www.who.int/whr/2001/en/whr01_en.pdf
27. Bernard M, Amigoni D, Munro L, Murray M, Rezzano J, Rickett M, Basten, R. Ages and stages: the place of theatre in representations and recollections of ageing. 2012. NDA findings 15. http://www.newdynamics.group.shef.ac.uk/assets/files/FINAL%20NDA%20Findings%2015%20(2).pdf).
28. Hallam S, Creech A, Gaunt H, Pincas A, Vavarigou M, McQueen H. Music for life project: the role of participation in community music activities in promoting social engagement and well-

being in older people. 2011. NDA Findings 9. http://www.newdynamics.group.shef.ac.uk/assets/files/NDA%20Findings_9.pd.
29. Warren L, Gott M, Hogan S, Richards N. Look at me! Images of women and ageing. 2012. NDA findings 10. http://www.newdynamics.group.shef.ac.uk/assets/files/NDA%20Findings_10.pdf).
30. World Health Organisation. Age friendly cities: a guide. 2007. Retrieved on 2nd March 2015. http://www.who.int/ageing/publications/Global_age_friendly_cities_Guide_English.pdf.
31. Phillipson C. Developing age-friendly cities: policy, challenges and options. 2007. Housing LIN, Viewpoint 37. Date retrieved: 30th November 2014. www.housinglin.org.uk.
32. The Audience Agency. An incredible journey: a review of Manchester's valuing older people cultural offer summary report. London: The Audience Agency; 2012. Retrieved on 8th June 2015. www.theaudienceagency.org.

Depression in Care Homes

13

Alisoun Milne

This chapter is in two main parts. The first part will offer an overview of the care home population including a profile of their mental health and what is known about the prevalence of depression amongst care home residents. The second half will focus on the assessment and management of depression in care homes, interventions to alleviate symptoms of depression and what more could be done to improve outcomes, including the contribution of primary care services.

13.1 The Care Home Sector in the UK

In the UK, approximately 420,000 older people [1] live in a care home; this represents 6 % of the older population. A distinction is generally made between residential care homes and homes providing nursing care (otherwise known as nursing homes). Residential care homes provide personal care with activities of daily living, such as washing, dressing and giving medication. Nursing homes offer nursing care to at least some of their residents, and although nursing homes tend to support people with higher dependency needs, in fact there is considerable overlap between the two types of home [2]. In this chapter the term 'care home' will be used to denote both types. Evidence about NHS continuing care facilities is not included. It is noteworthy that over the past 30 years, there has been a significant shift in the balance of provision in the UK. Care home services have transformed from a predominantly public sector activity in the mid-1970s to a predominantly private sector activity now. In 2010 the private sector accounted for three quarters of all long-stay bed capacity [3]. This trend looks likely to accelerate as local authorities seek to achieve economies in the face of public expenditure cuts.

A. Milne, BA, CQSW/Diploma ASS, MA, PhD
School of Social Policy, Sociology and Social Research, University of Kent,
Chatham Maritime, Kent, UK
e-mail: A.J.Milne@kent.ac.uk

© Springer International Publishing Switzerland 2016
C.A. Chew-Graham, M. Ray (eds.), *Mental Health and Older People:
A Guide for Primary Care Practitioners*, DOI 10.1007/978-3-319-29492-6_13

13.1.1 Profile of the Care Home Population

The vast majority of care home residents are women aged 75 years or over: most have multiple health problems [1]. It has been estimated that four fifths of care home residents have dementia and/or a hearing impairment, three quarters require assistance with mobility and/or activities of daily living, and three fifths have continence problems [4, 5]. In a 2004 study of 16,000 care home residents, over a quarter were immobile, cognitively impaired, *and* incontinent [6].

The biggest single health-related determinant of care home admission is dementia [7]. In people without dementia, high levels of dependency linked to physical ill health problems are common [8]. Having a co-resident carer had a strongly protective effect against admission to a care home – the risk of being admitted to a care home was 20 times higher in people who *do not* have a carer living with them [9]. A permanent move to a care home often follows some form of crisis, so tends to be relatively little time to plan the move or make informed choices [3]. The cause of the crisis may be the death of a spouse – or other long-term carer – or a hospital admission so, quite apart from the stress of giving up one's home, there will probably be additional losses to contend with. Other issues that prompt admission are poor or unsuitable housing, inadequate community-based care or a breakdown in care arrangements and other people's concerns about the older person's safety [10]. About a fifth of deaths in the UK occur in a care home. The average period between admission and death is around 2.5 years; a quarter of residents live for more than 3 years [11].

13.1.2 Depression Amongst Care Home Residents

Research suggests that there are very high levels of depression amongst care home residents. For major depressive disorders, prevalence figures range from 4 to 25 % and for minor depression – or the presence of depressive symptoms – 29–82 % [12]. This compares with an estimated prevalence of 9.3 % (for major depression) in the UK's community-based older populations (Table 13.1).

The course and nature of depression in care homes are incompletely understood, and current evidence is mixed: most studies suggest that symptoms tend to persist. For example, Sutcliffe et al. [12] found that almost half the residents with depression at admission were still depressed after 9 months; Scocco et al. [13] reported that the symptoms of those admitted with more serious depression increased over a 6-month period. In contrast, Payne et al. [14] found that, although 20 % of residents were depressed on admission, only 7.5 % were still depressed 12 months later. The

Table 13.1 Prevalence of depression in care home populations

Major depressive disorders: estimates range from 4 to 25 %
Minor depression or depressive symptoms: estimates range from 29 to 82 %
This compares with an estimated community-based prevalence of 9 %

incidence of new episodes of depression amongst care home residents is about 5 % per annum [16]. Suffering from depression nearly doubles the risk of a person being admitted to a care home [17].

A number of factors are correlated with depression in care home populations. Functional impairment appears to be an important independent risk factor, e.g. sensory loss, incontinence, loss of mobility and reduced capacity to perform activities of daily living. Other associations include physical health variables, such as dysphagia and heart disease; psychological variables, such as loneliness and neuroticism; and social variables, such as loss [18]. Loss is strongly associated with depression; personal loss includes grief over the death of loved ones and loss of home, pets, social support and close friends; loss of function and control over the body; loss of independence and autonomy; and loss of 'environmental mastery', i.e. the capacity to control one's life and surrounding world [19, 20]. Persistent pain is also a risk factor, from arthritis and pressure areas especially, and certain medications (e.g. antihypertensive/cardiac drugs, treatment for Parkinson's disease) may cause or worsen symptoms [21]. For residents without dementia, the risk of becoming or remaining depressed increases with length of stay and tends to be accompanied by a growing sense of hopelessness over health status and lack of autonomy [19] (Table 13.2).

Depression on admission is associated with increased mortality [13, 22], with one study suggesting that depressed residents were three times more likely to die than those without depression [23]. Depression is also implicated in suicide and attempted suicide [14, 24]. Deaths in care homes are usually heralded by gradual decline [25]. Depression is often overlooked and undertreated during the last months of life [26], though whether depressive symptoms actually increase at this time is not clear [27].

Up to half of care home residents with dementia also have depression [12]. Evidence suggests that people with both conditions have higher rates of disability and decline and higher rates of hospitalisation than people with dementia alone

Table 13.2 Risk factors for depression in care home populations

Physical factors
Functional impairment including sensory loss, mobility challenges, incontinence
Inability to perform activities of daily living
Chronic physical ill health such as heart disease
Persistent pain from conditions such as arthritis (some medications may amplify symptoms)
Psychosocial factors
Psychological issues primarily isolation and loneliness
Mental health problems including pre-existing depression
Multiple losses – loss of partner/spouse, loss of control over the body, loss of independence and autonomy and loss of environmental mastery
The depressogenic effect of 'institutional care' itself including limited opportunities for meaningful activity or social interaction, disempowerment, loss of privacy, noise, institutional furniture and odours and the constant presence of death

[28]. In terms of other mental health problems, anxiety symptoms are common in care home populations. Smalbrugge et al. [15] found that, in a sample of over 300 residents, 5.7 % had anxiety disorders, 4.2 % had sub-threshold anxiety disorders, and nearly 30 % had anxiety symptoms.

Whilst not specific to care home residents, there are also a set of intersecting risks that relate to the older person's life prior to admission. Clearly, older people arrive in a care home setting with a life history and a host of life course experiences; some of these will be relevant to enhanced risk of depression. As rates of depression are higher amongst women, being female is a primary risk. Living alone and having a low income are also risks: it is notable that both of these are more common features of the lives of older women than older men [29]. Experiences of abuse or trauma may also be relevant. There is no reason to suppose, for example, that childhood sexual abuse – which we know places younger adults at risk of depression – should not continue to influence mental health in later life and it is certainly a prominent aspect of an older resident's personal biography. It is interesting, but perhaps not unsurprising, that a number of the risks for developing depression are also primary triggers for admission to a care home.

The depressogenic effect of 'institutional care' itself is also noteworthy. Particular features identified in research are few opportunities for meaningful activity, disempowerment, minimal social interaction and being expected to live in a 'semi-public' environment [4, 30]. Other factors may include loss of privacy and frustration over sharing a room, noise, institutional furniture and odours, lack of stimulation or close relationships, high turnover rate of staff and cultural dissonance between residents and staff [19]. The medicalised environment of many care homes and the constant presence of death are also factors.

13.2 Assessment and Treatment of Depression Amongst Care Home Residents

As there is no doubt that depression has a significant adverse effect on residents' well-being and quality of life, it is important that it is identified, assessed and treated effectively.

A fundamental issue relates to care home staff's lack the knowledge and skills in identifying depression, especially if the main symptoms are changes in behaviour, such as withdrawal, aggressive behaviour or disruptive vocalization [31–33]. The fact that only 2 % of care staff receive in service training on depression is an obvious deficit [34]. A widespread assumption that depression is a 'normal' and 'untreatable' part of ageing compounds the problem. These combined barriers have led to the suggestion that residents should be screened for depression on admission and then regularly (re)assessed by primary or specialist health-care professionals [35]. This is an issue returned to below.

There are a number of difficulties in assessing depression amongst care home residents. Many residents cannot fully participate in interviews or complete a depression scale, because of dementia and/or communication problems [34].

Additionally, the instruments or measures used to assess levels of depression are often subject to confounding variables, such as physical symptoms, unrelated to depression per se. Even the Geriatric Depression Scale, which is widely used and trusted, contains items that could be endorsed by a care home resident even if they were not actually depressed (e.g. Do you prefer to stay at home, rather than going out and doing new things? Do you think it is wonderful to be alive now?). With a cut-off point of 5 or 6 (out of 15), it is easy to see how 'depression' could be over-diagnosed or simply mistaken for boredom, mourning or being close to death [36].

Antidepressants are the most common treatment for depression in care home residents, and research and National Institute for Health and Care Excellence (NIHCE) guidelines (90 and 91) suggest they are effective and should be included in the first-line treatment for major depression [37]. The choice of medication needs to be based on possible side effects, interactions with other medications and the resident's other illnesses (Refer to Chap. 9). Serotonin reuptake inhibitors are first-line drugs, recommended by NIHCE [38–40]. When tricyclic antidepressants are used, it is often for indications other than depression, such as chronic pain [41]. Related evidence suggests that those residents who are prescribed antidepressants (particularly when prescribed tricyclic antidepressants) are on subtherapeutic doses; this may be because the dosage is not reviewed often enough by GPs or other health-care professionals [42] (Table 13.3).

Table 13.3 Assessment and treatment of depression amongst care home residents

There are a number of difficulties in assessing depression amongst care home residents, including:
Many residents find it difficult (especially if they have advanced dementia) to participate in interviews or complete a 'depression scale' or measure
Depression measures are vulnerable to confounding variables, e.g. physical symptoms, and may contain questions that could be endorsed by a resident even if they were not depressed
Limited access to training amongst care home staff in being aware of symptoms of depression is a fundamental barrier
In terms of treatments and interventions:
Antidepressants are considered effective: serotonin reuptake inhibitors are first-line drugs, recommended by NIHCE
Many residents who are prescribed antidepressants are on subtherapeutic doses; this may be because the dosage is not reviewed often enough by health-care professionals
A number of psychological approaches are effective in reducing symptoms of depression including behavioural and cognitive therapies and life review approaches, although few residents are offered these in the UK
Psychosocial and recreational interventions such as exercise classes may reduce the symptoms of minor depression, and changes to the care homes environment are also effective, e.g. more homelike mealtimes
Whilst not an intervention per se, training of care home staff can lead to increased rates of detection of depression and to better quality of life for residents – it is also linked with reduced prescribing of antipsychotic medication and less use of physical restraint

Prevalence data about treatment for depression in care homes is patchy [13]. Although a 2007 study estimated that between 50 and 75 % of residents with depression received no treatment at all [43]. There is evidence that prescribing of antidepressants has increased dramatically in recent years [44]. This may be a response to concerns about antipsychotics but is probably also a recognition of the importance of treating depression in care home residents. There are concerns that whilst some residents are receiving appropriate treatment, it may also be the case that a number of those taking antidepressants are, in fact, not depressed. Prescribing patterns may also be influenced by the characteristics of the home rather than the clinical needs of residents per se [45].

A number of psychological approaches are effective in reducing symptoms of depression. Evidence from the USA suggests that behavioural and cognitive therapies and life review approaches are effective at treating depression amongst care home residents [46]. However, few residents are offered psychological therapy in the UK. Psychosocial and recreational interventions such as exercise classes may reduce the symptoms of minor depression, and changes to the care homes environment and culture are also effective, including more homelike mealtimes, less institutional lounge areas and accessible gardens [47].

13.2.1 Primary Care Support to Care Homes

Research demonstrates a long history of erratic and inequitable approaches to health-care delivery by both primary and secondary health-care services to care homes [48]. Although there are examples of innovation and good practice, these tend to be time limited, discretionary and locally determined; often they depend on an individual health practitioner's interest. Care home residents tend not to be seen as a priority. This is in part a consequence of residents receiving 24 hr care in the home; it is also a feature of care homes' 'off the radar' status.

Access to primary care services varies widely between care homes. One survey identified that 20 % of care homes 'had no regular support' from a GP [49]. Some homes pay a retainer to a primary care practice to ensure that they get reliable access to GP services, can secure the services of one GP for all residents and/or can arrange a 'clinic' or visits on set days of the week [50]. In 2010 this was the case for only 8–10 % of all care homes [48]. Other care homes encourage residents to register with a particular surgery close to the home or, in an attempt to maintain continuity of care, encourage them to remain registered with their 'old' practice. This may mean that residents in one care home are registered with a number of different practices, some of which may be some distance away from the home. A 2010 survey of care homes identified that most homes received GP support from more than one practice, a quarter had GPs providing regular clinics in the home, and a half received support from a community nurse [48].

Consistent regular primary health-care input to care homes is widely regarded as important by residents and care home staff. Where investment is made to develop

Table 13.4 Primary care support to care homes: reflective activity

Reflect on:
How might primary care services effectively support care home residents with depression?
Who else – other agencies and other professionals – might need to be involved in developing a 'system' that is sustainable?
What are the other elements of a 'support system' that may reduce depression and/or manage depressive symptoms?
How might consistent primary care support to care home residents help to assess, treat and manage depression amongst care home residents?
How can the NHS incentivise primary care services to engage to a greater degree with care homes?

this kind of support, outcomes can include earlier identification of preventable illness, earlier referral to specialist services and delayed or prevented hospital admission [48]. For example, 'actively managed primary care' with access to multidisciplinary team support has been shown to be effective in reducing hospital admissions with no adverse effects on mortality [51].

In terms of the management of depression, in-reach provision by primary care services is viewed as especially helpful. Routine screening, assessment and treatment for depression by a trusted primary care professional are consistently identified as desirable by care home staff; it would also encourage staff to identify possible symptoms of depression themselves [52]. A 2012 review by the Care Quality Commission (CQC) [53] found that a third of care homes were *not* provided with post-admission assessment of residents by GPs, a half said that these were both provided *and* paid for by the Clinical Commissioning Groups, and another 7 % said that they were provided by GPs but paid for by the care homes themselves.

There are a number of key challenges to providing good quality primary care to care homes. These include the fact that the care home sector is fragmented and there is limited sign up to embedding a 'system' of primary care support to care homes nationally, stretched NHS resources and piecemeal research investment in evidencing 'what works' and for whom. Barriers exist inside care homes too, including the limited capacity of residents themselves to request input from GPs, a high turnover of staff, limited access to staff training and lack of managerial commitment to partnership working with primary care services [54] (Table 13.4).

13.3 Improving the Management and Treatment of Depression in Care Homes

As depression is one of the most common conditions experienced by care home populations and it is, generally, poorly managed, it is important to explore what can be done to improve its management and treatment.

13.3.1 Transition into a Care Home

Moving into a care home is a life-changing decision often made in stressful circumstances. A well-managed transition can reduce the risk of an older person becoming (more) depressed [1]. A number of key findings emerge from research. Preparatory work with the person and their relatives before admission can help the older person feel they are part of the decision; their needs and biography can also be discussed and the person's wishes, views and tastes accommodated. On arrival in the home, the older person needs to feel supported by staff. This will include taking account of their feelings of guilt, loss, sorrow, grief and/or anger that may be associated with the move. The opportunity simply to talk to people may be the most important element in helping new residents to settle in satisfactorily [55]. Families have a major part to play in supporting this transition, as they occupy a role intermediate between the person and the care staff and can act as a bridge or conduit between life inside, and outside, the care home [56]. A move from acute hospital to a care home needs to be dealt with particularly sensitively as there are likely to have been fewer, if any, preparatory steps taken prior to admission [57].

This transition also offers a pivotal opportunity for a primary care professional to (re)assess any long-term conditions experienced by the resident – including depression – and reappraise the nature and objectives of any treatment(s). It may be the first time depression has been formally identified or discussed and/or the first time that an assessment of the persons medication(s) has been made. This may inform how the person is managed by staff and what types of support and monitoring they need.

13.3.2 Identification and Treatment

Identification and treatment of depression amongst care home residents needs to be implemented on a much more proactive and consistent basis if outcomes are to be improved [16].

In terms of sustainable impact, education and training of care home staff are of primary importance. This can lead to increased rates of detection of depression and to better quality of life outcomes for residents. For example, Proctor et al.'s [57] training intervention to improve care planning skills led to lower levels of depression in the 'intervention group' compared to the control group. Ray et al. [58] found a coherent programme of training resulted in reduced prescribing of antipsychotic medication and less use of physical restraint.

Improvement to the care home culture is also important [60]. A commitment to person-centred care with a particular focus on a biographical approach and staff spending time on developing relationships with residents is strongly linked to improved mental health [61]. Many of the tenets of person-centred care directly benefit residents with depression shifting the locus of care away from the 'functional' towards the social and psychological. Underpinning the delivery of care to residents with an appreciation that depression is (often) amenable to improvement is also important [62].

Reducing Depression Amongst Older People Living in a Care Home

Research has examined the impact of individualised, person-centred interventions on depression amongst older people living in care homes [63]. Eighty-seven participants with depression (GDS) were assigned care workers who were specifically trained to plan and carry out individualised interventions and support plans. Initially care workers undertook a detailed interview with the older participants in order to build up a picture of their life, biography, likes/dislikes, relationships, etc. They also sought to ascertain what improvements or changes the older person wished to make in their own life. Care plans were developed directly from the interviews to address individual needs and provide psychosocial support. Intervention goals included visits to the supermarket, review of hearing and hearing aid equipment, resuming attendance at church, going to football matches and being able to sit outdoors. Results suggested that, at follow-up, participants' mental health showed significant improvement including some having ceased to have clinical symptoms of depression. Improvement was greatest in those with the most severe symptoms at baseline.

Turning to primary care, a number of studies have investigated the impact of educating GPs about depression amongst care home residents. One study explored the impact of a single educational session with a group of Australian GPs; it led to improved recognition of depression [64]. In another Australian study, training of GPs and care staff in detecting and managing depression was one component of a multifactorial intervention which – overall – resulted in significantly reduced levels of depression [65, 66]. In the USA there is evidence that having a mandated screening tool improves recognition and initiation of treatment for depression amongst care home residents; regular assessment of mental health by primary care physicians also improves treatment outcomes for residents with depression [37].

13.3.3 Policy Issues and Care Homes

Recent policies, such as the National Dementia Strategy [7], have started to place more emphasis on the important contribution services external to care homes can, and should, make in supporting residents. It recognises that in order to achieve this care homes need: a well-trained specialist workforce, consistent and coherent access to NHS primary care and specialist mental health services and to be supported by an inspection regime that is committed to driving up quality [53].

In 2012 the National Institute for Health and Care Excellence (NIHCE) published a quality standard entitled 'The Mental Well Being of Older People in Care Homes' [66]. Two of the six quality standards are directly relevant to improving the identification and treatment of mental health problems amongst care home residents. Standard 3 states that: 'Older people in care homes have the symptoms and signs of mental health conditions recognised and recorded as part of their care plan'. Key recommendations in terms of achieving this standard include more training for care home staff on the recognition of symptoms and support for residents with mental health problems. Statement 6 states that, 'Older people in care homes have access to the full range of health-care services when they need them', including primary care services. NIHCE suggests that care homes develop good relationships with

GPs and other primary care professionals including developing effective referral arrangements so that services are available easily and without delay. The statement also identifies prevention as an important goal for primary care in working with care home residents and advises regular check-ups as a key way to ameliorate symptoms of conditions like depression. Regular reviews of medication for each resident are also important in alleviating distress and pain and in promoting well-being.

13.3.4 Research

The current evidence base is limited by small sample sizes, a lack of longitudinal data, few randomised controlled trials and differing outcome measures. More research is needed into the nature and course of depression amongst care home residents. Feeling sad or low may be a perfectly appropriate response to a change in circumstances, and to loss, and a balance needs to be struck between unhelpfully labelling people experiencing emotions within the normal range and failing to recognise and treat more intransigent symptoms of depression. That the 'natural history' of depression in care homes is little understood is additionally relevant; evidence is conflicting. We still do not really understand if we are dealing with a relatively mild and transient phenomenon or with a severe, enduring and disabling condition [41]. More longitudinal studies are also needed for a better understanding of which interventions are effective.

Limited attention has been paid to capturing the subjective experiences of care home residents including their perspectives on what influences their mental health [43]. The evidence we do have suggests that 'feeling well' and 'promoting health' are terms understood by care home residents to be as much about their capacity to (re)adjust and compensate to threats to their well-being as they are about treatment for 'symptoms'. The definitions underpinning health-care professionals interventions tend to be about what an older person 'cannot' do and what is 'wrong' with them and are rarely sufficiently individualised to take account of the older person's own perceptions, strengths and abilities. This is a challenge to the way that we construct 'care' including primary care support to care homes.

13.4 Conclusion

Despite its prevalence and profound impact on well-being, depression amongst care home residents is routinely under-identified and untreated. Much more needs to be done to identify, assess and treat depression in this population in both the short and longer term. Providing regular training to care home staff and managers and developing partnerships with primary care services have significant potential to improve outcomes for care home residents. Turning the provision of 'care' away from a task-focused activity to a person-focused one is also important, and a number of psychosocial interventions are evidenced as effective.

Primary care support to care homes tends to be highly variable; it is locally determined, often short term in tenure and/or is driven by a single committed individual.

Care home staff and residents welcome regular input from one or more primary care professionals with whom they can build trust relationships and call upon for advice and support. Although primary care input is evidenced as having considerable potential to identify, treat and monitor depression amongst care homes residents, they are not considered a priority by clinical commissioning groups (formally PCTs); thus, few specific services are commissioned. The fragmented nature of the care home 'sector' and funding complexities in relationship to who is responsible for providing, and paying, for health-care input to care homes compounds this situation. It is an issue that urgently requires coherent national attention including the development of systemic mechanisms that will facilitate sustained engagement of primary care services with care homes and care home residents with depression and other long-term conditions.

13.5 Case Study: Kathleen Jones

Kathleen Jones moved into the care home after her husband, John, died suddenly at home. The couple had been married for 45 years. They had no children, and this was a cause of great sadness for Kathleen as they tried to have a baby and Kathleen had several miscarriages. Now, Kathleen has memory difficulties, extensive osteoarthritis and very poor mobility. She also has high blood pressure and has had several TIAs, two of which resulted in brief periods in hospital. She relied on John for a great deal of informal care and day-to-day support, and after his death, Kathleen's sister arranged for her to move into the care home as she felt that Kathleen could not manage safely at home. Kathleen is self funding her care, and now her house has been sold by her sister who has power of attorney. She sees few people as the home is not in her old neighbourhood, and most of her friends are either dead or live away from the area. She has few surviving relatives and her niece lives in Australia. Her sister sees her every few months.

Kathleen is treated kindly at the home who tell her that this is her 'home' now. Kathleen knows that this is not her home, and she wishes that she had died with John. She is not eating or sleeping well and has lost weight. She appears generally disengaged and easily irritated by other residents. She avoids contact with people if at all possible and tells the staff that she prefers to be in her bedroom. The staff let her remain in her room for most of the time believing that this is good practice in demonstrating resident choice.

From the above history, Kathleen is likely to be at risk of developing a depressive illness. Depression is common amongst older people living in care homes [12]. A number of factors are likely to contribute to Kathleen's risk of being depressed – including her reduced mobility and its associated impact on her ability to undertake usual activities of daily living [15] and cognitive impairment will also impact. Critically, Kathleen's loss of her much loved husband and the abrupt loss of her home will doubtless impact on her emotional state and combine with feelings about changes in her sense of independence and autonomy [19, 20]. Kathleen's biography includes significant loss, and she had said to her husband that felt that she miscarried at a time when understanding of the emotional impact of miscarriage was very poor and women were expected to 'get on with it'. It is possible that unresolved loss and the trauma associated with miscarriage and failed fertility treatment have impacted over time on Kathleen's emotional state and her capacity for resilience in the face of further change and loss. The staff in the care home are kind but have given little attention to the circumstances of Kathleen's admission or to the possibility of her being emotionally distressed. Her financial circumstances mean that she has bypassed most formal services. Care staff training should include developing awareness of the emotional impact of loss and an awareness that a lack of time to prepare for a move can have profoundly upsetting consequences for an older person [55]. Training and leadership support should also challenge ageism, evidenced by, for example, an assumption that older people do not experience the same trauma as younger people do. Referral to Kathleen's General Practitioner may be helpful in identifying whether Kathleen has a depressive illness and to consider appropriate medical treatment and to ensure that Kathleen's care plan includes addressing her emotional needs as far as possible (e.g. having a named key worker; opportunities for linking with any external voluntary or befriending service). It is highly likely that there will be other residents living in the care home experiencing similar difficulties to Kathleen. Taking a broader view, CQC inspection will promote the value and importance of promoting emotional and mental health and well-being in care planning and in the culture of care in the care homes. This means, for example, encouraging care staff to support residents to engage in activities that are of interest and value and which support residents to do what they can for themselves. Visitors to the care home (e.g. primary care practitioners, social workers) should consider evidence of well-being amongst the care home population and identify and act upon evidence of ill being or poor care. Causes for concern should be acted upon. More generally, practitioners engaged in, for example, care reviews can encourage care homes to develop care practice which is aware of the potential for residents to experience emotional distress. Commissioners may encourage care homes to embrace the NIHCE quality standard 'The Mental Well Being and Older People in Care Homes' [66] through their commissioning practice.

13.6 Suggested Activities

Reflect on:

To what extent do you consider evidence of well or ill being amongst a care home population when you visit? What role do you have in identifying concerns about high levels of ill being?

When residents have multiple physical health problems and living in a care home, how often do you think about their emotional well-being? To what extent do you consider that they may have a depressive illness?

To what extent are you aware that care staff are regularly trained or receive leadership input which encourages them to think about and respond to mental health and well-being amongst the resident population?

What can you do in your role to encourage and support mental health and well-being amongst residents living in care homes?

> **Key Points**
> - Depression and anxiety are common in older people, especially when they live in residential care.
> - Depression amongst older people living with dementia in care homes is especially high.
> - There has traditionally been a poor recognition of the extent of depression amongst care home populations, and psychosocial interventions and access to specialist resources have been poor.
> - Evidence suggests that actively addressing mental health and well-being through care culture, care planning and effective primary care intervention can have a significant impact on well-being.

References

1. Dening T, Milne A. Care homes for older people. In: Dening T, Thomas A, editors. The Oxford Textbook of Old Age Psychiatry. Oxford: Oxford University Press; 2013. p. 343–58.
2. Bowman C, Whistler J, Ellerby M. A national census of care home residents. Age Ageing. 2004;33:561–6.
3. Laing and Buisson. Care of elderly people: market survey 2010–11. London: Laing and Buisson; 2010.
4. Alzheimer's Society. Home from home. London: Alzheimer's Society; 2008.
5. Cohen-Mansfield J, Taylor JW. Hearing aid use in nursing homes. Part 1: prevalence rates of hearing impairment and hearing aid use. J Am Med Dir Assoc. 2004;5:283–8.
6. Department of Health. Living well with dementia: a National Dementia Strategy. London: Department of Health; 2009.
7. Bharucha AJ, Pandav R, Shen C, Dodge HH, Ganguli M. Predictors of nursing facility admission: a 12-year epidemiological study in the United States. J Am Geriatr Soc. 2004;52:434–9.
8. Banerjee S, Murray J, Foley B, Atkins L, Schneider J, Mann A. Predictors of institutionalisation in people with dementia. J Neurol Neurosurg Psychiatry. 2003;74:1315–6.
9. Bowers H, Clark A, Crosby G, Eastbrook L, Macadam A, Macdonald R, Macfarlane A, Maclean M, Patel M, Runnicles D. Older people's vision for long term care. York: Joseph Rowntree Foundation; 2009.
10. Forder J., Fernandez, J. Length of stay in care homes. Discussion Paper 2769. Personal Social Services Research Unit, University of Kent, Canterbury; 2011.
11. Dow B, Xiaoping L, Tinney J, Haralambous B, Ames D. Depression in care homes. In: Dening T, Milne A, editors. Mental health and care homes. Oxford: Oxford University Press; 2011. p. 179–90.
12. Sutcliffe C, Burns A, Challis D, Mozley CG, Cordingley L, Bagley H, Huxley P. Depressed mood, cognitive impairment, and survival in older people admitted to care homes in England. Am J Geriatr Psychiatr. 2007;15:708–15.
13. Scocco P, Rapattoni M, Fantoni G, Galuppo M, De Biasi F, de Girolamo G, Pavan L. Suicidal behaviour in nursing homes: a survey in a region of north-east Italy. Int J Geriatr Psychiatry. 2006;21:307–11.

14. Payne JL, Sheppard JE, Steinberg M, Warren A, Baker A, Steele C, Brandt J, Lyketsos CG. Incidence, prevalence and outcomes of depression in residents of a long term care facility with dementia. Int J Geriatr Psychiatry. 2002;17:247–53.
15. Smalbrugge M, Pot AM, Jongenelis L, Gundy CM, Beekman AT, Eefsting JA. The impact of depression and anxiety on well being, disability and use of health care services in nursing home patients. Int J Geriatr Psychiatry. 2006;21:325–32.
16. Dening T, Milne A. Depression and mental health in care homes. Qual Ageing Spec Issue Depression Suicide Self-Harm Older Adults. 2009;10(2):40–6.
17. Seitz D, Purandare N, Conn D. Prevalence of psychiatric disorders among older adults in long-term care homes: a systematic review. Int Psychogeriatr. 2010;22:1025–9.
18. Hyer L, Carpenter B, Bishman D, Wu H-S. Depression in long term care. Clin Psychol Sci Pract. 2005;12:280–99.
19. Knight T, Davison TE, McCabe MP, Mellor D. Environmental mastery and depression in older adults in residential care. Ageing Soc. 2011;31:870–84.
20. Cipher DJ, Clifford PA. Dementia, pain, depression, behavioral disturbances, and ADLs: toward a comprehensive conceptualization of quality of life in long-term care. Int J Geriatr Psychiatry. 2004;19:741–8.
21. Barca ML, Engedal K, Laks J, Sellback G. A 12 months follow-up study of depression among nursing-home patients in Norway. J Affect Disord. 2010;120:141–8.
22. Ashby D, Ames D, West CR, MacDonald A, Graham N, Mann AH. Psychiatric morbidity as predictor of mortality for residents of local authority homes for the elderly. Int J Geriatr Psychiatry. 1991;6:567–75.
23. Suominen K, Hendrksson M, Isometsa E, Conwell Y, Heila H, Lonnqvist J. Nursing home suicides – a psychological autopsy study. Int J Geriatr Psychiatry. 2003;18:1095–101.
24. Bercovitz A, Gruber-Baldini AL, Burton LC, Hebel JR. Healthcare utilization of nursing home residents: comparison between decedents and survivors. J Am Geriatr Soc. 2005;53:2069–75.
25. Evers MM, Samuels SC, Lantz M, Khan K, Brickman AM, Marin DB. The prevalence, diagnosis and treatment of depression in dementia patients in chronic care facilities in the last six months of life. Int J Geriatr Psychiatry. 2002;17:464–72.
26. Cuijpers P, van Lammeren P. Secondary prevention of depressive symptoms in elderly inhabitants of residential homes. Int J Geriatr Psychiatry. 2001;16:702–8.
27. Godfrey M, Denby T. Depression and older people: towards securing wellbeing in later life. Bristol: Policy; 2005.
28. Milne A. Mental well being in later life. In: Williamson T, editor. Older people's mental health today: a handbook. Brighton: Mental Health Foundation & Pavilion Publishing; 2009.
29. Clare L, Rowlands J, Bruce E, Surr C, Downs M. The experience of living with dementia in residential care: an interpretive phenomenological analysis. Gerontologist. 2008;48(6):711–20.
30. Dwyer M, Byrne GJ. Disruptive vocalization and depression in older nursing home residents. Int Psychogeriatr. 2000;12:463–71.
31. Menon AS, Gruber-Baldini AL, Hebel JR, Kaup B, Loreck D, Itkin Zimmerman S, Burton L, German P, Magaziner J. Relationship between aggressive behaviors and depression among nursing home residents with dementia. Int J Geriatr Psychiatry. 2001;16:139–46.
32. Bartels SJ, Horn SD, Smout RJ, Dums AR, Flaherty E, Jones JK, Monane M, Taler GA, Voss AC. Agitation and depression in frail nursing home elderly patients with *dementia*: *treatment characteristics and service use*. Am J Geriatr Psychiatr. 2003;11:231–8.
33. Bagley H, Cordingley L, Burns A, Mozley CG, Sutcliffe C, Challis D, Huxley P. Recognition of depression by staff in nursing and residential homes. J Clin Nurs. 2000;9:445–50.
34. Cohen CI, Hyland K, Kimhy D. The utility of mandatory depression screening of dementia patients in nursing homes. Am J Psychiatr. 2003;160:2012–7.
35. Brühl KG, Hendrika JL, Martien TM. Nurses' and nursing assistants' recognition of depression in elderly who depend on long-term care. J Am Med Dir Assoc. 2007;8:441–5.

36. American Geriatrics Society and American Association for Geriatric Society. Consensus statement on improving the quality of mental health care in US nursing homes: management of depression and behavioural symptoms associated with dementia. J Am Geriatr Soc. 2003;51:1287–98.
37. Borson S, Scanlan J, Doane K, Gray S. Antidepressant prescribing in nursing homes: is there a place for tricyclics? Int J Geriatr Psychiatry. 2002;17:1140–5.
38. National Institute for Health and Care Excellence. Depression in adults: the treatment and management of depression in adults CG90. London: NIHCE; 2009. https://www.nice.org.uk/guidance/cg90.
39. National Institute for Health and Care Excellence. Depression in adults with a chronic physical health problem: treatment and management CG91. London: NIHCE; 2009. https://www.nice.org.uk/guidance/cg91.
40. National Institute for Health and Care Excellence. Depression in adults, Quality Standard 8. London: NIHCE. 2011. https://www.nice.org.uk/guidance/qs8.
41. Brown MN, Laplace KL, Luisi AF. The management of depression in older nursing home residents. J Am Geriatr Soc. 2002;50:69–76.
42. George K, Davidson TE, McCabe M, Mellor D, Moore K. Treatment of depression in low level residential care facilities for the elderly. Int Psychogeriatr. 2007;13:107–20.
43. Dening T, Milne A, editors. Mental health and care homes. Oxford: Oxford University Press; 2011.
44. Lapane KL, Hughes CM. Which organizational characteristics are associated with increased management of depression in US nursing homes? Med Care. 2004;42:992–1000.
45. Hyer L, Yeager CA, Hilton N, Sacks A. Group, individual, and staff therapy: an efficient and effective cognitive behavioral therapy in long-term care. Am J Alzheimers Dis Other Dementias. 2008;23:528–39.
46. Snowden M, Sato K, Roy-Byrne P. Assessment and treatment of nursing home residents with depression or behavioral symptoms associated with dementia: a review of the literature. J Am Geriatr Soc. 2003;51:1305–17.
47. Goodman C, Davies S. Good practice outside the care home. In: Dening T, Milne A, editors. Mental health and care homes. Oxford: Oxford University Press; 2011. p. 297–312.
48. O'Dea G, Kerrison H, Pollock MP. Access to health care in nursing homes: a survey in one English Health Authority. Health Soc Care Community. 2000;93:180–5.
49. Glendinning C, Jacobs S, Alborz A, Hann M. A survey of access to medical services in nursing and residential homes in England. Br J Gen Pract. 2002;52(480):545–9.
50. Joseph A, Boult C. Managed primary care of nursing home residents. J Am Geriatr Soc. 1998;46(9):1152–6.
51. Goodman C, Robb N, Drennan V, Woolley R. Partnership working by default: district nurses and care home staff providing care for older people. Health Soc Care Community. 2005; 13(6):553–662.
52. Care Quality Commission. Health care in care homes. London: CQC; 2012.
53. Davies S, Goodman C, Dickinson A. The approach survey: integrated working between care homes and the health care service, Centre for Research in Primary and Community Care, Hatfield: University of Hertfordshire; 2010.
54. Andersson I, Petterson E, Sidenvall B. Daily life after moving into a care home-experiences from older people, relatives and contact persons. J Clin Nurs. 2007;16:1712–8.
55. Kellett U. Seizing possibilities for positive family caregiving in nursing homes. J Clin Nurs. 2007;16:1479–87.
56. Care Quality Commission. Cracks in the pathway. London: CQC; 2014.
57. Proctor R, Burns A, Powell H, Tarrier N, Faragher B, Richardson G, Davies J, South B. Behavioural management in nursing and residential homes: a randomized controlled trial. Lancet. 1999;354(9172):26–9.
58. Ray WA, Taylor J, Meador KG, Lictenstein MJ, Griffin MR, Fought R, Adamsn ML, Blazer DG. Reducing antipsychotic drug use in nursing homes: a controlled trial of provider education. Arch Intern Med. 1993;153(6):713–21.

59. Milne A, Adams A. Enhancing critical reflection amongst social work students: the contribution of an experiential learning group in care homes for older people. Soc Work Educ. 2014. doi:10.1080/02615479.2014.949229.
60. Brooker D. Promoting health and well-being: good practice inside the care home. In: Dening T, Milne A, editors. Mental health and care homes. Oxford: Oxford University Press; 2011. p. 279–96.
61. Ray M, Bernard M, Phillips J. Critical issues in social work with older people. Basingstoke: Palgrave MacMillan; 2009.
62. Lyne KJ, Moxon S, Sinclair I, Young P, Kirk C, Ellison S. Analysis of care planning intervention for reducing depression in older people in residential care. Aging Ment Health. 2006;10(4):394–403.
63. Davidson S, Koritsas S, O'Connor DW, Clarke D. The feasibility of a GP led screening intervention for depression among nursing home residents. Int J Geriatr Psychiatry. 2006;21:1026–30.
64. Llewellyn-Jones RH, Snowden J. Depression in nursing homes, ensuring adequate treatment. CNS Drugs. 2007;21:627–40.
65. Llewellyn-Jones RH, Baikie KA, Smithers H, Cohen J, Snowden J, Tennant CC. Multifaceted shared care intervention for late life depression in residential care: randomised controlled trial. Br Med J. 1999;319:676–82.
66. National Institute for Health and Care Excellence. The mental well being of older people in care homes. London: NIHCE; 2012. http://www.nice.org.uk/guidance/qs50.
67. Milne A. Living with dementia in a care home: a review of research evidence. In: Dening T, Milne A, editors. Mental health and care homes. Oxford: Oxford University Press; 2011. p. 53–65.

Part III
Delirium

Delirium

14

Rashi Negi and Valentinos Kounnis

14.1 Historical Context

The Latin verb 'delire' (to be deranged, crazy, out of one's wits) appears in the Coventry mystery plays in 1400. Other accounts from literature include Shakespeare's death of Falstaff (a babbled of green fields), Lady Macbeth sleepwalking and Tolstoy's depiction of Anna Karenina's post-partum delirium [1].

14.2 Core Features

Many terminologies have been used interchangeably for delirium, such as 'acute confusional state', 'acute organic brain syndrome', 'acute brain failure' and 'postoperative psychosis'. The definitions may embrace all varieties of acute organic reactions, sometimes referring to the degree of overt disturbance or confine the term to a clinical picture with specific features. The Oxford English dictionary defines delirium as a 'disordered state of the mental faculties resulting from disturbances of the functions of the brain, and characterized by incoherent speech, hallucinations, restlessness and frenzied or manic excitement'. The NICE guideline for delirium [2] describes delirium as a 'common clinical syndrome characterized by disturbed consciousness, cognitive function or perception, which has an acute

---

R. Negi, MBBS, MD, MRCPsych, MSc Med (✉)
Department of Old Age Psychiatry, South Staffordshire and Shropshire Foundation Trust, Lichfield, Staffordshire, UK
e-mail: rashi.negi@sssft.nhs.uk

V. Kounnis, MD, MSc, PhD
Department of Oncology, Oxford University Hospitals NHS Foundation Trust, University of Oxford, Oxford, Oxfordshire, UK
e-mail: valentinos.kounnis@oncology.ox.ac.uk

© Springer International Publishing Switzerland 2016
C.A. Chew-Graham, M. Ray (eds.), *Mental Health and Older People: A Guide for Primary Care Practitioners*, DOI 10.1007/978-3-319-29492-6_14

onset and fluctuating course.' It emphasises that delirium is a serious condition and associated with poor outcome, but that it could be prevented and treated if dealt with urgently.

The broad characteristics of delirium have been well documented: wakefulness with ability to respond verbally, increased psychomotor activity, pronounced disturbance of affect, defective reality testing or symptoms such as delusions and hallucinations [2]. In the UK, delirium predominately has been used to describe patients suffering with acute confusion and who present with disturbed or disruptive behaviour; however, not all patients with delirium present with these symptoms, and patients can be quiet with dulling of senses: hence the use of terminologies like 'hypoactive' or 'mixed' state. The consciousness is not merely quantitatively reduced in delirium, but also qualitatively changed. The patient becomes preoccupied with his own inner world and commonly has illusions, hallucinations and delusions. The clinical condition typically fluctuates, and even though awareness of external events is impaired, arousal may be high, enabling these productive symptoms to occur. It has been also suggested that toxic and metabolic disturbances are more likely to be associated with listlessness and apathy, whereas infective processes and alcohol withdrawal are associated with hyperactivity, fearfulness and prominent hallucinations [3].

14.3 Prevalence of Delirium

A number of studies have investigated the incidence and prevalence of delirium in older patients on medical wards. It has been reported that 11–24 % patients present, at the time of admission, with symptoms of delirium, while these symptoms may develop in another 5–35 % of patients during their inpatient admission [4]. Delirium has been documented in 16–62 % of patients following hip surgery [5] and as high as 70–87 % patients in intensive care units [6]. The incidence of delirium occurs at a higher frequency in patients with pre-existing cognitive impairment amongst hospitalised patients. In the community, the prevalence of delirium has been reported to be 0.4–1.1 % of elderly patients living in residential care home settings [7].

Delirium can have adverse consequences; thus, the diagnosed patients in general hospitals have overall high morbidity and mortality due to a high risk of dehydration, malnutrition, falls, continence problems and pressure sores. The in-hospital diagnosed delirium has a 1-year mortality of 35–40 %, high readmission rate and increased risk of admission to residential care (47 % vs. 18 %) [8, 9]. Approximately a quarter of elderly medical patients with delirium will die within 1 month of its onset [10]. This risk of mortality increases by 11 % for every additional 40 h of non-treated delirium [11]. Delirium may also be an accelerating and possibly a casual factor in the development of dementia (Fig. 14.1).

The National Institute for Health and Care Excellence highlights that the reporting of delirium is poor. They also suggest that there are two areas of improvement which are: raising awareness of delirium amongst clinicians and the need for reporting delirium when identified.

Fig. 14.1 "Stop delirium!" project [39] (Courtesy of Dr. Najma Siddiqi)

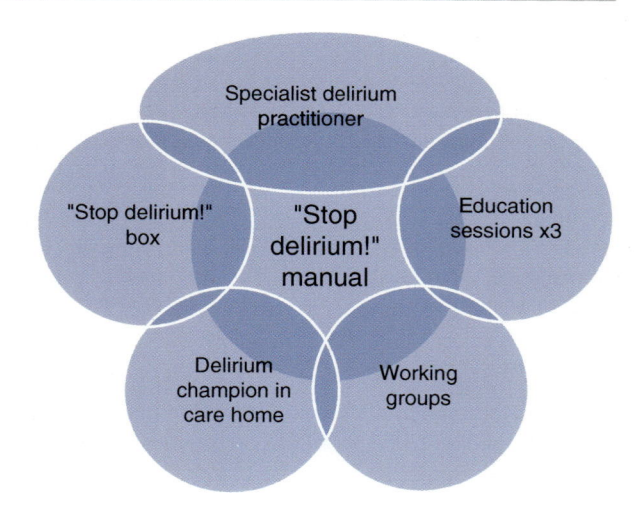

14.4 Identification and Assessment of Delirium

The clinical presentation of delirium incorporates a range of clinical features that are listed in Table 14.1, while its two core symptoms are cognitive impairment and disturbance of the sleep-wake cycle [1].

Although "clouding of consciousness" has been described as a classical sign, in clinical practice its importance is questioned, as old people can be drowsy if they are uninterested in their environment, have been awake overnight or are/had been sedated [1]. It may be difficult to separate "clouding of consciousness" from impaired cognition.

Perceptual disturbances are usually present in the form of visual hallucinations (such as insects, strange people, shadowy presence, fronds that cannot be brushed away) or illusions (e.g., flecks on the wall, or a pattern on the bedclothes being perceived as mites, moving ants or beetles) [1].

Patients may experience distortions, with either increased, diminished or distant sights and/or sounds. Furthermore disturbances of body image are not uncommon, with patients complaining that some body parts have shrunk or enlarged, or there may be a sensation of floating. The sense of time is also distorted, as a day may seem like a week and a week like a few hours. What complicates the whole picture is that a patient may have insight into their symptoms and fear that they may be regarded as 'mad'.

Logic, reason and judgement are all jeopardised by delirium and 'getting hold of the wrong end of the stick' is the basis for the development of paranoid delusions. Conversations that could almost make sense under normal circumstances often may be hard for a patient with delirium to follow. Speech may be rapid, hard to follow, hesitant, repetitive, stammering, laboured and not articulated well and may resemble that of a drunk person [1].

Table 14.1 Clinical features of delirium: ICD10

Disorientation in time, place and person
Symptoms have rapid onset and show fluctuations over the course of the day
At least one of the following psychomotor disturbances is present: rapid, unpredictable shifts from hypoactivity to hyperactivity; increased reaction time; increased or decreased flow of speech; enhanced startle reaction
Disturbance of sleep or the sleep-wake cycle, manifest by at least one of the following: insomnia, which in severe cases may involve total sleep loss, with or without daytime drowsiness or reversal of the sleep-wake cycle; nocturnal worsening of symptoms; disturbing dreams and nightmares, which may continue as hallucinations or illusions after awakening

Many patients experience memory impairment in the acute phase of delirium, with registration being affected, due to the inattention and distractibility. The recent memory appears to be more affected than the remote, and this contributes to the disorientation found in delirium.

Psychomotor disturbances can be in the form of excitement or agitation, but more commonly the patient becomes apathetic and inactive especially in old age. In the hyperactive state, patients may appear hyperalert, scanning their environment and demonstrating agitated behaviour which can make care difficult, for example, pulling out intravenous lines and catheters, and even striking out at staff. A patient in a hypoactive state will be less alert with slowed motor movements, decreased pace of cognition and verbal responsiveness [12].

Delirium most commonly presents as mixed state, with periods of both hypoactivity and hyperactivity within a matter of minutes or hours [13, 14], and furthermore the hypoactive delirium is associated with a poor outcome [14]. The hypoactive (reduced psychomotor activity) subtype is more common than the hyperactive subtype and is often under-recognised. The obvious lack of noticeable agitation, psychosis and disruptive behaviour may mean that an observer or a carer may take little notice of an elderly patient who is causing no management problem.

Table 14.2 illustrates a useful mnemonic to illustrate the clinical features of delirium.

Emotional disturbances in the form of apathy are the most commonly described; however, anger, irritation, terror, apprehension, bewilderment and even euphoria can also be seen. The fluctuation in symptoms, severity and level of arousal is common and makes the diagnosis challenging. Symptoms are often at their worst in the evening and at night and might be referred to as 'sun-downing', particularly in individuals with underlying dementia [15].

Disorganised thinking and disturbance of perception in the form of illusions and hallucinations are common and can occur in up to 40 % of patients. Hallucinations are usually visual, ranging from dreamlike experiences to terrifying visions of dangerous animals and bizarre images. Less frequently, hallucinations involving other modalities can be present such as auditory or taste. Delusions are typically of paranoid in theme, for example, the patient is commonly worried that the staff are poisoning them or intending them harm.

Table 14.2 Physical: mnemonic for the clinical features of delirium

Perplexity: due to acute onset of delirium, the patient is often bemused and bewildered, which may better distinguish it for dementia than, say, clouding of consciousness
Hallucination: mainly visual
Yawning: by day, due to lack of sleep at night
Suspicion: misapprehensions and frank delusions, secondary to cognitive disorder
Illusions: distorted perceptions
Cognitive impairment: memory, communications, comprehension, judgement
Apathy or **A**gitation: psychomotor disturbances
Lability of mood: laughter, tears, anger, terror

Adopted from "Seminars in old age psychiatry" with permission [52]

14.5 Aetiology of Delirium

The development of delirium, results from complex interwoven multifactorial pathophysiological factors as illustrated in Table 14.3.

These factors include, brain insults, e.g., hypoxia with aberrant stress response and excess cortisol along with exaggerated central nervous system inflammation. Relative cholinergic deficiency and dopaminergic excess can partly explain why one person will suffer from delirium, but not another. However, whether these are predisposing or precipitating factors or merely an epiphenomenon requires further clarification.

It was shown that existing neurodegenerative pathology is associated with greater susceptibility to delirium secondary to an exaggerated response to systemic and CNS inflammatory signals due to factors such as microglial, priming and synaptic loss at key areas of the brain (such as the hippocampus), which in turn are associated with heightened and more prolonged transcription of inflammatory mediators [16]. Biomarkers can provide better understanding of the pathophysiology of delirium, and they also allow more accurate detection and assessment of the illness severity as well as monitoring the response to treatment. Studies so far have taken into account other confounding factors such as age, prior cognitive function impairment, including dementia and severity of morbidity, hence aiming in identifying people at risk of developing delirium in any setting. In the literature, EEG has been described as being potentially helpful in identifying delirium suggestive neuro-electrical activity; however, practicalities of doing an EEG on a delirious patient limit its widespread use [17].

14.6 Diagnosis of Delirium

There is a common consensus that delirium is under-diagnosed in clinical practice [2, 18]. It is suggested that between one and two thirds of delirium cases do not get recognised and diagnosed [19], mainly because, the hypoactive form of delirium

Table 14.3 Predisposing factors

Ageing or neurodegenerative disease of the brain
Impairment of vision and hearing
Reduced synthesis of neurotransmitters (especially acetylcholine)
Changes in pharmacokinetics and pharmacodynamics
High prevalence of chronic diseases and high susceptibility to acute illness

Adopted from "Seminars in old age psychiatry" with permission [52]

can be easily missed; the clinical appearance of the syndrome may fluctuate and there could be an overlap with dementia. Clinicians may lack awareness of delirium, particularly on general medical and surgical wards, and may not possess the skills to diagnose and manage delirium. In addition, multiple ward transfers, staff shift patterns and understaffing can all contribute to delirium being underdiagnosed. Delayed detection or failure to diagnose are both associated with poor outcomes including high mortality [20].

Improving delirium detection should focus particularly on increasing staff awareness of less obvious presentations, such as those that involve hypoactivity, as they are easily mistaken for 'fatigue' or 'frailty' in the seriously unwell or post-operative patients. The acute phase of delirium is preceded by what is described in the literature as "prodromal phase" during which early detection and prevention of transition to full syndrome illness can be achieved [21]. This prodromal phase could include symptoms like anxiety, general malaise and a variety of non-specific complaints, deterioration in cognitive function, reduced pain tolerance and simply 'patients not being themselves' [21–26]. This shows the importance of knowing the patient's pre-morbid personality.

The importance of eliciting a good collateral history cannot be over-emphasised, as the observation of the people around this seems to be more important, since the patient may not be able to give a clear account of their problems. Observing, monitoring and recording the patients' overall level of arousal throughout the interaction could be considered equally important as baseline vital signs observations.

In general, delirium detection is a two-stage process involving initial screening with the help of a brief, simple and sensitive instrument as described below, followed by a formal diagnosis using the ICD10 code which is of high specificity for identifying delirium. Simple tests which have high sensitivity and relative specificity for diagnosing delirium, such as attention, digital spatial span, "serial seven" or naming months backward, can all be used as initial screening tools [27]. The second stage of assessment involves the confusion assessment method which is a delirium-specific tool and includes a series of parameters like the acute onset inattention, disorganised thinking, altered level of consciousness, disorientation, memory impairment, perceptual disturbances, psychomotor agitation or retardation and altered sleep-wake cycle as its main components [28–30]. This could be followed by formal assessment for delirium by applying ICD-10/DSM-IV for patients who screen positive from the first stage.

Cognitive tests for delirium (CTD) and delirium rating scales (DRS) tools, have been proven to be very useful in distinguishing delusion from other neuro-phychiatric conditions such as depression and dementia [31, 32]. Other structured cognitive screening tests such as the MMSE or the abbreviated mental score can also be used to test patients' cognition; however, often patients find it difficult to engage and complete these tests. There are some other tests of attention that can be used, such as asking patients to name the months of the year, or the days of the week in reverse, or asking the patient to spell their last or first name backwards, or to perform a serial subtraction (counting backwards) from 100. Deficit in attention, recall and orientation in the setting of an acute change in mental state is very suggestive of delirium. Gathering collateral information from the family, relatives, spouses or other carers is vital. Comprehensive physical examination may uncover signs suggestive of an underlying cause for the delirium, and it is also important to remember that patients, particularly the frail and elderly ones, may have multiple causes of delusion, active at the same time.

Investigations such as full blood count, urea and electrolytes, blood glucose, liver function and thyroid function tests, an MSU (midstream specimen of urine) and, possibly, a chest X-ray may be indicated for diagnosing any underlying acute illness contributing to the development of delirium. Other investigations may be considered on an individual case basis such as blood culture, arterial oxygen saturation, toxicology screening or more advanced tests such as EEG (electroencephalogram) or CT (computerised tomography) and MRI (magnetic resonance imaging) scanning.

14.7   Management of a Patient with Delirium

The diagnosis and management of delirium remains challenging, because it usually presents with other complex multi-morbidity; hence, it is often being treated as a symptom rather than a syndrome and is therefore not addressed as a condition in its own therapeutic right. What is clear though is that delirium has a highly predictable occurrence and hence should be amenable to primary prevention. 'Delirium readiness' has been described, where the interaction of a range of predisposing factors with acute precipitants results in the emergence of delirium [33]. Innouye and Charpentier [34] identified a set of predisposing and precipitating factors such as male, age >65, baseline cognition, hearing and visual impairment, polypharmacy, any coexisting medical or surgical conditions, pain, constipation, frailty and sleep deprivation as predisposing on the one hand and the use of restraints, bladder catheterization, malnutrition, addition of a new drug the previous day and any major iatrogenic event as the precipitating factors on the other hand which together increase the risk of developing delirium substantially.

The combination of all these factors predicted a 17-fold increase in the relative risk of older medical inpatients developing delirium. Subsequent work has validated this model in older patients undergoing hip surgery [35].

The NICE guideline [2] describes a range of recommendations to prevent delirium, suggesting that a patient with delirium needs to be cared by a multidisciplinary team and that team members should be trained and competent in delirium prevention and management.

Interventions to prevent symptoms such as dehydration and constipation, to manage pain, or current illness (e.g. infections) and to review polypharmacy are important strategies in prevention. NICE also highlights the importance of sensory impairment and poor sleep pattern as factors which could also increase the risk of developing acute delirium [2].

14.8 Delirium in Care Homes

Delirium is common in elderly, frail residents in care home settings, who may already be suffering from dementia, along with other precipitating factors, such as infections, medication interactions, polypharmacy and environmental changes [36].

There is a great number of preceding symptoms that could be observed by the care home staff over days and weeks leading up to the development of more obvious clinical symptoms of delirium such as those comprising the "clouding of consciousness" entity [37]. Apart from being obviously confused, residents can become quiet and sleepy, or agitated and disorientated. Delirium increases the risk of admission in hospitals, falls, development or worsening of dementia and eventually death [38]. Care home staff are in a unique position of identifying subtle changes that often precede a full-blown episode of delirium; however, due to factors such as high staff turnover, or poor training and inexperience, lead to, poor identification and recognition of important prodrome signs and symptoms of delirium [39].

Delirium contributes to increased healthcare costs when admission to hospital occurs: preventing these admissions is thus a focus for policy-makers and commissioners.

Hospital admission could be prevented by adopting simple strategies by care home staff, such as better lighting to improve orientation, avoiding unnecessary use of catheters and medications that potentially could increase delirium risk. Is worth highlighting the recent Cochrane review which assessed the role of two major interventions which included adequate hydration and review by a pharmacist to adjust or stop medications that could potentially increase the risk of delirium [36].

The results of a recent project (at the time of writing this chapter) called "Stop Delirium" [39], were promising. This is a feasibility study to develop and evaluate a complex intervention, aimed at delirium prevention and management in care homes. The aim was to develop an enhanced educational package to improve delirium care for older people. The package had interactive teaching for staff, encouraging them to take ownership of the project with individuals to 'champion' the change and a 'delirium practitioner' working with staff.

14.9 "STOP DELIRIUM" Project

The study included a survey to explore staff's perception and experience of integrating delirium prevention and management activities into their daily care routine.

The main outcome of the project showed that the care home staff were more aware of the common triggers of delirium like infection, constipation, medication effects, dehydration, falls and moving to a noisy or new environment. Interestingly this project resulted in broadening care workers' répertoire in managing confusion and increasing their confidence in identifying early signs.

The *culture* of a care home also influences the quality of relationships between staff and residents [40]; thus, staff may perceive aggressive and unpredictable behaviours as indicating that the resident is deliberately not cooperating [41]. Interestingly this project resulted in broadening care workers' répertoire in managing confusion and increased their confidence in identifying early signs.

14.10 Management of Patients with Delirium in Primary Care

Most patients with delirium can be managed in primary care if the symptoms and signs are identified early enough. As most common causes of delirium are related to common infections, such as those of urinary and respiratory tract, localised or generalised pain due to degenerative causes like osteoarthritis or drug interactions. The primary care clinician needs to identify the cause of delirium, if possible at the 'prodromal', or early stage, with the help of carers if a patient is at home, or staff in residential homes.

In more severe cases, where the patients' behaviour poses a risk to either the patients themselves or their carers, they may then need to be removed from their usual surroundings to a safe place, which usually means hospital admission is required. Alternatively, if the primary care clinician has access to an *Intermediate Care* scheme, where a step-up in nursing care can be provided, in the patient's home, this may be a more appropriate option. It is important to bear in mind that confused, frail elderly patients are likely to get more confused in unfamiliar and new settings, hence admission to hospital should only be considered as the last resort, where more complex problems have developed and expert management is required or when patient safety is compromised.

Prevention of delirium by non-pharmacological intervention has a key role in the overall management of this syndrome. There is strong evidence to suggest incidence of delirium can be reduced, and its severity and duration can be controlled by implementing simple management interventions [42]. These include assisting orientation, enhancing efficacy, promoting sleep-wake cycle, pain relief and optimising physiological parameters (hydration, electrolyte balance) [42]. Delirium is a complex syndrome, hence rigid protocols and guidelines have limited impact, and an individualised approach is vital [43, 44].

Interventions targeting at reducing the incidence of delirium should also be focused on minimising polypharmacy, and preventing dopamine-acetylocholine imbalance. Regular reviews of patients' medications, and prescribing only the essential ones in the lowest minimum doses, should be the initial clinical intervention before any other pharmacological agent is to be considered to treat troublesome symptoms of delirium. Sudden withdrawal of certain medications, together with administration of deliriogenic drugs and benzodiazepines or anticholinergic agents, have been implicated in across population [45]. The anticholinergic side effects of many commonly prescribed medications are not acknowledged by a great proportion of clinicians [46]. However, it is well known that under-treatment of common pathological issues like pain is linked to an increased incidence of delirium [47].

Acetylcholine-dopamine imbalance or neurochemical theory exploring pharmacological prevention has focused upon agents that either diminish dopaminergic or enhance cholinergic functions [48–50]. The role of these medications in co-morbid dementia is unclear though, and prescription of these agents has been aiming to treat distressing symptoms or to provide sedation in the event of an uncontrolled and difficult to manage crisis.

Management of a patient with delirium also includes ensuring their personal safety, orienting them with clocks and ensuring the room is light in the daytime and dark at night. Pharmacological treatment may become necessary to treat behavioural and psychotic symptoms of delirium; haloperidol has been shown to be effective for the treatment of behavioural symptoms of delirium. The Cochrane database systemic review has shown low-dose haloperidol, less than 3 mg, being effective in reducing the degree and duration of behavioural symptoms of delirium in elderly post-operative patients [51]. Haloperidol is as effective as atypical antipsychotic medications, but causes more side effects in higher doses. NICE [2] also refers to the use of haloperidol or olanzapine; however, haloperidol can potentially cause life-threatening complications in patients suffering from Parkinson's disease or Lewy body dementia. Hence, it is best to be avoided, especially in the initial stages, as the symptoms of this condition may not be obvious during this time.

A study [48] reported the efficacy of various agents in reducing the behavioral symptoms of delirium. Risperidone and olanzapine at doses of 0.5–4 mg and 2.5–11 mg showed effectiveness of 80–85 % and 70–75 % respectively; however, based on the author's (RN) experience as an old-age specialist psychiatrist, lower doses than the ones mentioned above may be sufficient. Thus, most patients will respond up to 2 mg of risperidone or 7.5 mg of olanzapine, without experiencing any major adverse effects. It is important to note that most atypical antipsychotic medications lose their pharmacological benefits at higher doses. It is worth mentioning that there are currently no high-quality double-blind trials available for this population of patients with these behaviour symptoms of delirium. The CSM [31, 32] issued a warning; highlighting an increased risk of cerebrovascular events in the patients suffering with delirium, with background dementia, who were treated with risperidone or olanzapine. Interestingly it was also found that the majority of antipsychotics have a potential to increase that risk. Benzodiazepines are usually considered when delirium is associated with withdrawal from alcohol, and where sedation is required, such as in cases of Lewy body dementia (DLB). Short-acting lorazepam is usually the preferred choice as it has a rapid onset, shorter duration of action and sedative properties. In suspected cases of DLB, rivastigmine has been found to be more effective than placebo [50]. It is important that these medications are reviewed regularly by the prescriber and should be discontinued after one week of continuous treatment if delirium has resolved.

14.11 Case

Mrs. A is an 86-year-old widow who has been a resident of a care home for the past 6 months. She had a history of diabetes, myocardial infarction, osteoarthritis and treated hypertension. There was no prior history of involvement with psychiatric services. She was placed in the residential home as she was struggling to look after herself after the death of her husband one year ago. Her GP had treated her for depression with antidepressants for a few months, but then she had suffered a number of falls and felt to be unsafe living alone.

The care home manager was informed by the staff that Mrs. A was increasingly confused with paranoid ideas – telling her family that the staff were poisoning her food and had been stealing her clothes. The manager called the GP who visited and talked to both Mrs. A, and the staff on duty. Mrs. A told the GP that she could see a man in her room at nights, and that frightened her. The GP examined Mrs. A and asked for an MSU (midstream specimen of urine) to be sent for microscopy and cultures, after the staff reported that Mrs A's urine had an offensive smell.

The GP suggested that Mrs. A might have had a urine infection and prescribed empirically a course of trimethoprim, and also suggested that the antihypertensive agent (ramipril) should be reduced as her blood pressure was as low as 100/60. Blood sample for basic laboratory investigations was obtained (FBC, U&Es, BS and HbA1C), and arranged to see Mrs. A in a couple of days, but Mrs. A had been unwell overnight and the staff contacted the general practice and reported that the patient had been shouting all night and was trying to take the bedclothes off, as there were 'ants on the bed'. She seemed frightened by something, and the staff reported that they were not able to manage her.

The GP visited the care home again and found Mrs. A in a very agitated state, crying and talking about 'the man in the corner'. The doctor telephoned Mrs. A's daughter who reported that her mother had been forgetful prior to her admission to the care home, and she was worried that Mrs A. had not been eating enough as she had seemed to have forgotten how to cook. The GP suggested that they should try to manage Mrs. A in the care home and gave advice about how to support and monitor her, and prescribed risperidone (0.5 mg to use at night). A few days later the MSU result confirmed a urinary tract infection, sensitive to trimethoprim. The following week, the GP contacted the care home to review Mrs. A's progress, and the manager reported that no risperidone had been given for the previous three nights. However, although Mrs. A was found to be less confused and agitated, the manager said she was very forgetful and asked if she could be referred for an old age psychiatry assessment. A domiciliary visit was arranged and the psychiatrist elicited collateral information from her daughter, which suggested memory problems for previous 2 years. Mrs. A scored 66/100 on a cognitive test (ACE 3). The psychiatrist suggested then that a CT scan was needed to identify cerebrovascular disease and to exclude a subdural haematoma or any space-occupying lesion, and the relevant referral was made.

The psychiatrist gave advice to the staff about how to manage future episodes of delirium and confusion, and asked the GP to re-prescribe risperidone for use on a

"PRN" basis until the results of the CT scan became available. The psychiatrist indicated that the community psychiatric nurse from the local old-age community mental health team should visit and support Mrs. A and the care home staff.

14.12 Suggested Activities

14.12.1 Reflections

Consider the case of Mrs. A and what your role would have been in her management. Would you do anything differently?

What is the role and the risks of prescribing antipsychotic medications in older people?

What services are available in your area to support older people to remain in their own home/residential home?

14.12.2 Audit: Prevention of Delirium

Aim and Objectives
To set up strategies to prevent new cases of delirium
   Primary outcome would be to investigate whether these strategies could improve the incidence of delirium and aiming at cultivating awareness and to increase the confidence of the staff involved in recognizing the early signs of delirium.

Background
Delirium in elderly in care homes is common but preventable. This proposed audit is to explore a review strategy setting up in care homes with the help of a local pharmacist, also regular dipstick, pain and bowel movement review and eliciting any change in the behaviour of the residents. There is extensive bibliographic evidence available to support these strategies are effective in reducing the incidence of delirium.

Method
This would be a prospective audit with data collection spanning over an 8-week period. The standards are medication review, urine dipstick, pain, bowel movement monitoring and exploration of change in the resident's behaviour. The standards should be set at 100 % as all residents would have these monitored.

Data Collection
- Proforma:
    - Initials
    - Age
    - Sex
    - Known diagnosis
    - Current meds
    - Physical status

- Week 1–8
  - Medications review
  - Urine dipstick
  - Pain chart
  - Bowel movement
  - Observation of behaviour

Conclusions

Delirium is a serious public health problem with a high incidence and prevalence across all care settings. Age and cognitive impairment are the major predisposing factors of delirium, and infections, vascular, metabolic, drugs and anoxia are common precipitants. Delirium carries a serious risk of mortality, much greater than dementia. Despite this, delirium is frequently under-recognised and under-treated.

Delirium is common in care home settings and potentially preventable with the right strategies; this may not happen routinely due to lack of knowledge and inadequate training of the health care professionals. An organisational approach is essential to prevent this condition developing, with education of everyone delivering care as an essential component.

Key Points

Delirium is common and highly prevalent in hospitals and care homes, but is also seen in primary care.

Due to its complex aetiology and presentation, is often under-recognised and under-treated.

Early identification and prevention is crucial in improving patients' outcome.

The mainstay of treatment of delirium is to identify and manage effectively the underlying cause.

The management of a patient with delirium should adopt a holistic multi-disciplinary approach.

References

1. Pitt RBB. Seminars in old age psychiatry. London: RCPsych Publications; 1998.
2. NICE guideline. Delirium: diagnosis, prevention and management. NICE clinical guideline 103. Available at www.nice.org.uk/CG103. 2010.
3. Lishman WA. Organic psychiatry: the psychological consequences of cerebral disorder. 3rd ed. Oxford: Blackwell Science; 1997. 922 p.
4. Levkoff SE, Evans DA, Liptzin B, Cleary PD, Lipsitz LA, Wetle TT, et al. Delirium. The occurrence and persistence of symptoms among elderly hospitalized patients. Arch Intern Med. 1992;152(2):334–40.
5. O'Keeffe ST, Ni Chonchubhair A. Postoperative delirium in the elderly. Br J Anaesth. 1994;73(5):673–87.
6. Barclay L. Delirium predicts mortality for ICU patients on ventilators. JAMA. 2004;291:1753–62.

7. Folstein MF, Bassett SS, Romanoski AJ, Nestadt G. The epidemiology of delirium in the community: the Eastern Baltimore Mental Health Survey. Int Psychogeriatr/IPA. 1991;3(2):169–76.
8. George J, Bleasdale S, Singleton SJ. Causes and prognosis of delirium in elderly patients admitted to a district general hospital. Age Ageing. 1997;26(6):423–7.
9. Inouye SK, Rushing JT, Foreman MD, Palmer RM, Pompei P. Does delirium contribute to poor hospital outcomes? A three-site epidemiologic study. J Gen Intern Med. 1998;13(4):234–42.
10. McCusker J, Cole M, Abrahamowicz M, Primeau F, Belzile E. Delirium predicts 12-month mortality. Arch Intern Med. 2002;162(4):457–63.
11. Gonzalez M, Martinez G, Calderon J, Villarroel L, Yuri F, Rojas C, et al. Impact of delirium on short-term mortality in elderly inpatients: a prospective cohort study. Psychosomatics. 2009;50(3):234–8.
12. Neufeld KJ, Thomas C. Delirium: definition, epidemiology, and diagnosis. J Clin Neurophysiol: Off Publ Am Electroencephalogr Soc. 2013;30(5):438–42.
13. Han JH, Zimmerman EE, Cutler N, Schnelle J, Morandi A, Dittus RS, et al. Delirium in older emergency department patients: recognition, risk factors, and psychomotor subtypes. Acad Emerg Med: Off J Soc Acad Emerg Med. 2009;16(3):193–200.
14. Meagher DJ, Leonard M, Donnelly S, Conroy M, Adamis D, Trzepacz PT. A longitudinal study of motor subtypes in delirium: relationship with other phenomenology, etiology, medication exposure and prognosis. J Psychosom Res. 2011;71(6):395–403.
15. Bachman D, Rabins P. "Sundowning" and other temporally associated agitation states in dementia patients. Annu Rev Med. 2006;57:499–511.
16. Murray C, Sanderson DJ, Barkus C, Deacon RM, Rawlins JN, Bannerman DM, et al. Systemic inflammation induces acute working memory deficits in the primed brain: relevance for delirium. Neurobiol Aging. 2012;33(3):603–16. e3.
17. Thomas C, Hestermann U, Kopitz J, Plaschke K, Oster P, Driessen M, et al. Serum anticholinergic activity and cerebral cholinergic dysfunction: an EEG study in frail elderly with and without delirium. BMC Neurosci. 2008;9:86.
18. Inouye SK, Foreman MD, Mion LC, Katz KH, Cooney Jr LM. Nurses' recognition of delirium and its symptoms: comparison of nurse and researcher ratings. Arch Intern Med. 2001;161(20):2467–73.
19. Siddiqi N, House AO, Holmes JD. Occurrence and outcome of delirium in medical in-patients: a systematic literature review. Age Ageing. 2006;35(4):350–64.
20. Kakuma R, du Fort GG, Arsenault L, Perrault A, Platt RW, Monette J, et al. Delirium in older emergency department patients discharged home: effect on survival. J Am Geriatr Soc. 2003;51(4):443–50.
21. Hakim SM, Othman AI, Naoum DO. Early treatment with risperidone for subsyndromal delirium after on-pump cardiac surgery in the elderly: a randomized trial. Anesthesiology. 2012;116(5):987–97.
22. van Eijk MM, Roes KC, Honing ML, Kuiper MA, Karakus A, van der Jagt M, et al. Effect of rivastigmine as an adjunct to usual care with haloperidol on duration of delirium and mortality in critically ill patients: a multicentre, double-blind, placebo-controlled randomised trial. Lancet. 2010;376(9755):1829–37.
23. Kaneko T, Takahashi S, Naka T, Hirooka Y, Inoue Y, Kaibara N. Postoperative delirium following gastrointestinal surgery in elderly patients. Surg Today. 1997;27(2):107–11.
24. de Jonghe JF, Kalisvaart KJ, Dijkstra M, van Dis H, Vreeswijk R, Kat MG, et al. Early symptoms in the prodromal phase of delirium: a prospective cohort study in elderly patients undergoing hip surgery. Am J Geriatr Psychiatry: Off J Am Assoc Geriatr Psychiatry. 2007;15(2):112–21.
25. Fann JR, Alfano CM, Burington BE, Roth-Roemer S, Katon WJ, Syrjala KL. Clinical presentation of delirium in patients undergoing hematopoietic stem cell transplantation. Cancer. 2005;103(4):810–20.

26. Duppils GS, Wikblad K. Delirium: behavioural changes before and during the prodromal phase. J Clin Nurs. 2004;13(5):609–16.
27. Hall RJ, Meagher DJ, MacLullich AM. Delirium detection and monitoring outside the ICU. Best Pract Res Clin Anaesthesiol. 2012;26(3):367–83.
28. Inouye SK, van Dyck CH, Alessi CA, Balkin S, Siegal AP, Horwitz RI. Clarifying confusion: the confusion assessment method. A new method for detection of delirium. Ann Intern Med. 1990;113(12):941–8.
29. Gaudreau JD, Gagnon P, Harel F, Tremblay A, Roy MA. Fast, systematic, and continuous delirium assessment in hospitalized patients: the nursing delirium screening scale. J Pain Symptom Manage. 2005;29(4):368–75.
30. Schuurmans MJ, Shortridge-Baggett LM, Duursma SA. The delirium observation screening scale: a screening instrument for delirium. Res Theory Nurs Pract. 2003;17(1):31–50.
31. Hart RP, Levenson JL, Sessler CN, Best AM, Schwartz SM, Rutherford LE. Validation of a cognitive test for delirium in medical ICU patients. Psychosomatics. 1996;37(6):533–46.
32. Trzepacz PT, Baker RW, Greenhouse J. A symptom rating scale for delirium. Psychiatry Res. 1988;23(1):89–97.
33. Henry WD, Mann AM. Diagnosis and treatment of delirium. Can Med Assoc J. 1965;93(22):1156–66.
34. Inouye SK, Charpentier PA. Precipitating factors for delirium in hospitalized elderly persons. Predictive model and interrelationship with baseline vulnerability. JAMA. 1996;275(11):852–7.
35. Kalisvaart KJ, Vreeswijk R, de Jonghe JF, van der Ploeg T, van Gool WA, Eikelenboom P. Risk factors and prediction of postoperative delirium in elderly hip-surgery patients: implementation and validation of a medical risk factor model. J Am Geriatr Soc. 2006;54(5):817–22.
36. Clegg A, Siddiqi N, Heaven A, Young J, Holt R. Interventions for preventing delirium in older people in institutional long-term care. Cochrane Database Syst Rev. 2014;(1):CD009537.
37. Peacock R, Hopton A, Featherstone I, Edwards J. Care home staff can detect the difference between delirium, dementia and depression. Nurs Older People. 2012;24(1):26–30.
38. Fick DM, Agostini JV, Inouye SK. Delirium superimposed on dementia: a systematic review. J Am Geriatr Soc. 2002;50(10):1723–32.
39. Siddiqi N, Young J, House AO, Featherstone I, Hopton A, Martin C, et al. Stop delirium! A complex intervention to prevent delirium in care homes: a mixed-methods feasibility study. Age Ageing. 2011;40(1):90–8.
40. Cook G, Brown-Wilson C. Care home residents' experiences of social relationships with staff. Nurs Older People. 2010;22(1):24–9.
41. Brodaty H, Draper B, Low LF. Nursing home staff attitudes towards residents with dementia: strain and satisfaction with work. J Adv Nurs. 2003;44(6):583–90.
42. Marcantonio ER, Flacker JM, Wright RJ, Resnick NM. Reducing delirium after hip fracture: a randomized trial. J Am Geriatr Soc. 2001;49(5):516–22.
43. Young LJ, George J. Do guidelines improve the process and outcomes of care in delirium? Age Ageing. 2003;32:525–8.
44. Gagnon P, Allard P, Gagnon B, Merette C, Tardif F. Delirium prevention in terminal cancer: assessment of a multicomponent intervention. Psychooncology. 2012;21(2):187–94.
45. Clegg A, Young JB. Which medications to avoid in people at risk of delirium: a systematic review. Age Ageing. 2011;40(1):23–9.
46. Campbell N, Boustani M, Limbil T, Ott C, Fox C, Maidment I, et al. The cognitive impact of anticholinergics: a clinical review. Clin Interv Aging. 2009;4:225–33.
47. Morrison RS, Magaziner J, Gilbert M, Koval KJ, McLaughlin MA, Orosz G, et al. Relationship between pain and opioid analgesics on the development of delirium following hip fracture. J Gerontol Ser A Biol Med Sci. 2003;58(1):76–81.
48. Larsen KA, Kelly SE, Stern TA, Bode Jr RH, Price LL, Hunter DJ, et al. Administration of olanzapine to prevent postoperative delirium in elderly joint-replacement patients: a randomized, controlled trial. Psychosomatics. 2010;51(5):409–18.

49. Prakanrattana U, Prapaitrakool S. Efficacy of risperidone for prevention of postoperative delirium in cardiac surgery. Anaesth Intensive Care. 2007;35(5):714–9.
50. Wang W, Li HL, Wang DX, Zhu X, Li SL, Yao GQ, et al. Haloperidol prophylaxis decreases delirium incidence in elderly patients after noncardiac surgery: a randomized controlled trial*. Crit Care Med. 2012;40(3):731–9.
51. Mac Sweeney R, Barber V, Page V, Ely EW, Perkins GD, Young JD, et al. A national survey of the management of delirium in UK intensive care units. QJM. 2010;103(4):243–51.
52. Butler R, Pitt B. Seminars in old age psychiatry. London: Gaskell; 1998.

Part IV
Psychosis

Psychosis in the Elderly

15

Salman Karim and Kimberley Harrison

15.1 Introduction

Psychosis is a particularly distressing psychiatric illness for sufferers and their carers, and it can feel especially difficult for practitioners dealing with its uncertain course whilst trying to instil hope. Although assessing and managing a patient with psychosis in primary care can be daunting, the majority of patients should also receive input from mental health services. Psychotic symptoms are found in a wide range of medical and psychiatric conditions. Patients with psychosis in later life can be divided into three groups: those with pre-existing schizophrenia, new diagnoses of schizophrenia ('late-life schizophrenia', also known as 'late paraphrenia') and other conditions producing hallucinations or delusions (dementia, delirium, mood disorders, delusional disorder, paranoid personality disorders). As the population ages and treatments improve, the first group is getting significantly larger and making up a greater proportion of mental illness in older people. The prevalence of all psychotic disorders over 65 years of age is 4–6 %, rising to 10 % over 85 years. However, a large proportion of these cases are related to dementia. True schizophrenia or delusional disorder in the over-65s has a prevalence of 0.5–1.0 %. There is a female preponderance, with a ratio of female to males of 5:1, which is partly because the onset of schizophrenia tends to be later in females. Sixty per cent of older people

S. Karim, MBBS, MSc, MD, FCPS
Central Lancashire Memory Assessment Service, Lancashire Care NHS Trust,
Preston, Lancashire, UK
e-mail: salman.karim@manchester.ac.uk

K. Harrison, MBBS, BSc, MRCPsych (✉)
ST6 in Old Age Psychiatry, Woodlands Hospital,
Greater Manchester West Mental Health Foundation Trust, Meadowsweet Lane,
Little Hulton, Manchester M28 0FE, UK
e-mail: kwoodhouse@doctors.org.uk; kimberleyharrison1@nhs.net

© Springer International Publishing Switzerland 2016
C.A. Chew-Graham, M. Ray (eds.), *Mental Health and Older People:
A Guide for Primary Care Practitioners*, DOI 10.1007/978-3-319-29492-6_15

with psychosis have paranoid schizophrenia, 30 % delusional disorder and only 10 % all other forms of psychosis [1].

15.2 Symptoms and Classification

Psychosis is best conceptualised as a syndrome with delusions and hallucinations as its core features [2] (Table 15.1). A delusion is a fixed, false belief that is out of keeping with one's social, religious and cultural background. Hallucinations are perceptions in the absence of stimuli and can occur in any of the sensory modalities. An illusion is a distortion or misinterpretation of a stimulus and is not considered to be a psychotic phenomenon. A psychotic patient will often experience more than just the core symptoms of psychosis.

Auditory hallucinations can be classified further into second or third person, command, running commentary and by the nature of the content, for example, derogatory or complimentary. Other symptoms associated with psychosis include *thought interference,* i.e. thought echo, insertion, withdrawal and broadcast, and *thought disorder* where breaks in the train of thought lead to illogical speech content. Although these symptoms are included in the diagnostic criteria for schizophrenia, they are not pathognomonic for the condition. There are no pathognomonic symptoms of schizophrenia but characteristic distortions of thinking and perception and inappropriate or blunted affect are considered to be core features [3].

Psychiatrists refer to 'positive' and 'negative' psychotic symptoms especially in relation to schizophrenia. 'Positive' symptoms refer to the core psychotic features, i.e. delusions and hallucinations, whereas negative symptoms are marked apathy, social withdrawal and blunting of affect [3].

A decline in social and occupational functioning often reflects the severity. The onset of psychosis can occur in younger adult life with the sufferer 'graduating' into old age with their psychotic illness or symptoms can present for the first time in old age.

15.2.1 Functional and Organic Psychoses

Broadly speaking psychosis can be divided into functional and organic. The term 'organic' indicates a detectable physiological or structural change, resulting in a

Table 15.1 Symptoms of psychosis

Core symptoms	Delusions, hallucinations
Behavioural changes	Apathy, aimlessness, self-absorbed attitude
Mood symptoms	Depression, anxiety
Vegetative changes	Energy, sleep, appetite
Motor changes	Excitement, posturing, stupor
Cognitive symptoms	Planning, reasoning, problem solving, working memory

disturbance of normal functioning, and is commonly due to delirium (psychiatric manifestation of an underlying medical condition characterised by changes in consciousness and cognition) and neurodegenerative disorders, for example, dementia and Parkinson's disease. Other examples are during the use of, and following withdrawal from, alcohol and psychoactive substances and from brain damage [3]. A predominance of olfactory, tactile, gustatory and visual hallucinations point towards an 'organic' cause for the psychosis. The word 'functional' applies to conditions where there is no identifiable physiological or anatomical change to explain the symptoms, and from a psychiatric perspective, this includes psychotic, affective and neurotic disorders. When psychotic symptoms are present in nonpsychotic disorders, for example, depression, it often reflects the severity of the underlying primary condition.

15.2.2 Primary Psychotic Disorders

The term 'primary psychotic disorder' refers to a heterogeneous group of 'functional' disorders. In the World Health Organization's International Statistical Classification of Diseases and Related Health Problems (ICD-10), which are the main psychiatric diagnostic guidelines in the UK, schizophrenia, schizotypal disorder, schizoaffective disorder, persistent delusional disorders, induced delusional disorders, acute and transient psychotic episodes and 'other non-organic psychotic disorders' are considered to be primary psychotic disorders. The term 'other non-organic psychotic disorders' is assigned to psychotic symptoms that don't meet the criteria for the mentioned psychotic disorders or any other psychiatric disorder.

Schizophrenia is further classified as either paranoid (which is the commonest type), hebephrenic, catatonic, residual, undifferentiated or simple schizophrenia. 'Schizotypal disorder' is grouped with schizophrenia due to a probable genetic link and the similarities in anomalies of thinking, odd behaviour and affect [3]. In schizoaffective disorder, both affective (mood) and schizophrenic symptoms are prominent in the same episode. There are essentially two types: manic and depressive [3].

Persistent delusional disorders are characterised by long-standing delusions which cannot be explained by schizophrenia, an affective disorder or an organic process. Delusions must be present for at least 3 months. Induced delusional disorder is a rare condition whereby two or more people with close emotional links share the same delusion [3].

'Acute and transient psychotic disorders' include acute polymorphic (highly variable) psychosis with or without symptoms of schizophrenia, acute schizophrenia-like psychosis and an acute predominantly delusional psychosis [3].

15.2.3 Late-Onset Schizophrenia

Historically late-onset psychoses have sat uncomfortably in their relation to schizophrenia due to the existence of both significant similarities and differences and perhaps a tendency to attribute late-onset psychoses to organic causes. Interestingly, neither ICD-10 or the American Psychiatric Association's fifth edition of the Diagnostic and Statistical Manual of Mental Disorders (DSM-V) contain 'codeable' separate diagnoses for late-onset schizophrenia which means that the diagnosis is made by meeting the diagnostic criteria for schizophrenia irrespective of age. Although the first onset of schizophrenia, for the majority of suffers, occurs in late adolescence and early adult life, there is a small, but nonetheless significant, proportion of people who have their first onset of schizophrenia in middle or old age [4]. Meesters et al. revealed the 1-year prevalence of early-onset, late-onset and very late-onset schizophrenias to be 0.35 %, 0.14 % and 0.05 %, respectively [5].

Due to this debate, there was an international consensus in 1998 which closely examined existing research, and it was agreed that the word schizophrenia should be used for both early- and late-onset cases. Late-onset schizophrenia was divided further into late and very late onset representing onset after the age of 40 and 60 years, respectively [4].

15.2.4 Similarities and Differences Between Early- and Late-Onset Schizophrenias

The similarities between early- and late-onset schizophrenias include genetic risk, the presence and severity of positive symptoms, early psychosocial maladjustments and subtle brain abnormalities revealed by imaging. Late-onset schizophrenia, as compared to the early-onset subtype, has fewer negative symptoms and suffers tend to perform better on neuropsychological testing and respond better to antipsychotic medication [6, 7].

15.2.5 Risk Factors for Psychosis in Older People

Risk factors for psychosis in older people include frontal and temporal cortical degeneration, neurochemical changes associated with ageing, social isolation, sensory deficits, cognitive decline, pharmacokinetic and pharmacodynamic changes associated with age and polypharmacy [6, 8, 9].

15.3 Assessment of the Patient

Psychotic symptoms should be routinely and specifically enquired about because they won't necessarily be reported. Physical conditions can produce psychotic symptoms, for example, in delirium; therefore, one must undertake a thorough medical assessment which includes a collateral history from a carer or family member and a full physical examination to rule out and treat any underlying causative medical pathology. A thorough physical examination and full set of blood tests (to exclude metabolic causes for symptoms) are considered essential. This assessment

Table 15.2 Medications potentially causing psychotic symptoms

Antihistamine	Cimetidine
Anti-Parkinson drugs	Levodopa, amantadine, bromocriptine and procyclidine
Anti-arrhythmics	Digoxin, propranolol, quinidine, procainamide
Anti-inflammatory drugs	Aspirin, indomethacin
Anticonvulsants	Phenytoin, primidone, carbamazepine
Steroids	Prednisolone
Other drugs	Benzodiazepines and anticancer drugs

From Wood et al. [33] with permission

should be carried out in primary care, the Emergency Department (when a patient has presented acutely and been taken to the ED), on a medical ward, if the patient has been admitted, or by the old age psychiatrist.

A medication review is another important part of the investigation of psychotic symptoms as there are a number of medications that can cause psychotic symptoms (Table 15.2) during their use or withdrawal.

Whilst GPs and hospital doctors should be able to assess a patient, and identify symptoms suggestive of a psychosis, the diagnosis will usually be made by an old age psychiatrist.

15.4 Management of Psychosis in Older People

Following diagnosis of psychosis, the old age psychiatrist should negotiate a management plan with the patient, their carer (if appropriate), and communicate this to the primary care physician.

15.4.1 NICE Guideline

A guideline from the National Institute for Health and Care Excellence (NICE) [10] addresses the management and treatment of primary psychotic disorders in adults under the age of 60 years, but there are no similar published guidelines for the over 60 age group. There are however general principles which can be applied to the over 60 years age group.

The NICE guideline recommends working in partnership with the service user and their carer in an 'atmosphere of hope and optimism' [10]. There is a strong emphasis on the management of both mental and physical health, the role and needs of carers and the recovery model leading to optimal social functioning.

The NICE guideline (2014) recommends a prompt referral to mental health services if a distressed person, with an associated decline in social functioning, has transient or attenuated psychotic symptoms, other experiences or behaviour suggestive of possible psychosis or a first-degree relative with psychosis or schizophrenia. The guideline stipulates that the assessment should be carried out by a consultant psychiatrist or a trained specialist with experience in at-risk mental states [10].

Mental health services should now be offering carers, an assessment of their needs forming the basis of an annually reviewed care plan which should be received by their GPs. Carers should also be advised about their statutory rights to a formal carer's assessment from social care services and how to access it. With the service user's permission, carers are to be included in decision-making and be offered a 'carer-focused education and support programme' [10], which has a positive message about recovery.

Oral antipsychotic medication and psychological input, namely, family intervention and cognitive behavioural therapy, are the mainstays of treatment. Psychological interventions are not recommended on their own.

The management of psychosis in older people requires special consideration especially with respect to prescribing medication but also to the legal framework under which treatment is administered. It is not uncommon for treatment decisions to be made in a patient's best interests under the Mental Capacity Act 2007 when they lack capacity to consent for themselves, for example, when managing BPSD in dementia, or to use the Mental Health Act 2007 when assessment and treatment are necessary to manage risk to the patient or others.

15.4.2 Antipsychotic Medication

Antipsychotic drugs are amongst the most commonly prescribed psychotropic medications and are the mainstay of treatment for psychotic symptoms. Second-generation antipsychotics, also known as *atypicals*, are generally preferred over first-generation antipsychotics, also known as conventional and typical antipsychotics, and are considered first-line treatments internationally [11]. The most popular second-generation antipsychotics are risperidone, olanzapine, quetiapine, aripiprazole and clozapine. There are few well-conducted trials on antipsychotic use in the elderly with the most evidence existing for risperidone.

Antipsychotics should not be initiated in primary care, for a first presentation of psychosis, unless on the advice of a consultant psychiatrist.

Prescribing psychotropic medication in the elderly requires special consideration; one must take into account medical co-morbidities and polypharmacy and the altered pharmacodynamics and pharmacokinetics associated with ageing.

A prescriber not only needs to be mindful of drug interactions and the increasing frequency and severity of side effects [12], compared to a younger adult population, but also needs to bear in mind that older patients may be more susceptible to developing the more serious side effects of psychotropic medication, for example, stroke with antipsychotics [13] and agranulocytosis [14] and neutropenia with clozapine [15]. There is a slower rate of drug absorption, due to reduced gut motility and reduced gastric acid secretion, resulting in a somewhat delayed onset of action although the same amount of the drug is eventually absorbed [16].

Although liver size is reduced in the elderly, this is only significant in the presence of hepatic disease or significantly reduced hepatic blood flow, meaning there is no significant reduction in metabolic capacity associated with ageing per se which is fortuitous since the majority of drugs are metabolised by the liver [12]. The second-generation antipsychotic sulpiride and the mood stabiliser lithium are notable examples of drugs that do not undergo hepatic metabolism before renal secretion. As renal function decreases with age, one can assume that all elderly patients have at most two-thirds of normal renal function, with e-GFR (estimated glomerular filtration rate) being the best measure of renal function [17]. There is a greater loss in renal function associated with co-morbidities such as heart disease, diabetes and hypertension [12]. This age-related decline in renal function can lead to toxicity and side effects of drugs that are primarily excreted via the kidney.

Many drug interactions occur because some drugs inhibit or induce liver enzymes, meaning a drug can affect the metabolism of another drug indirectly. The appendices in the British National Formulary (the BNF) contain details on drug interactions.

It should be emphasised that drugs should only be prescribed when absolutely necessary. A common prescribing principle in old age psychiatry is 'start low and go slow' [18] but avoid the temptation to undertreat by prescribing a subtherapeutic dose; some drugs require the full adult dose in order to achieve the full therapeutic effect [12]. General principles, aimed at reducing drug-related risk in the elderly, include once daily administration, finding an alternative medication when a patient experiences side effects instead of treating the side effects with another medication and to 'avoid, if possible, drugs that block alpha 1 adrenoceptors, have anticholinergic side effects, are very sedative, have long half-lives or are potent inhibitors of hepatic metabolising enzymes [12].

A 'trial' of an antipsychotic is considered to be medication at the optimum dose for 4–6 weeks. Individualised treatment and care plans are promoted with decisions about antipsychotic medication informed by their side effect profiles [10].

Baseline investigations, before prescribing antipsychotics, include weight, waist circumference, pulse and blood pressure, fasting blood glucose, HbA1c, lipid profile and prolactin levels and assessment of any movement disorders. NICE now recommend the assessment of nutritional status, diet and level of physical activity. These parameters require regular monitoring. ECGs are indicated if specified by the summary of product characteristic (SPC), cardiovascular risk has been identified from the physical examination (e.g. hypertension), the patient has a history of cardiovascular disease or the service user is being admitted to a psychiatric unit [10].

Until at least the first 12 months, or until the patient has stabilised, whichever is longer, the responsibility for monitoring physical health lies primarily with the secondary care team. After this time, under shared care agreements, physical health monitoring can be transferred to primary care [10]. Physical health monitoring is a pertinent focus of clinical audit.

Side Effects of Medication (Table 15.3)

Generally speaking, first-generation (*typical*) antipsychotics are more likely to cause extrapyramidal side effects (EPSEs), anticholinergic effects and sedation at

Table 15.3 Common side effects of antipsychotics

Extrapyramidal	Acute dystonia, pseudoparkinsonism, akathesia, tardive dyskinesia
Anticholinergic	Urinary hesitancy, constipation, blurred vision, dry mouth, delirium
Gastrointestinal	Nausea, constipation, diarrhoea
Liver	Cholestatic jaundice, raised transaminases
Cardiovascular	QTc prolongation
Endocrine and metabolic	Weight gain, diabetes mellitus, hyperlipidaemia, hyperprolactinaemia, sexual problems
Other	Postural hypotension, sedation, hypersalivation, epilepsy, cerebrovascular events (TIAs, stroke)

Adapted from Karim and Byrne [6] with permission

higher doses. Second-generation antipsychotics (*atypical*) are more likely to cause metabolic side effects and cerebrovascular adverse events although at higher doses EPSEs and sedation do occur. However as a class, atypical antipsychotics should not be viewed as a homogenous group in terms of their ability to treat symptoms and their side effects [19]; therefore, the potential risks and benefits of a specific drug should be considered on an individual basis [20].

There is concern that atypical antipsychotics increase the risk of stroke compared to typical antipsychotics. In 2004, there was a Committee on Safety of Medicines (CSM) alert issued by the Medicines and Healthcare products Regulatory Agency (MHRA) [21] because manufacturer data showed an increased risk of cerebrovascular adverse events (transient ischaemia attacks, strokes) with risperidone and olanzapine. The CSM data suggested a threefold risk. Those at the highest risk seem to be people over the age of 80 years and presumably those with vascular risk factors although this is not yet proven. Mental healthcare providers are now recommended to offer 'a combined healthy eating and physical activity programme' [10] for people with psychosis especially those taking antipsychotics. Smokers should be offered help to stop smoking irrespective of previous failed attempts but be mindful of the impact of reducing or stopping smoking on olanzapine and clozapine levels. This is due to the hydrocarbons in cigarette smoke, not the nicotine, and a reduction in smoking can lead to an increase in the plasma levels of these drugs.

Interestingly, a 2004 American retrospective population-based cohort study of patients over 66 years old taking either risperidone or olanzapine concluded that olanzapine and risperidone were not associated with a statistically significant increase of stroke compared to typical antipsychotics [22].

15.4.3 Behavioural and Psychological Symptoms in Dementia (BPSD)

BPSD is a descriptive concept, not a diagnostic entity, encompassing a mixed group of noncognitive symptoms and behaviours, which includes psychotic symptoms, when they occur in the context of a dementia syndrome [23]. BPSD is a clear indication for referral to mental health services, and it forms a significant part of the workload of old age psychiatry teams, yet it is a somewhat neglected area of research [24]. It is estimated that about two-thirds of dementia sufferers experience BPSD at any given time [24], and this figure rises to over two-thirds for dementia patients living in care homes [25]. Early identification leads to a better quality of life for suffers and their families: BPSD is a major risk factor for carer burden [26] and institutionalisation [27] and can also result in neglect and even elder abuse [28].

BPSD is likely to be a complex interplay between mental illness, physical illness, medication and the environment; therefore, environmental manipulation and behavioural treatments should be first-line management options especially in milder cases. This is an important but somewhat neglected area of research which is surprising given the controversy surrounding antipsychotic prescribing in dementia.

Despite being used for decades, antipsychotic use in the management of BPSD is a contentious issue and the subject of enduring debate due to their adverse effects and lack of properly conducted studies. Currently, risperidone is the only licensed antipsychotic in the UK for BPSD [12] although there is evidence to support the efficacy of other atypical antipsychotics: olanzapine, risperidone, quetiapine, aripiprazole and amisulpride [12]. There is some evidence to suggest that the cholinesterase inhibitors donepezil, galantamine and rivastigmine, which are ordinarily used as cognitive enhancers in Alzheimer's dementia, can also ameliorate psychotic symptoms in the disease [29, 30]. The Royal College of Psychiatrists advocates the '3T' approach; target, titration and time, i.e. drug treatments have a specific symptom target, the starting dose should be low and titrated upwards, and they should be time limited. Although more research is needed to establish the natural course of BPSD, a 2004 study [31] suggests that withdrawal from treatment after a 3-month symptom-free period can be successful.

Both the National Institute for Health and Care Excellence (NICE) and Royal College of Psychiatrists have issued guidance on BPSD. Arguably, old age psychiatrists view the NICE guidelines as too restrictive for their purposes with too great an emphasis on the associated risks and unrealistic expectations of resources, and the Royal College guidelines are perceived as more useful. A survey completed by 31 % of career old age psychiatrists indicated that the average number of their patient's prescribed antipsychotics was 40 % with a range of 5–90 %. The most common reason for prescribing was psychosis at 93.3 %. The most commonly prescribed antipsychotic by far was quetiapine, and the first-generation antipsychotic haloperidol was the second most popular choice [32].

15.4.4 Subsequent Acute Episodes of Psychosis and Referral in Crisis

Crisis resolution and home treatment teams (CRHTT) should now be the single point of access to *acute* community and inpatient mental health services. It is also the first-line service to support people who are too unwell (severity of symptoms and high risk to self and/or others) to be managed by other community mental health teams and should always be considered as an alternative to inpatient admission. They also play a key role in early discharge from hospital. Again, oral antipsychotic medication and psychological interventions are the mainstay of treatment for acute exacerbations or recurrent symptoms [10].

Service users should be told there is a high risk of relapse if medication is stopped in the first 1–2 years. Monitoring for signs of relapse is necessary at least 2 years following the withdrawal of antipsychotic medication [10].

15.4.5 Psychological and Psychosocial Interventions

According to the 2014 NICE guideline, CBT and family interventions can be started in the acute phase, including inpatient settings, or later. Consider offering art therapies to people with psychosis or schizophrenia, and again this can be started during the acute phase of the illness or later. Group art therapies, which promote creative expression, should be provided by a Health and Care Professions Council registered art therapist. Therapies commenced during an inpatient admission should continue after discharge. Supportive psychotherapy and counselling should not be routinely offered as specific interventions, but service user preference should be taken into account especially if more efficacious therapies (CBT, family interventions and art therapies) are not available locally. Similarly, it is not recommended to offer adherence therapy or social skills training. Family therapy is particularly useful following a recent relapse or for someone who is at risk of relapse and also for persistent symptoms [10].

15.4.6 Return to Primary Care

The current recommendations for mental health services are to 'offer people with psychosis or schizophrenia whose symptoms have responded effectively to treatment and remain stable the option to return to primary care for further management' [10]. Physical health monitoring becomes the responsibility of primary care following the transfer of such responsibility and requires annual review with the recommendation that the care coordinator and psychiatrist receive a copy of these results.

15.4.7 Relapse and Re-referral to Secondary Care

When a patient with an established diagnosis is showing signs of relapse, one should refer to the 'crisis' section of the care plan. Referral should also be considered if the patient has poor response to treatment, non-compliance to medication, intolerable side effects, substance misuse or risk to self or others. Depot antipsychotics (long-acting injectable preparations) can be offered for patient preference and to aid compliance. Clozapine is offered for treatment resistant schizophrenia, i.e. following an inadequate response to at least two sequential trials of different antipsychotic drugs of which at least one should be an atypical antipsychotic [10].

15.5 Case Study

Mrs Barbara Taylor is an 85-year-old widow who lives alone in a semi-detached property. She has no children, but she receives visits from her great-niece every 2 months. Mrs Taylor had begun repeatedly accusing her neighbour of trying to poison her cat by leaving contaminated cat food in her garden and of 'piping gas' into the house when she was sleeping. She had grabbed her neighbour by his shirt threatening to get her own back on him. She could also hear her neighbours making negative comments about her at night time, and sometimes she heard a running commentary of her actions which was impacting on her sleep. Her neighbour, who was becoming increasingly intolerant, spoke to her niece who took Mrs Taylor to her GP. She was referred urgently to mental health services following an 'organic screen' which included a physical examination, medication review, a full set of bloods (FBC, U&Es, LFTs, TFTs, CRP, B12, folate, glucose, bone profile, lipids) and a urine microscopy, culture and sensitivity.

Mrs Taylor received a course of antidepressants 30 years ago following the death of her husband, but there was no other psychiatric history including no history of deliberate self-harm. She also had no history of harm to others or a forensic history. There was no family history of mental illness that she could recall.

Mrs Taylor wears hearing aids and takes bisoprolol for essential hypertension and simvastatin for hypercholesterolemia, and occasionally she takes co-codamol 8/500 mg tablets for arthritis.

Mrs Taylor does not have any history of ischaemic heart disease or cerebrovascular disease. She has never had any brain imaging.

Mental state examination revealed a pleasant lady who was easy to engage. She was appropriately dressed and kempt. Her speech was fluent, spontaneous, coherent and relevant, and she was able to give a good account of herself. Her mood was euthymic with a reactive and congruent affect. She exhibited persecutory delusions about her neighbour poisoning her and her dog, but there was no formal thought disorder or thoughts plans or intent to harm herself or others. There was also no thought interference. There were no auditory hallucinations during the assessment; however, she described derogatory third-person auditory hallucinations which were sometimes running commentary in nature, but there were no perceptual disturbances in the other sensory modalities. Her insight was impaired, but she agreed to take antipsychotic medication as it might help with her sleep.

A baseline ECG was taken (her QTc interval was within normal range), and she was started on olanzapine, as an outpatient, with her consent following a discussion about side effects. She responded well to the olanzapine and received occupational therapy input which enabled her to attend a day centre twice a week. Unfortunately, she developed impaired glucose tolerance (polydipsia, polyuria, fatigue) and she was changed to aripiprazole with continued improvement.

Mrs Taylor received a diagnosis of very late-onset schizophrenia. Characteristic features of very late-onset schizophrenia, as compared to the early- and late-onset varieties, includes an increased likelihood of sensory impairment, social isolation, visual hallucinations and a greater risk of developing tardive dyskinesia. Significantly more women are affected than men. Formal thought disorder, affective blunting and family history are less likely.

15.6 Suggested Activity

A potentially neglected area of clinical practice is the monitoring of physical health for patients on antipsychotics and is an ideal topic for audit because patients with psychosis on treatment are arguable doubly disadvantaged; firstly because their psychosis may hinder their ability to look after their health and secondly due to the side effects of antipsychotic medication. Older people are also more likely to have physical co-morbidities because of their age. An audit of the physical healthcare of older people with psychosis may lead to system changes in your practice and improve patient care.

> **Key Points**
> - Psychotic symptoms in older people are not uncommon but may not be apparent.
> - Diagnosis can be difficult, as patients may not volunteer their symptoms. A collateral history from family or carers is important.
> - For suspected late-onset psychosis, it is important to undertake a physical examination and investigations and prompt referral to specialist services will allow patients access to diagnosis, treatment and support.
> - Clinicians should take a holistic approach when assessing the needs of their older patients with psychosis and routinely involve relatives and the multidisciplinary team.
> - Pharmacological and psychological treatments are recommended but unacceptable variations in service provision in CBT exist.
> - Management of psychosis in older people requires special consideration especially with respect to the legal framework under which treatment is administered.

References

1. Geddes P. McKnight psychiatry, 4th ed. Oxford: Oxford University Press; 2012. ISBN 978-0-19-923396-0.
2. Cowen P, Harrison P. The shorter Oxford textbook of psychiatry, 6th ed. Oxford: Oxford University Press; ISBN 9780199605613.

3. The World Health Organization. The ICD-10 classification of mental and behavioural disorders: clinical descriptions and diagnostic guidelines. Geneva: World Health Organization; 1992.
4. Howard, et al. Late-onset schizophrenia and very-late-onset schizophrenia-like psychosis: an international consensus. Am J Psychiatry. 2000;157:172–8.
5. Meesters, et al. Schizophrenia spectrum disorders in later life: prevalence and distribution of age at onset and sex in a Dutch catchment area. Am J Geriatr Psychiatry. 2012;20(1):18–28.
6. Karim S, Byrne E. Treatment of psychosis in elderly people. Adv Psychiatr Treat. 2005;11:286–96.
7. Palmer, et al. Schizophrenia in late life: findings challenge traditional concepts. Harv Rev Psychiatry. 2001;9:51–8.
8. Targum SD. Treating psychotic symptoms in elderly patients. Prim Care Companion J Clin Psychiatry. 2001;3:156–63.
9. Targum SD, Abbott JL. Treating psychotic symptoms in the elderly: a spectrum of disorders. J Clin Psychiatry. 1999;60 Suppl 8:4–10.
10. National Institute for Health and Care Excellence, Guidelines (CG178), psychosis and schizophrenia in adults: treatment and management, February 2014.
11. Gaebel W, Weinmann S, Sartorius N. Schizophrenia practice guidelines: international survey and comparison. Br J Psychiatry. 2005;187:248–55.
12. Taylor et al. The Maudsley, prescribing guidelines in psychiatry, 11th ed. West Sussex, UK: Wiley-Blackwell; 2012. 978-0-470-97948-8.
13. Douglas, et al. exposure to antipsychotics and risk of stroke: self controlled case series study. Br Med J. 2008;337:a1227.
14. Munro, et al. Active monitoring of 12,760 clozapine recipients in the UK and Ireland. Beyond Pharmacovigilance. Br J Psychiatry. 1999;175:576–80.
15. O'Connor, et al. The safety and tolerability of Clozapine in aged patients: a retrospective clinical file review. World J Biol Psychiatry. 2010;11:788–91.
16. Mayersohn M. Special pharmacokinetic considerations in the elderly. In: Evans WE, Schentag JJ, Jusko WJ, editors. Applied pharmacokinetics principles of therapeutic drug monitoring. Spokane: Applied Therapeutics; 1986. p. 229–93.
17. Morris R, et al. Lithium and eGFR: a new routinely available tool for the prevention of chronic kidney disease. Br J Psychiatry. 2008;193:93–5.
18. Gurwitz JH. Start low and go slow: dosing of antipsychotic medications in elderly patients with dementia. Arch Intern Med. 1995;155(18):2017–8.
19. Davis JM, Chen N, Glick ID. A meta-analysis of the efficacy of second-generation antipsychotics. Arch Gen Psychiatry. 2003;60:553–64.
20. Ucok, Gaebel. Side effects of atypical antipsychotics: a brief overview. World Psychiatry. 2008;7(1):58–62.
21. Medicines & Healthcare products Regulatory Agency, atypical antipsychotic drugs and stoke, 9th Mar 2004, mhra.gov.uk.
22. Herman, et al. Atypical antipsychotics and risk of cerebrovascular accidents. Am J Psychiatry. 2004;161:1113–5.
23. Lawlor B. Managing behavioural and psychological symptoms in dementia. Br J Psychiatry. 2002;181:463–5.
24. Lyketsos, et al. Mental and behavioural disturbances in dementia: findings from Cache County Study on Memory and Aging. Am J Psychiatry. 2000;157:708–14.
25. Margallo-Lana, et al. Prevalence and pharmacological management of behavioural and psychological symptoms amongst dementia suffers living in care environments. Int J Geriatr Psychiatry. 2001;16:39–44.
26. Coen, et al. Behaviour disturbance and other predictors of carer burden in Alzheimer's disease. Int J Geriatr Psychiatry. 1997;12:331–6.
27. O'Donnell, et al. Incontinence and troublesome behaviours predict institutionalisation in dementia. J Geriatr Psychiatry Neurol. 1992;5:45–52.

28. Steele, et al. Psychiatric symptoms and nursing home placement of patients with Alzheimer's disease. Am J Psychiatry. 1990;147:1049–51.
29. Finkel SI. Effects of rivastigmine on behavioural and psychological symptoms of dementia in Alzheimer's disease. Clin Ther. 2004;26:980–90.
30. Wynn ZJ, Cummings JL. Cholinesterase inhibitor therapies and Neuropsychiatric manifestations of Alzheimer's disease. Dement Geriatr Cogn Disord. 2004;17:100–1008.
31. Ballard, et al. A 3 month randomized, placebo-controlled, neuroleptic discontinuation study in 100 people with dementia: the neuropsychiatric inventory median cut off is a predictor of clinical outcome. J Clin Psychiatry. 2004;65:114–9.
32. Haw, et al. Guidelines on antipsychotics for dementia—are we losing our minds? Psychiatry Bull. 2009;33:57–60.
33. Wood KA, Harris MJ, Morreale A, Rizos AL. Drug-induced psychosis and depression in the elderly. Psychiatry Clin North Am. 1988;11(1):167–93.

Part V

The Dementias

Dementia: Introduction, Epidemiology and Economic Impact

16

Perla Werner, George M. Savva, Ian Maidment,
Jochen René Thyrian, and Chris Fox

Dementia is a syndrome of progressive cognitive and functional impairment. It is caused by one or more neurodegenerative diseases, the most common of which are Alzheimer's disease (AD) and cerebrovascular disease (leading to vascular dementia). People with dementia suffer from diverse impairments and symptoms that affect them in different ways depending on dementia subtype and their personal and social circumstances. Memory is characteristically affected in Alzheimer's disease, but other dementias may present with behavioural or mood changes, communication or perceptual difficulties. Dementia onset may be sudden or it may be preceded by a stage of sub-dementia cognitive deficits, often termed mild cognitive impairment.

Cost-of-illness studies aim to assess the economic burden of a disease [1] and highlight the impact of the disease on society and provide important knowledge and

---

P. Werner, PhD
Department of Community Mental Health, University of Haifa, Haifa, Israel
e-mail: werner@research.haifa.ac.il

G.M. Savva, PhD
School of Health Sciences, University of East Anglia, Norwich, UK
e-mail: g.savva@uea.ac.uk

I. Maidment, PhD
School of Life and Health Sciences, Aston University, Birmingham, UK
e-mail: i.maidment@aston.ac.uk

J.R. Thyrian, PhD, Dipl-Psych
Site Rostock/Greifswald, German Center for Neurodegenerative Diseases (DZNE), Greifswald, Germany
e-mail: rene.thyrian@dzne.de

C. Fox, MB, BS, MMedsci, MRCPsych MD (✉)
Department of Clinical Psychology, Norwich Medical School, Norwich, Norfolk, UK
e-mail: Chris.Fox@uea.ac.uk

© Springer International Publishing Switzerland 2016
C.A. Chew-Graham, M. Ray (eds.), *Mental Health and Older People:
A Guide for Primary Care Practitioners*, DOI 10.1007/978-3-319-29492-6_16

guidance to decision-makers in prioritising their decisions regarding healthcare and prevention policies.

There is increasing interest in examining the costs of dementia, and yearly reports are published regarding the worldwide cost [2]. These reports synthesise the knowledge emerging from the studies assessing the cost of the disease in individual countries and show that, geographically, the majority of the studies are conducted in high-income countries, with 70 % being conducted in Western countries, mainly Europe and North America [2]. More studies need to be conducted in low-income countries, because the prevalence of dementia in such countries is expected to significantly increase [3].

Dementia is accompanied by a loss of occupational function and progressive dependence on others for basic activities of daily living. This gradual loss of personhood is distressing for the person with dementia, places a large strain on caregivers, often spouses or other family members, and commonly leads to institutionalisation. Almost 70 % of care home residents have dementia [4], although the majority of people with dementia live in the community. The life expectancy from onset of dementia to death, although dependent on age at onset, is 4.8 years [5]. Prevalence increases rapidly with age, and one in three people currently aged 65 or older will die with dementia [6]. As more people survive into old age, and fertility rates fall, the prevalence of dementia worldwide is likely to rise [7].

16.1 Studying Dementia in Populations

Epidemiology is the study of disease in a population. Epidemiological studies can be classified into one of four basic designs [8, 9], depending on whether they focus on the *prevalence* of a disease at any given time or its *incidence* over a time period and hence its risk factors and whether participants are sampled on the basis of their disease status (e.g. using a case-control study) or not (e.g. using a cohort or cross-sectional study). Sampling without reference to disease status is preferable for studies of dementia as this avoids bias caused by factors that determine access to routine diagnostic services. Random sampling from a population also means that people are captured from a wide range of socioeconomic groups and across the spectrum of disease severity. Epidemiological studies also do not typically exclude participants on the basis of age or comorbidity, thereby leading to estimates of the effects of risk factors and impacts of disease that are genuinely applicable to populations.

16.1.1 Case Study

Mrs S, aged 50 and married, is primary carer for her mother who has moderate dementia. Her mother receives a letter from a university saying that she has been selected to participate in a dementia survey, and seeking consent for a researcher to visit, conduct an interview with them both and to perform tests, which might take several hours. Mrs S thinks that this might be too demanding and upsetting for her mother and in any case does not have the time to participate and so is inclined to refuse on her mother's behalf.

What effect might this refusal have on estimates of dementia prevalence and impact derived from this survey?

What could be done to encourage Mrs S to participate?

What other approach could be taken to include Mrs S in the survey?

Conducting studies of the prevalence, incidence and impact of dementia is difficult for a number of reasons. People with dementia or at risk of dementia are often vulnerable, leading to issues of access, capacity and informed consent. Ethical concerns surround the disclosure or non-disclosure of dementia to a survey participant. Participation rates of surveys have fallen in recent years, and rates of around 60 % are now typical. Participation is less likely among people with cognitive impairment. Dementia is difficult to diagnose even in a clinical setting and often relies on repeat visits, neuroimaging and the professional judgement of a specialist. Applying a rigorous diagnostic process to a sample of thousands is difficult, and epidemiological diagnoses are usually made on the basis of a one-off assessment conducted by a lay interviewer, nurse or technician which is interpreted by a clinical team at a later date. Ascertaining contextual information from participants is complicated by memory and communication difficulties, and recall bias will be high when assessing previous exposures. Finally, attrition rates can be high, and large population representative samples are needed to derive estimates with reasonable precision.

Despite these difficulties, a growing number of high-quality epidemiological studies of dementia do now exist. High-quality systematic reviews of these have been conducted, and here we will draw on these to provide an overview of the epidemiology and economic impact of dementia.

16.2 Prevalence of Dementia

16.2.1 Global Prevalence of Dementia

A recent systematic review of dementia prevalence included papers published up to March 2009, including all studies where fieldwork was started during or after 1980 [10]. This is used as the basis for current World Health Organization estimates of dementia prevalence and includes 135 studies of sufficient quality to accurately estimate the prevalence of dementia in their respective communities. Findings from these were synthesised using meta-analysis and modelled to update age-specific dementia prevalence estimates for each of the 21 regions defined by the 2010 Global Burden of Disease.

Table 16.1 is adapted from this review and shows an exponentially increasing dementia prevalence rate with increasing age across all world regions. There is a small but consistently higher prevalence of dementia among women compared to men at all ages.

Among high-income and middle-income countries, the age-standardised prevalence of dementia is similar, between 5 % and 7 % when standardised to the age and sex structure of the Western European population aged 60 and older. In African regions, the prevalence at all ages is much lower, albeit with estimates based on far less reliable data.

Table 16.1 (a) The prevalence of dementia (%) in Western Europe by age and sex estimated using a 2009 meta-analysis of 52 studies conducted since 1980 and (b) a more recent estimate from England based on a 2008–2011 survey (Cognitive Function and Ageing Study II [4])

Age group	Alzheimer's Disease International Meta-analysis (a)			CFAS II (b)
	Male	Female	All	All
60–64	1.4	1.9	1.6	–
65–69	2.3	3.0	2.6	1.2
70–74	3.7	5.0	4.3	3.0
75–79	6.3	8.6	7.4	5.2
80–84	10.6	14.8	12.9	10.6
85–89	17.4	24.7	21.7	12.8
90+	33.4	48.3	43.1	17.1

Survey methods have a large impact on prevalence estimates, so when making comparisons between studies, it is important to bear these in mind. For example, surveys using an informant interview often report higher prevalence than those that rely solely on patient examination, and there can often be little overlap between people identified as having mild dementia using different diagnostic criteria [11, 12].

16.2.2 Dementia Subtypes

Dementia can be classified into subtypes based on the underlying pathology. The prevalence of dementia subtypes has been reported but should be treated with caution as making differential diagnosis without neuroimaging or autopsy data is difficult, particularly in an epidemiological setting.

The most common subtypes are AD, vascular dementia (VaD), dementia with Lewy bodies (DLB) and frontotemporal dementia (FTD), although many cases are discovered at autopsy to be mixed or unknown cause and neuropathology does not often correlate well with clinical dementia, particularly in the oldest old [13]. Alzheimer's Disease International reports that AD accounts for around 50–75 % of cases, VaD for 20–30 %, FTD for 5–10 % and DLB for less than 5 %, while acknowledging the high prevalence of mixed pathology and likely synergistic effects when more than one pathology is present [14]. Estimates of the relative frequencies of subtypes vary depending on population and setting. Among men and younger people, DLB and VaD are over-represented, while AD is more common among older people with dementia and women.

16.2.3 Prevalence of Dementia Among Specific Population Groups

While these dementia prevalence estimates are applicable to populations in general, specific subgroups of the population are at greater risk. In particular, people from deprived areas or low socioeconomic status are thought to be at greater risk of dementia.

Poor health is a risk factor for dementia (see below) and so those at risk of poor health are likely to be at elevated risk of dementia. Cognitive test scores are lower in people with lower education, but whether this translates into an increased dementia risk is controversial with mixed findings from epidemiologic studies [15]. A study from the United States found a higher incidence of dementia among black compared to white older adults but that this was almost entirely explained by adjustment for demographics, socioeconomic status and other lifestyle-related risk factors [16]. Those in prison are at particularly high risk of dementia owing to risk factors present in that environment including low activity levels, poor health, poor mental health and poor healthcare [17] as well as an ageing prison population.

Dementia is more common among those with intellectual disability. In particular, people with Down syndrome have a higher prevalence of Alzheimer's disease than the general population, up to one in three among those aged 50 and older and one in two in those aged 60 and older [18] although estimates are imprecise.

16.2.4 Case Study

Mrs S notices that her husband has become more likely to forget things since he retired. Mr S has not noticed the change, but Mrs S worries that he might have early-stage dementia. Mrs S does not bring it up with the doctor as she does not want to upset her husband and she believes from her previous experience of caring that nothing can be done to help and at the moment they are managing well.

16.2.5 Under-Recognition of Dementia in Primary Care

Many people with dementia, particularly those with mild dementia, are not formally diagnosed. Comparison of prevalence estimates with numbers of known cases suggests that in Western populations, around 50 % of people with dementia lack a formal diagnosis [19] although this varies significantly with dementia severity and the vast majority of severe cases are diagnosed. Epidemiological surveys consistently find that people with mild dementia, men, those living alone, the oldest old and those without behavioural problems are less likely to be diagnosed [20]. Many older people are likely to have mild cognitive deficits or early dementia, and they or their carers might believe that their symptoms are a normal part of ageing or that there is little point in seeking help as nothing can be done for them. Information campaigns and active case finding in recent years have helped to increase diagnosis rates in many countries and further efforts could increase rates further. However, recently focus has changed from an emphasis on 'early' to 'timely' diagnosis, in recognition that where people are coping well, a diagnosis of dementia might not benefit them and that formal diagnosis should be made at the right time for the individual.

16.3 Incidence of Dementia

Estimating the incidence (the rate of occurrence of new cases) of dementia is difficult as vulnerable cohorts must be followed for a period of time, and sufficient new cases must arise during that period for precise estimates to be calculated. A recent systematic review discovered 34 high-quality dementia incidence studies conducted since 1986, 21 of which were conducted in Western Europe or North America [21]. In high-income countries, the incidence of dementia was estimated to double every 5.8 years, from 3.4 per 1,000 person years among those aged between 60 and 64 to 100 per 1,000 person years at age 90–94. Whether this risk continues to increase into very old age is debated as study findings have been mixed, but in any case, the absolute numbers of very old people (aged 95 and older) with dementia are relatively small.

16.3.1 Risk Factors for Dementia and Primary Prevention

Observational studies of dementia incidence have suggested many modifiable risk factors for dementia, but none have been successfully targetted in prevention trials.

Cerebrovascular disease is a common cause of dementia. There is an increased incidence of dementia among people with heart disease [22], stroke [23] and diabetes [24], and an association with atrial fibrillation is suggested [25]. Modifiable lifestyle factors known to affect health are also associated with dementia risk including smoking [26], poor diet [27], low physical activity [28] and vitamin D deficiency [29]. Pharmacoepidemiological studies suggest that the use of medication to control diabetes [30], blood pressure [31] and cholesterol [32] is linked with lower dementia risk, but these findings have not been consistently replicated. While it is difficult to distinguish VaD from AD in epidemiological studies, moderate associations have also been shown between poor cardiovascular health and pathology associated with Alzheimer's disease as well as with VaD and 'all-cause' dementia.

Lifestyle is also hypothesised to moderate the relationship between neuropathology and cognitive function. The link between more years of education and lower dementia incidence suggests that mental activity throughout life might build up a 'cognitive reserve' to protect against dementia [33]. Increased social activity in midlife to late life has been linked to lower incidence of dementia and loneliness to an increased risk [34], although this finding has not been consistently replicated. Affective disorders, in particular depression, are likely to be prodromes of and risk factors for dementia [35]. Sleep loss is also suggested to be both a cause and consequence of Alzheimer's disease [36].

Thus, there are three plausible mechanisms whereby poor health and lifestyle might increase dementia risk: first through worsening vascular health, second by decreasing cognitive reserve and finally by increasing Alzheimer's and other neurodegenerative disease pathology. Each of these pathways suggests that usual advice of living a healthy active lifestyle should protect against dementia and that the risk of dementia could be used in promoting a healthy lifestyle. A review of preventable risk factors estimated that around 50 % of dementia is potentially attributable to preventable factors, and with reasonable reduction of 25 % in risk factor exposure around 9 % of cases could be prevented [37]. Yet, despite consistent evidence of associations from observational studies, no modifiable risk factors have been 'validated' using large-scale primary prevention trials. Control of diabetes and hypertension and cholesterol has failed to prevent cognitive decline or dementia in randomised controlled trials, [38, 39] although limitations of trials including short follow up times could account for these failures [40]. Dementia prevention research is in its infancy, but major research efforts are now underway to test primary and secondary prevention interventions.

16.4 Impact of Dementia

People with dementia have complex care needs and other common health problems can be exacerbated by dementia. Comorbidity is common in older people generally and hence among people with dementia [41]. Behavioural and psychological symptoms affect almost all people with dementia at some stage in the disease and are an important and potentially modifiable cause of distress for people with dementia and their caregivers [42].

Dementia is increasingly recognised as a cause of death, but it is not often recorded as a main or underlying cause. Dementia increases mortality, with mortality rates consistently around twice as high as those without dementia once age and comorbidity are taken into account. In the United Kingdom, median survival from dementia onset is 4.8 years (IQR 2.5–7.6 years), varying from 10.7 years (25th centile 5.6 years) among those who develop dementia aged 65–69 to 3.8 years (IQR 2.3–5.2) among those who develop dementia aged 90 or older [5] Life expectancy from diagnosis is lower, reflecting the time taken to diagnose dementia [43].

16.5 Ageing Populations and Trends in Health

Western cohorts born in the middle of the last century enjoyed better health and education than those born in the preceding decades, as well as improved healthcare, particularly cardiovascular preventive health. Consequently, those coming into old age now are generally in better health than previous older cohorts. Dementia is linked to many aspects of health and to educational attainment so we should expect a consequent improvement in cognitive health and reduction in age-specific dementia prevalence and incidence. This has been demonstrated in Western European and North American populations by comparing findings from surveys using identical methods conducted over periods of years or decades [4]. Most notably, the Cognitive Function and Ageing Studies showed a reduction in age-specific dementia prevalence of around 20 % between 1990–1992 and 2008–2011, based on surveys using the same recruitment method and diagnostic criteria at both time points [4]. Table 16.1 shows UK prevalence estimates from 2008 to 2011 alongside Alzheimer's Disease International consensus estimates derived from Western European prevalence studies conducted between 1980 and 2009, illustrating this

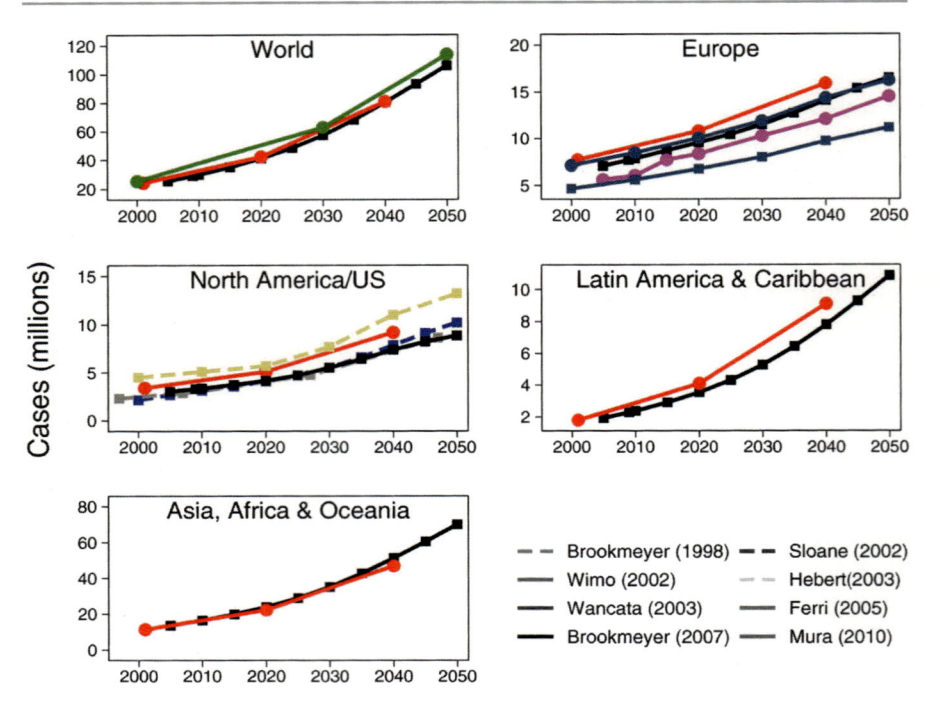

Fig. 16.1 Dementia projections. *Lines with circle* markers indicate dementia; *lines with square markers* indicate Alzheimer's disease; *dashed lines* indicate projection is for the United States only. The figure shows projections from previously published projections by continent (From Norton et al. [7] with permission)

decline. Conversely, improved healthcare for those with dementia could lower mortality which would increase prevalence relative to incidence and may explain why a reduction in prevalence has not been observed in all populations [44].

The projected increase in the number of older people and the relative increase in the numbers of older people to those of working age have led to alarming predictions of a dementia 'time bomb' over the next few decades. The increase will disproportionately affect developing countries that have not previously experienced significant numbers of older people, as seen in Fig. 16.1 which compares different projections of the absolute numbers of older people across different regions. As with prevalence estimates projection estimates also depend on methodology, and most projections do not take into account the recent evidence of possible reductions in age-specific incidence [7].

16.6 Economic Impact of Dementia

Conceptually, the majority of the latest studies assessing the cost of AD [45, 46] are based on a societal perspective. This is the most comprehensive perspective used in cost-of-illness studies because it includes direct and indirect costs, allowing a more complete examination of the costs incurred by a disease at the society level. Indeed, a recent review of cost-of-illness studies in AD, found that 14 out of the 17 studies included assessed direct and indirect medical costs as well as informal costs [47].

The most common direct costs examined include hospital inpatient, physician inpatient, physician outpatient, institutional care, specialists' care and other professionals' care, diagnostic tests, prescription drugs and medical supplies. The most common indirect cost examined is informal care, usually based on the replacement approach [45], which values care by using the cost of an equivalent service purchased in the market.

16.6.1 Methodological Issues

Studies assessing costs of dementia vary in the estimation procedures used, instruments used for the assessment of costs and sensitivity analyses performed.

Estimation Procedures
Studies have used a variety of methods to estimate the cost of dementia. In recent years, a number of studies have used a bottom-up approach [48], which calculates the resources used and loss of productivity in individuals with the health problem in question. The mean per-person costs are then extrapolated to the whole population with relevant epidemiological data [46]. Studies using this approach collected their data either prospectively or retrospectively and recruited their participants from memory clinics or from other specialised units and therefore might not be representative as they tend to exclude people with dementia treated by primary physicians or not identified by the healthcare system.

Three studies [45, 48, 49] used a mixture of bottom-up and top-down methods to estimate the cost of dementia. The top-down approach estimates costs by using aggregated data on mortality, morbidity, hospital admissions, and general practice consultations, etc. The aggregated data were taken from national healthcare statistics, patient registers, insurance database, or from large representative samples (such as the Health and Retirement Study or the National Longitudinal Caregiver Study).

Although sensitivity analyses are recommended for cost-of-illness studies as a way of testing the robustness of the results, only several of the studies assessing costs of AD performed it.

Instruments Used
Many of the studies assessing cost of dementia fail to use a structured, validated instrument. When such instruments are used, the resource utilisation in dementia (RUD) instrument is the most common one. The RUD is a standardised instrument that captures the utilisation of a range of community care resources, special accommodation, inpatient care and informal care (time spent by the primary non-professional caregiver on personal and instrument ADL tasks and supervision during the last months [2]).

16.7 Findings About Costs and Its Correlates

Aside from their conceptual and methodological characteristics, several interesting and consistent results emerge from the studies examining cost of dementia relating to the cost of the disease and its correlates.

Regardless of the methodology used, all studies show that the economic burden of dementia is very high. The global cost of dementia increases steadily – from $315 billion in 2005 to $422 billion in 2009 (an increase of 34 %) and to $604 billion in 2010 (an increase of 43 %), probably as a consequence of the increase in the prevalence rates. The total cost varies widely across countries, from 0.24 % of GDP in low-income countries to 1.24 % in high-income countries, and the distribution between direct costs and informal care costs also varies considerably across countries – with low-income countries having small direct social care costs and high informal care costs.

In Western countries, informal care costs account for a large proportion of the overall cost of the disease – from 44 % in Switzerland [50] to 56 % in Sweden [51]. This is not surprising since AD is associated with substantial burden on family members who are usually required to provide unpaid care to their cognitively impaired relative [47].

Regardless of the methodological difficulties in making comparisons across studies, two main factors emerge as clear correlates of cost in the area of AD: cognitive deterioration and difficulties in the performance of ADL and IADL [48].

Limitations of studies in this area include failing to clarify the perspective of analysis, small samples and selection bias, lack of sensitivity analysis and lack of controls. Another key issue is that many studies fail to assess comorbidities. This is especially important in the area of AD, since due to the high prevalence of dementia among the elderly, the co-occurrence of other chronic conditions is frequent. Indeed, studies have shown that patients with dementia attending primary care have on average 2.4 chronic conditions and receive 5.1 medications [52].

16.8 Opportunities for Reflection

- How many of the patients you come into contact with (your practice, your caseload) are likely to have dementia?
- Given the age and sex distribution of the people you see/your registered population, how many new cases of dementia should you see each year?
- Is there anything about your local population that make dementia more likely in some people?
- Which patients are most at risk?
- What might prevent patients affected by dementia seeking help?
- Would these people benefit from a diagnosis?
- What steps could you take to facilitate early diagnosis?
- What help is there for people with dementia in your local area?

Key Points
- Dementia affects the person with dementia, their caregivers, immediate family and wider society.
- The prevalence of dementia increases with age.
- People from deprived areas or low socioeconomic status are thought to be at greater risk of dementia.
- People with dementia may have a number of physical and psychological comorbidities.
- Current policy highlights the need for a 'timely' diagnosis of dementia, taking account of the context of the patient and family.
- The economic burden of dementia is high, so dementia is an important public health issue.

References

1. Rice DP. Cost of illness studies: what is good about them? Inj Prev. 2000;6:177–9. European Neuropsychopharmacology, 21, 718–779.
2. Wimo A, Gustavsson A, Jonsson L, Winblad B, Hsu MA, Gannon B. Application of Resources Utilization in Dementia (RUD) instrument in a global setting. Alzheimers Dement. 2013;9:429–35.
3. Wu YT, Matthews FE, Brayene C. Dementia: time trends and policy responses. Maturitas. 2014;79(2):191–5.
4. Matthews FE, et al. A two-decade comparison of prevalence of dementia in individuals aged 65 years and older from three geographical areas of England: results of the Cognitive Function and Ageing Study I and II. Lancet. 2013;382(9902):1405–12.
5. Xie J, et al. Survival times in people with dementia: analysis from population based cohort study with 14 year follow-up. BMJ: Br Med J. 2008;336(7638):258–62.
6. Brayne C, et al. Dementia before death in ageing societies—the promise of prevention and the reality. PLoS Med. 2006;3(10):e397.
7. Norton S, Matthews FE, Brayne C. A commentary on studies presenting projections of the future prevalence of dementia. BMC Public Health. 2013;13(1):1.
8. Greenland S, Morgenstern H. Classification schemes for epidemiologic research designs. J Clin Epidemiol. 1988;41(8):715–6.
9. Pearce N. Classification of epidemiological study designs. Int J Epidemiol. 2012;41(2):393–7.
10. Prince M, et al. The global prevalence of dementia: a systematic review and metaanalysis. Alzheimers Dement. 2013;9(1):63–75.e2.
11. Fichter MM, et al. Dementia and cognitive impairment in the oldest old in the community. Prevalence and comorbidity. Br J Psychiatry. 1995;166(5):621–9.
12. Erkinjuntti T, et al. The effect of different diagnostic criteria on the prevalence of dementia. N Engl J Med. 1997;337(23):1667–74.
13. Savva GM, Wharton SB, et al. Age, neuropathology, and dementia. N Engl J Med. 2009;360(22):2302–9.
14. Alzheimer's Disease International. World Alzheimer report 2009: the global prevalence of dementia. 2009. https://www.alz.co.uk/research/files/WorldAlzheimerReport.pdf
15. Sharp ES, Gatz M. The relationship between education and dementia: an updated systematic review. Alzheimer Dis Assoc Disord. 2011;25(4):289–304.

16. Yaffe K1, Falvey C, Harris TB, Newman A, Satterfield S, Koster A, Ayonayon H, Simonsick E. Health ABC Study. Effect of socioeconomic disparities on incidence of dementia among biracial older adults: prospective study. BMJ. 2013 Dec 19;347:f7051. doi:10.1136/bmj.f7051.
17. Maschi T, et al. Forget me not: dementia in prison. Gerontologist. 2012;52(4):441–51.
18. Stanton LR, Coetzee RH. Down's syndrome and dementia. Adv Psychiatr Treat. 2004;10(1):50–8.
19. Health and Social Care Information Centre. NHS Outcomes Framework. 2013. Available at: http://www.hscic.gov.uk/catalogue/PUB13054. Accessed 24 June 2014.
20. Mitchell AJ, Meader N, Pentzek M. Clinical recognition of dementia and cognitive impairment in primary care: a meta-analysis of physician accuracy. Acta Psychiatr Scand. 2011;124(3):165–83.
21. World Health Organisation. Dementia: a public health priority, World Health Organisation. 2012. Available at: http://whqlibdoc.who.int/publications/2012/9789241564458_eng.pdf.
22. Justin BN, Turek M, Hakim AM. Heart disease as a risk factor for dementia. Clin Epidemiol. 2013;5:135–45.
23. Savva GM, Stephan BCM. Epidemiological studies of the effect of stroke on incident dementia: a systematic review. Stroke; J Cereb Circ. 2010;41(1):e41–6.
24. Biessels GJ, et al. Risk of dementia in diabetes mellitus: a systematic review. Lancet Neurol. 2006;5(1):64–74.
25. Kwok CS, et al. Atrial fibrillation and incidence of dementia: a systematic review and meta-analysis. Neurology. 2011;76(10):914–22.
26. Anstey KJ, et al. Smoking as a risk factor for dementia and cognitive decline: a meta-analysis of prospective studies. Am J Epidemiol. 2007;166(4):367–78.
27. Lourida I, et al. Mediterranean diet, cognitive function, and dementia: a systematic review. Epidemiology (Cambridge, Mass). 2013;24(4):479–89.
28. Lövdén M, Xu W, Wang H-X. Lifestyle change and the prevention of cognitive decline and dementia: what is the evidence? Curr Opin Psychiatry. 2013;26(3):239–43.
29. Littlejohns TJ, et al. Vitamin D and the risk of dementia and Alzheimer disease. Neurology. 2014. doi:10.1212/WNL.0000000000000755.
30. Cheng C, et al. Type 2 diabetes and antidiabetic medications in relation to dementia diagnosis. J Gerontol A Biol Sci Med Sci. 2014;69(10):1299–1305. doi:10.1093/gerona/glu073.
31. Yasar S, et al. Antihypertensive drugs decrease risk of Alzheimer disease: Ginkgo Evaluation of Memory Study. Neurology. 2013;81(10):896–903.
32. Swiger KJ, et al. Statins and cognition: a systematic review and meta-analysis of short- and long-term cognitive effects. Mayo Clin Proc. 2013;88(11):1213–21.
33. Valenzuela MJ, Sachdev P. Brain reserve and cognitive decline: a non-parametric systematic review. Psychol Med. 2006;36(8):1065–73.
34. Wilson RS, et al. Loneliness and risk of Alzheimer disease. Arch Gen Psychiatry. 2007;64(2):234–40.
35. Da Silva J, et al. Affective disorders and risk of developing dementia: systematic review. Br J Psychiatry: J Ment Sci. 2013;202(3):177–86.
36. Ju Y-ES, Lucey BP, Holtzman DM. Sleep and Alzheimer disease pathology – a bidirectional relationship. Nat Rev Neurol. 2014;10(2):115–9.
37. Barnes DE, Yaffe K. The projected effect of risk factor reduction on Alzheimer's disease prevalence. Lancet Neurol. 2011;10(9):819–28.
38. McGuinness B, Todd S, et al. Blood pressure lowering in patients without prior cerebrovascular disease for prevention of cognitive impairment and dementia. In: Cochrane Database Syst Rev. Wiley. 2009. Available at: http://onlinelibrary.wiley.com/doi/10.1002/14651858.CD004034.pub3/abstract. Accessed 27 Aug 2014.
39. McGuinness B, Craig D, et al. Statins for the prevention of dementia. In: Cochrane Database Syst Rev. Wiley. 2009. Available at: http://onlinelibrary.wiley.com/doi/10.1002/14651858.CD003160.pub2/abstract. Accessed 27 Aug 2014.
40. Williamson JD, et al. Cognitive function and brain structure in persons with type 2 diabetes mellitus after intensive lowering of blood pressure and lipid levels: a randomized clinical trial. JAMA Intern Med. 2014;174(3):324–33.

41. Poblador-Plou B, et al. Comorbidity of dementia: a cross-sectional study of primary care older patients. BMC Psychiatry. 2014;14(1):84.
42. Black W, Almeida OP. A systematic review of the association between the behavioral and psychological symptoms of dementia and burden of care. Int Psychogeriatr. 2004;16(03):295–315.
43. Rait G1, Walters K, Bottomley C, Petersen I, Iliffe S, Nazareth I. Survival of people with clinical diagnosis of dementia in primary care: cohort study. BMJ. 2010 Aug 5;341:c3584. doi:10.1136/bmj.c3584.
44. Mathillas J, Lövheim H, Gustafson Y. Increasing prevalence of dementia among very old people. Age Ageing. 2011;40(2):243–9.
45. Hurd MD, et al. Monetary costs of dementia in the United States. N Engl J Med. 2013;368(14):1326–34.
46. Gustavsson A, Jonsson L, Rapp T, Reynish E, Ousset PJ, Andrieu S, Cantet C, Winblad B, Vellas B, Wimo A . On Behalfe of The ICTUS Study Group. Differences in resource use and costs of dementia care between European countries: Baseline data from the ICTUS study. J Nutr Health Aging. 2010;14(8): 648–54.
47. Costa N, Derumeaux H, Rapp T, Garnault V, Ferlicoq L, Gillette S, Vellas B, Lamure M, Grand A, Molinier L Methodological considerations in cost of illness studies on Alzheimer disease. Health Econ Rev. 2012;2(18): 1–12.
48. Delavande A, Hurd MC, Martorell P, Langa KM. Dementia and out-of-pocket spending on health care services. Alzheimers Dement. 2013;9:19–29.
49. Connolly S, Gillespie P, O'Shea E, Cahill S, Pierce M. Estimating the economic and social costs of dementia in Ireland. Dementia. 2014;13(1):5–22.
50. Kraft E, Marti M, Werner S, Sommer H. Cost of dementia in Switzerland. Eur J Med Sci. 2010. doi:10.4414/smw.2010.13093.
51. Wimo A, et al. The worldwide economic impact of dementia 2010. Alzheimers Dement: J Alzheimers Assoc. 2013;9(1):1–11.e3.
52. Schubert CC, Boustani M, Callahan CM, et al. Comorbidity profile of dementia patients in primary care: are they sicker? J Am GeriatrSoc. 2006;54(1):104–9.

Timely Diagnosis of Dementia in Ireland: Recent Policy Developments

17

Suzanne Cahill

17.1 Introduction

Dementia is a progressive condition that generally affects older people. It is the umbrella term used to describe a group of disorders that have common symptoms but different causes. A wide range of diseases cause dementia, but by far the majority of all dementias are caused by Alzheimer's disease. The second most common cause of dementia is vascular disease, and the third is a combination of both Alzheimer's disease and vascular dementia. Increasingly, those risk factors associated with cardiovascular disease such as smoking, hypertension, heavy alcohol consumption, high cholesterol, obesity, diabetes and lack of exercise have also been identified as contributing to several of the more frequently presenting dementias [1].

17.2 Prevalence Rates

The application of EuroCode age-/gender-specific dementia prevalence rates to the 2011 Census of Population in Ireland suggests that there are approximately 48,000 Irish people currently living with Alzheimer's disease or a related dementia [2]. An estimated 4000 of these men and woman have young onset dementia (YOD) [1]. Our best estimates (although generated from a number of different sources) have suggested that in addition, approximately 700 people in Ireland diagnosed with Down syndrome will also have Alzheimer's disease [1]. Like in other European

---

S. Cahill, B.Soc.Science, M.Soc.Science, PhD
The Dementia Services Information and Development Centre, St. James's Hospital and Trinity College Dublin, St. James's Street, Dublin, Ireland
e-mail: scahill@stjames.ie

© Springer International Publishing Switzerland 2016
C.A. Chew-Graham, M. Ray (eds.), *Mental Health and Older People: A Guide for Primary Care Practitioners*, DOI 10.1007/978-3-319-29492-6_17

and overseas countries, most Irish people with dementia live at home and are cared for in the community by family members. Pending where they live and the severity of their dementia, some people will also receive support from health and social care services.

17.3 Proportion of Irish People Diagnosed

It is not known what percentage of Irish people living with dementia receive a clinical diagnosis or indeed a differential diagnosis, nor is any valid or reliable data available on where diagnosis occurs if it takes place. Like in other countries, we suspect diagnosis probably occurs in a variety of settings including primary care, hospital outpatient departments and Memory Clinics. It needs to be remembered too that family members may be complicit with their relatives and despite worrying signs and symptoms of cognitive and memory loss, they may actively avoid pursuing a diagnosis, because of stigma and a desire to deny or disguise the extent of their relatives' cognitive and memory problems.

17.4 The Role and Responsibility of Primary Care Practitioners in Dementia Diagnosis and Disclosure

The role and responsibility of primary care practitioners in the diagnosis and disclosure of dementia is not clear-cut in Ireland, although this issue is not unique to Ireland. The first and only national survey of Irish GPs conducted over 10 years ago, involving a large sample size ($N=600$), revealed that the vast majority (90 %) had never undergone specialist training in dementia and 83 % of these Irish GPs claimed they would welcome upskilling in this area [3]. In the same study, GPs reported that they diagnosed an average of four new cases of dementia annually. Whilst about one third believed, they themselves were responsible for the late presentation of dementia in primary care and smaller numbers blamed their patients, their families and the health-care system [4], many GPs reported they were reluctant to diagnose. The key barriers to diagnosis cited by them were therapeutic nihilism, stigma, diagnostic uncertainties, lack of confidence, risk avoidance and concerns about clinical and professional competencies.

Several GPs mentioned the difficulties encountered differentiating normal age-associated memory problems from the signs and symptoms of dementia. In the same survey, when questioned about disclosure patterns, less than 20 % reported they often or always disclosed news of the diagnosis to their patients, and 41 % stated that they rarely or never disclosed the diagnosis to their patients. At the time, these low Irish disclosure rates contrasted sharply with those reported elsewhere, for example in the UK and Scandinavian countries, patient disclosure was much more likely. A follow-up study (cross-national) has more recently supported these earlier research findings showing, once again, GP's reluctance to be proactive in dementia diagnosis and disclosure [5]. Interestingly however in this more recent small-scale qualitative study, although Swedish GPs were more likely to have undergone dementia training in their undergraduate and later postgraduate training, several were also reluctant to disclose.

17.5 Timely Diagnosis and the Irish National Dementia Strategy

The diagnosis of dementia is said to be a complex medical and social practice [6], and unlike several other major illnesses, no definitive test exists to diagnose – indeed it is said that diagnosis tends to be more one of exclusion conducted by a process of elimination and undertaken in different distinct stages [7]. The need to make Irish GPs more dementia aware and engage them more formally in the diagnostic process and for significant policy development in this area has recently been highlighted in the National Dementia Strategy for Ireland [8]. The latter is a 5-year government programme for dementia service reform and development. When implemented, it will mean that ring-fence funding matched by philanthropic monies will be utilised to improve and expand services for people living with dementia.

Priority areas have been identified in this long-awaited National Dementia Strategy, one of which is timely diagnosis in primary care. As part of the implementation of this priority area, an educational needs analysis of GPs and Allied Health Professionals regarding training needs and preferred referral pathways is currently taking place. The Strategy emphasises the need for a timely rather than an early diagnosis, meaning that diagnosis should be made at a time most opportune for both the individual, for his/her family members and for the clinician. From the medical practitioners' point of view, timeliness inevitably involves balancing a wide range of judgments and should not be experienced in terms of chronological notions of time [6].

It is argued that medical uncertainty and reluctance to diagnose can be reduced by the dissemination of clinical practice guidelines [9] and by educational programmes designed to tackle therapeutic nihilism, increase knowledge and bring about attitudinal change. Being aware of the absence of clinical guidelines, a new Irish reference guide for the diagnosis of dementia in primary care has recently been published [10] through the Irish College of General Practitioners, and based on these new guidelines, e-learning modules will soon become available to all GPs across Ireland. To date, no information is available on the take-up of the guidelines and on the extent to which this new reference guide has helped increase dementia diagnostic rates in Ireland in primary care.

17.6 The Need to Incentivise General Practitioners

The issue of incentivising primary care practitioners to be more proactive in the area of dementia diagnosis has been the subject of much recent debate and criticism in the UK. In Ireland, some of the most vocal critiques of such a policy are younger people themselves who argue they have a right to a clinical diagnosis [11]. Outrage has been expressed at what is perceived to be the unnecessary requirement to incentivise GPs by paying them extra to diagnose dementia in primary care. Interestingly, in certain geographical areas in the UK in an effort to improve diagnostic rates in primary care, Memory Clinic specialist staffs have been working more directly with primary care practitioners. Preliminary findings reveal that such an approach has resulted in higher detection and diagnostic rates [12]. This practice has not been trialled in Ireland and represents yet another approach to upskilling GPs. A recent survey of the directors of Irish Memory Clinics revealed significant variability across the country regarding the availability and numbers of patients assessed at such specialist resources. When asked for their views on standards for Memory Clinics, results were equivocal. Directors of Memory Clinics were ambivalent about the prospects of introducing standards because of insufficient resources, some expressing concerns that if such a policy was to be introduced, their services might have to close down [13].

17.7 Recent Development in Primary Care Education

As mentioned earlier some of these identified deficits in the Irish primary care landscape are currently being addressed by a new and extensive programme of research led by the Department of General Practice at University College Cork. This research programme forms part of several major work streams aligned to the implementation of the Irish National Dementia Strategy. Primary Care Education, Pathways and Research of Dementia (PREPARED) is a Cork-based 3-year general practice-led initiative, funded by the Health Service Executive and by the Atlantic Philanthropies. The programme is designed to upskill primary care practitioners and support them to make a timely diagnosis of dementia and to adhere to dementia care management guidelines. It contains three distinct phases, namely, (i) a needs analysis of general practitioners' and primary care team members' knowledge and educational needs; (ii) the design and delivery of bespoke interventions including education materials, the development of integrated care pathways and decision support software; and (iii) programme evaluation. The evaluation will investigate primary outcomes such as reaction to the intervention, knowledge base and behaviour and will include a qualitative review of health-care professionals' attitudes, behaviour and practice. A quantitative component will also be used to assess change in coding, dementia registers, work-up screening and referrals.

17.8 Young Onset Dementia and Primary Care Practitioners

Although as stated earlier, dementia is a disease by and large affecting older people, the complex and unique needs of young people with dementia (those aged less than 65) should not be overlooked since in this age cohort, dementia can have exceptionally serious consequences. YOD has a prevalence rate of between 54 and 260 cases per 100,000 population. It presents a more complex diagnosis challenge, and it is more often associated with a delay in diagnosis and misdiagnosis both in primary care and elsewhere. Indeed the structure and organisation of YOD services in Ireland is especially problematic since care pathways for this vulnerable group are irregular and poorly aligned within mental health, older people or disability services. People with suspected YOD can be referred to neurology services in hospitals, but waiting times can be very long at a time when families are under enormous stress. There is limited research conducted on the topic of YOD in primary care in Ireland, and the only Irish research [14] available on the topic has shown that less than two fifths of the 61 people interviewed in the study availed of any service.

17.9 Dementia Diagnosis in Residential Care

The importance of providing older people resident in long-stay residential care with opportunities for dementia diagnosis has also been flagged in the Irish National Dementia Strategy. There are no accurate recent estimates of dementia in long-stay care in Ireland, and in the absence of a substantive audit of nursing homes, prevalence rates noted have varied from between 33 % and over 60 % [8]. A study conducted some years ago [15] revealed that in one metropolitan area, where four nursing homes were randomly sampled and 100 residents (25 in each facility) screened, up to 89 % of all of residents were shown to have a cognitive impairment. By far the majority were moderately to severely impaired, suggesting a probable dementia. In the same study, when directors of nursing were interviewed in depth about their residents' cognitive status, many either underestimated or conversely overestimated their residents' cognitive deficit. This study's findings have important ramifications as where dementia remains undetected and unrecognised in long-term care, such may adversely affect the quality of care and quality of life of the resident.

17.10 Conclusion

Ireland is currently implementing a 5-year National Dementia Strategy for the approximate 48,000 Irish men and women believed to be living with dementia. This National Strategy has prioritised three core areas for immediate action: (i) community awareness and understanding of dementia, (ii) timely diagnosis and the upskilling and support of primary care health-care professionals and (iii) improved in-home services.

Whilst as argued in this chapter, significant advances have occurred in Irish dementia policy in recent years and as a direct result, primary care practitioners will in the future probably be better equipped and supported to diagnose dementia, population trends and increased prevalence rates will mean that dementia diagnosis will need to occur in a variety of settings and not just in primary care. It is for this reason that there is a need for more efficient and effective use of primary, secondary and acute care services and for more dementia-specific guidelines to be established regarding appropriate referral pathways. Questions such as who is the most appropriate health service provider (the GP, the geriatrician, the old age psychiatrist or Memory Clinic staff) to assess and diagnose dementia pending the individual's age, symptoms and circumstances need to be addressed more systematically and a more structured approach taken to general versus more specialist referral pathways. There is also a need for protocols to be shared between primary care and secondary care services around diagnosis, referral and interventions. There is a need for dementia diagnostic services to be readily available to both younger people and to all those residents in long-stay care who may have a suspected dementia and who like others have a right to a differential diagnosis. Finally, there is a need for research to be conducted on disclosure patterns to find out the optimal way by which news of a life-threatening illness like dementia should be conveyed to patients. GPs need to be trained not just to diagnose but also how best to disclose this type of sensitive and often highly distressing information about a greatly feared illness to their patients and family members.

17.11 Points for Reflection

1. What are the key barriers in primary care to openly communicating a diagnosis to a person living with dementia and their families?
2. How might specialist dementia training support GPs in discussing/disclosing information about diagnosis?
3. What factors influence the notion of 'timely' diagnosis as distinct from 'early' diagnosis?

References

1. Cahill S, O'Shea E, Pierce M. Creating excellence in dementia care: a research review for Ireland's National Dementia Strategy. Dublin: Trinity College Dublin and the National University of Ireland Galway; 2012.
2. Pierce M, Cahill S, O'Shea E. Planning services for people with dementia in Ireland: prevalence and future projections of dementia'. Ir J Psychol Med. 2013;30(1):13–20.
3. Cahill S, Clark M, Walsh C, O'Connell H, Lawlor B. Dementia in primary care: the first survey of Irish general practitioners'. Int J Geriatr Psychiatry. 2006;21:319–24.
4. Cahill S, Clarke M, O'Connell H, Lawlor B, Coen R, Walsh C. The attitudes and practices of general practitioners regarding dementia diagnosis. Int J Geriatr Psychiatry. 2008;23:663–9. doi:10.1002/gps.1956.
5. Moore V, Cahill S. Diagnosis and disclosure of dementia: a comparative qualitative study of Irish and Swedish general practitioners'. Aging Ment Health. 2013;17(1):77–84.
6. Dhedhi S, Swingelhurst D, Russell J. Timely diagnosis of dementia- what does it mean? A narrative analysis of General Practitioners' accounts. Br Med J. 2014;4:E 004439. doi:10.1136/bmjopen-2013-004439.

7. Lindesay J. New treatment for Alzheimer's disease: questions answered, a prescriber guide. Guilford: Interface; 1999.
8. Department of Health. The Irish national dementia strategy. Dublin: Government of Ireland; 2014.
9. Fortinsky R, Zlateva L, Delaney C, Kleppinger A. Primary care physicians' dementia care practices; evidence of geographic variation. The Gerontologist. 2010;50(2):179–91.
10. Foley T, Swanick G. Reference guide for dementia diagnosis. Dublin: Irish College of General Practitioners; 2013.
11. Rochford-Brennan H. My journey through dementia. Key note address at conference titled "Young Onset Dementia", Dublin Castle, Nov 27th, 2014.
12. Burns, A. Lessons from the United Kingdom's National Dementia Strategy. Paper presented at Alzheimer Society of Ireland Seminar titled "Dementia Strategies, An Opportunity to Transform? Dublin Castle, Nov 12th, 2014.
13. Cahill S, Pierce M, Moore V. A National survey of memory clinics in Ireland. Int Psychogeriatr. 2014;26:1–9. doi:10.1017/S104161021300238X.
14. Haase T. Early onset dementia: the needs of younger people with dementia in Ireland. Dublin: The Alzheimer Society of Ireland; 2005.
15. Cahill S, Diaz-Ponce A, Coen RF, Walsh C. The under-detection of cognitive impairment in nursing homes in the Dublin area: the need for on-going cognitive assessment. Age Ageing. 2010;38(1):128–30.

Person-Centred Care and Dementia

18

Mo Ray

18.1 Background

Person-centred approaches in dementia, based on the concept of personhood, have undoubtedly provided a fulcrum to challenging and changing traditional approaches to dementia care. Over the past two decades, there has been a significant growth in awareness of dementia and a developing discourse on the potential to fundamentally change the experience of living with dementia. The growing visibility and voice of people living with dementia has offered an important challenge to the systematic marginalisation and invisibility that has long been a characteristic experience. There have been some real achievements in changing awareness, attitude and approaches to the care and support of people living with dementia, and arguably, a more positive view of dementia has been achieved. The message that it is possible to 'live well' with dementia is included at least in its general message, in the national dementia strategy for England. Yet, it is evident that structural, social and interpersonal factors continue to negatively impact on and shape the lived experience of people with dementia. This chapter argues that despite the fundamentally important role that person-centred approaches have played, and will doubtlessly continue to play, it is inevitably limited in addressing structural and social processes which influence the experience of living with dementia.

M. Ray, PhD
Gerontological Social Work and Programme, School of Social Science and Public Policy,
Keele University, Keele, Staffordshire, UK
e-mail: m.g.ray@keele.ac.uk

18.2 Traditional Perspectives: Dementia as a Diagnosis of Hopelessness

Traditionally, people diagnosed with dementia were perceived and treated as being effectively consumed by their condition. Their identity, personality, skills and attributes – or personhood – were assumed to be irrevocably 'lost' in the progression of an untreatable condition. These assumptions supported the belief that nothing could be reasonably done to support a person to retain personhood and individual identity.

Kitwood [1] in his critical re-examination of dementia and approaches to care observed that the overwhelming assumption of the loss of personhood in dementia both supported and reinforced negative social and interpersonal processes, or a 'malignant social psychology' (Table 18.1) commonly employed in interaction with a person with dementia. People living with dementia were at best physically tended – kept warm, dry and fed – with little recognition of the individual person. The emphasis on deficit and loss systematically disempowered people living with dementia and marginalised and undermined human rights, dignity and respect [2]. It was assumed, for example, that the expression of emotion and most behaviour such as, social withdrawal, remonstrance, anger and sadness were caused by dementia, rather than recognising the possibility that such expression could be authentic emotional responses to objectively difficult, frightening, oppressive and marginalising experiences.

Table 18.1 Examples of malignant social psychology and its impact on dementia care

Treachery – using deception to coerce or cajole a person to doing something that you want them to do
Disempowerment – preventing a person from continuing to use their skills, attributes, strengths and resources
Infantilisation – talking to the person in a childlike way; making assumptions about how a person should be addressed; believing that living with dementia makes a person childlike
Intimidation – introducing fear via threats or intimidation. Intimidating can be overt or more subtle, for example, using personal power or authority to achieve compliance
Labelling – using labels as a definition of the person, for example, 'poor historian'
Stigmatisation – being perceived or treated as a person of less worth or value as a result of living with dementia
Outpacing – engaging with a person with dementia at a speed or pace faster than the person can process/cope with
Invalidation – failing to value or validate the feelings, experiences or perceptions of a person living with dementia
Banishment – excluding or removing a person or people with dementia
Objectification – treating a person as an object
Ignoring – carrying on, for example, a conversation 'over the head' of a person with dementia

From Kitwood [1] with permission

18.3 Redefining Personhood

Kitwood's [1] analysis of traditional approaches to personhood with its emphasis on rationality and capacity led him to propose person-centred dementia care in which personhood was redefined and reclaimed. The redefinition of personhood moved away from narrow conceptualisations based on characteristics such as insight, rationality and memory. His inclusive definition proposed personhood as: "A standing or status which is bestowed on one human being, by others, in the context of relationship and social being. It implies recognition, respect and trust" [1]. It feels unremarkable now to think in terms of person – first and foremost – who happens to live with dementia. However, at the time, Kitwood's work constituted a very significant challenge to established practice and a ground shift in thinking and attitude from ruined 'non' person overtaken by dementia to a focus on the person, as a moral being with agency and rights, and with a unique identity and biography. To this end, person-centred care became a crucial contributor to challenging established cultures of practice and care, to supporting people to express, retain and develop identity and to take seriously individual lived experience. Other practitioners and researchers have developed Kitwood's earlier formations; for example, Brooker [3] has developed the 'VIPS' approach to person-centred dementia care which highlights the importance of *v*aluing people and promoting the rights of the person, *i*ndividualised care and support, appreciating and working from the *p*erspective of the person living with dementia and facilitating a *s*upporting social environment. Brooker's work has significantly and positively impacted on realising the implications of working towards person-centred care.

18.4 Key Routes to Person-Centred Care

Recognising the importance of biography draws attention to the importance of a life course perspective. This has a number of benefits including:

- Recognising each person as a unique individual with their own strengths, resources and capabilities
- Challenging the tendency to homogenise individual experience into the 'dementia experience'
- Contextualises the experience of dementia within a whole life course – the life lived as well as a person's present and their future
- Supports the recognition of potential, as well as actual, strengths and resources
- Encourages consideration of life course inequalities which influence the resources a person may be able to draw upon
- Highlights the importance of relationships and reciprocity

Biographical approaches include the construction of life history, life review and reminiscence work and constituted a significant development in dementia [4]. Actively engaging with individual biography is reported to enhance peoples' ability to recognise people living with dementia as unique human beings with individual life course experiences [5]. Crucially underpinning support and care with understanding of individual biography may provide opportunities for personalising care and support and as an important memory aid and support to individual identity, when autobiographical memory changes in the progression of dementia. Research has highlighted the importance of formal and informal carers understanding individual biographical experience such as occupational identity, people who are important to the person living with dementia and significant life events in supporting sensitive understanding of behaviour or communication, which may at first appear difficult to understand or interpret [4].

The 'struggle for empowerment' is cited as something which people living with dementia experience in many aspects of their lives – often from the point of diagnosis – when others 'relegate their qualities, skills and capabilities behind their deficits, struggles and difficulties' [2]. Experiences of disempowerment characterised by experiences of loss of agency may be further perpetuated by age-based discrimination which reinforce particular assumptions about old age and ageing [6]. A person-centred approach supports the view that a person living with dementia should not be disadvantaged or discouraged from the right to make decisions and choices about their life. Early research [7] supported this assertion and showed that people living with complex needs in dementia capably evaluated and expressed their feelings about and experiences of the care and support they received. Whilst balancing rights to make choices and decisions against worries about risk is complex, person-centred approaches should offer a challenge to ill-founded paternalistic actions based on a presumption that 'we' know best what is in a person's 'best interests' and invite critical review of how risks are defined and constructed.

Communication is fundamental to human life and to being in relationship with other people [8]. People living with dementia have traditionally experienced exclusion from communication on the grounds that communication skills are lost, rendering meaningful communication impossible. As well as being underpinned by assumptions about the loss of personhood in dementia, these assumptions also highlight the deeply ingrained importance we attach to the use of words and conventions of language and speech [9]. People with dementia who do not communicate using expected language convention may be perceived as different or 'other'. If meaning cannot be quickly determined, it is perhaps easier to assume that meaningful communication cannot take place and the person may be labelled as non-communicative or difficult to engage with. In other words, **our problem** becomes the problem of the person living with dementia. Killick and Allen make the point that by '…. labelling the individual and withdrawing them from normal interactions, we can precipitate the kinds of features and behaviours which we then consider evidence of the dementia. This in turn magnifies our own distorted responses, which triggers deeper distress and disorganisation in the individual and so it goes on' [8]. Supporting personhood implies being in relationship with a person living with dementia, and thus communication is a fundamental aspect of the relationship. From the late 1990s when Malcolm Goldsmith published the ground-breaking book, 'Hearing the Voice of People with Dementia', the possibility of communication – widely defined, and regardless of the apparent complexity of a person's experience of dementia – is emphasised [10]. Further work has uncovered, for example, the importance of creativity in communication [9] that behaviour is a means of communication [8]; the importance of starting where the person living with dementia is in their communication [11]; the value of sensory approaches to communication with people with high support needs and the role of nonverbal communication [8]. These examples promoted by person-centred thinking and practice provide compelling evidence of the importance of communication in dementia and point to the need for 'us' – to challenge our own assumptions and prejudices about what communication is or should be and the need to devote energy to helping an individual remain in communication (Refer to Chap. 26) and thus support the maintenance and growth of self [12].

The importance of emotional attachments, relationships and the comfort and security we gain (and give) from people we love and care for and about us is crucial to our ongoing sense of who we are. We know however, that people living with dementia may experience both a heightened need for reliable sources of comfort and security and, at the same time, a reduction in the potential resources and sources that those people that they may draw from. Social network research [13] has demonstrated a reduction in sources of social contact for a person living with dementia over time, caused by a combination of factors including people withdrawing from the person with dementia. Older people living with dementia may experience the loss of key social and emotional relationships through successive bereavement, and at the time of writing, it is estimated that one third of people living with dementia also live alone [14]. Interventions geared to support people living with dementia, such as moving to a specialist residential facility, may effectively remove the person from their community and thus challenge the continuance of existing relationships or activities such as church attendance or local citizenship roles. Person-centred approaches have highlighted the importance of biography and person-centred, individualised support planning in identifying people who are important and how, where and why a person may have need for extra comfort and security and how best to support the person to meet those needs.

Similarly, opportunities for occupation and being included in everyday life are core to our biography and identity as well as providing structure and a counterpoint for periods of inactivity or rest [8]. The benefits of engaging in personally enjoyable and stimulating activities are considerable as Table 18.2 shows.

Occupational identity in dementia care, and indeed in gerontological care in general, was traditionally overlooked and considered to be unimportant or less relevant to a person living with dementia. Indeed, it remains the case that many assessments fail to have serious regard of a person's occupational preferences, interests and aspirations. Perrin [15] has highlighted the importance of developing approaches to occupation that are both relevant to a person who has experienced deterioration in their ability to engage with long-established interests and skills and also reflect their current abilities, interests and aspirations. We cannot assume that a person who has been, for example, a magnificent baker will be content to sit on the side lines and watch others bake if they are no longer able to do what they used to do. How might a person remain involved in a way that is congruent with their sense of self? What

Table 18.2 Potential benefits of enjoyable/personally meaningful activity

Physical benefits of activity, for example:
Maintains joint mobility/prevents stiffness
Improves sleep quality
Improves appetite
Heart and lung function
Weight control
Coordination, balance and reaction
Physical strength
Mental benefits of activity, for example:
Enhances/improves mood
Opportunities to experience success, mastery and enjoyment
Improves confidence
Relieves boredom
Supports coping strategies
Supports identity, esteem and self-image
Improves orientation
Improves social engagement and opportunities for social connection
Supports agency/control
Reasons for getting up
Purpose
Opportunities for reciprocity and exchange
Social benefits, for example:
Facilitates companionship and new friendships
Decreases social isolation
Promotes continued involvement and participation
Promotes a sense of usefulness, belonging and purpose
Increases life satisfaction
Decreases boredom
Restores role and may support dignity
Reduces preoccupation with worries and problems
Improves independence and autonomy
Participation in personal hobbies and associated networks/groups
Teaches new skills/widens horizons
Maintains communication skills
Provides a change of pace and scenery

other valued and valuable opportunities might be offered in its stead? Person-centred approaches – including the active collaboration of people living with dementia – have effectively pushed our rather limited horizons on the issue of activity and occupation. The impact of artistic and creative activity by people living with dementia begins to demonstrate impact in areas such as personal/spiritual fulfilment, relationship development, social inclusion, skill and mastery, new learning and sharing expertise and ability with others – and simple enjoyment [9, 16–18].

Opportunities to remain involved in everyday life, including housework, gardening and cooking may provide important sources of validation and support for people to use existing strengths and abilities. Undertaking citizenship activities such as intergenerational work, peer support, co-research and voluntary work is increasingly visible and challenges conventional understanding of what a person living with dementia may be able to achieve or do.

18.5 Discussion

Despite some improvement in individual dementia care with some outstanding examples of what can be achieved to support people to live well, negative social processes continue to exert influence on people living with dementia. As a result, people living with dementia continue to experience a sense of being 'othered' and treated as an inferior group.

Evidence suggests that the experience of stigma and its association with discrimination remain a persistent experience with significant impact on peoples' lives [19, 20]. Bamford and her colleagues argue that whilst stigma is recognised to some extent, 'we still have much to understand about why dementia remains outside the realm of acceptable everyday conversation even as the profile of dementia rises' [20]. Data from a survey exploring attitudes to, and knowledge of dementia in Northern Ireland [21], found that from a sample of 1,200 people, 83 % agreed that 'all you could do was keep a person (with dementia) clean, healthy and safe', and 73 % agreed with the statement that 'people with dementia are like children and need to be cared for as you would a child'. Whilst national dementia campaigns offer important opportunities to raise awareness and insight, communicating the complexity of the message can be problematic. Dementia Awareness Week 2015 achieved considerable and diverse media coverage. The coverage included interviews, which without context risked unwittingly reinforcing the negative perceptions and associated stigma that the campaign sought to challenge. This was manifested in narratives from celebrities who often shared the personal pain and experience of the death of a much loved relative from dementia and in so doing expressed a belief that personhood was effectively lost – the person 'gone'. Attention-grabbing headlines such as 'I have a death pact with my sister' underlined by 'I do not want to be a burden' were used to summarise an interview published in a national newspaper with Sir Cliff Richard about his experience of dementia [22]. This kind of reporting doubtlessly continues to fuel and reinforce the common belief that dementia becomes *the* fundamental aspect of a person's life. Our focus on autonomy, independence and self-responsibility as the only goals which merit attention and reinforce has the potential for people living with dementia – often perceived as different – to be effectively subsumed into what Milne [6] has described as a single stigmatised identity.

The focus of person-centred care has brought about a fundamentally important change in understanding personhood in dementia and has undoubtedly challenged traditional care cultures resulting in areas of change with a real and significant impact on the lives of people living with dementia. But as the example briefly cited above illustrates, dementia remains a difficult, troubling topic for society, and public narrative remains significantly characterised by fear and anxiety. Critical perspectives informed by social perspectives which seek to unsettle and problematize taken for granted assumptions are argued to be more pertinent in challenging societal understanding and constructions of dementia. A growing number of commentators have pointed to the role of social perspectives in illuminating understanding in the way dementia is perceived and understood. The Joseph Rowntree Foundation [23] in a viewpoint paper asks 'How can/should society adapt to dementia?' They argue from a social model of disability that the responsibility to adjust to dementia rests with society rather than with individuals who live with dementia [23]. Recognising that dementia is influenced by socio-political contexts is more likely to offer important insights about the power of social barriers which persistently impact the lives of people living with dementia [24]. For example, an analysis of the societal importance placed on economic productivity to measure human value and worth, combined with the contemporary policy focus on self-management and self-responsibility, may illuminate the way in which people living with dementia are often constructed as passive recipients of care or as people who 'fail' to remain independent/become a burden. The relationship between dementia and ageing highlights the importance of thinking about relationships, for example, between the way dementia is constructed and endemic ageism that permeates our thinking about older age [19]. Bartlett and O'Connor [24] argue the need to 'go beyond care issues and to see men and women with dementia in a much more contextualised and dynamic way….having multiple social positions, as opposed to that simply of care recipient'. This argument in no sense precludes the importance of individual personhood or understanding the complexities and challenges of living with declining cognitive powers and its impact on individual people. Nor does it – or should it – preclude the reality that people living with dementia are likely to need support and care as we all do to some extent or another at various points in the course of our lives. Rather Bartlett and O'Connor and others such as the Joseph Rowntree Foundation challenge us to 'expand imagination in the dementia debate' [24] especially towards unsettling our assumptions. These arguments constitute vitally important elements in challenging the persistently negative focus on dementia which effectively homogenises the experience of dementia. The potential to offer new theoretical insights, which may disturb long-established assumptions, is timely.

18.6 Questions for Reflection

1. How can you evidence a commitment to person-centred approaches in your organisation to the support of individual people living with dementia and their families?
2. What impact have these commitments had on the experience of people living with dementia and their families?

3. To what extent does your service/organisation recognise the person beyond their diagnosis?
4. What examples can you identify of the ways in which people living with dementia are socially disadvantaged by institutional barriers, attitudes and behaviours?

References

1. Kitwood T. Dementia reconsidered. Buckingham: Open University Press; 1997.
2. Morris G, Morris J. The dementia care workbook. Buckingham: Open University Press; 2010.
3. Brooker D. Person centred dementia care: making services better. London: Jessica Kingsley; 2006.
4. Gibson F. The past in the present: using reminiscence in health and social care. London: Health Professions Press; 2004.
5. McKeown J, Clarke A, Repper J. Life story work in health and social care: a systematic literature review. J Adv Nurs. 2006;55(2):237–47.
6. Milne A. The 'D' word: reflections on the relationship between stigma, discrimination and dementia. J Ment Health. 2010;19(3):227–33.
7. Allan K. Communication and consultation: exploring ways for staff to involve people with dementia in developing services. York: Joseph Rowntree Foundation; 2001.
8. Killick J, Allan K. Communication and the care of people with dementia. Buckingham: Open University; 2001.
9. Killick J. You are words. London: Hawker; 1997.
10. Goldsmith M. Hearing the voice of people with dementia: opportunities and obstacles. London: Jessica Kingsley; 1996.
11. Sheard DM. Growing: training that works in dementia care. London: Alzheimer's Society; 2008.
12. Sabat SR, Harré R. The construction and deconstruction of self in Alzheimer's disease. Ageing Soc. 1992;12:443–61.
13. Wenger CG. Support networks and dementia. Int J Geriatr Psychiatry. 1994;9(3):181–94.
14. Alzheimer's Society. People with Alzheimer's living alone. 2014. http://www.alzheimers.org.uk/site/scripts/documents_info.php?documentID=550. Accessed 10 June 2015.
15. Perrin T, May H, Milwain M. Wellbeing in dementia: an occupational approach for therapists and carers. London: Elsevier Ltd.; 2006.
16. Greenland P. Dance: five minute love affairs. J Dement Care. 2009;17(1):30–1.
17. Benson S. Ladder to the moon: interactive theatre in care settings. J Dement Care. 2009;5:15–6.
18. Stenhouse R, Tait J, Hardy P, Sumner T. Dangling conversations: reflections on the process of creating digital stories during a workshop with people with early stage dementia. J Psychiatr Ment Health Nurs. 2013;20:134–41.
19. Milne A, Peet J. Challenges and resolutions to psychosocial wellbeing for people in receipt of a diagnosis of dementia: a literature review. London: Mental Health Foundation/Alzheimer's Society; 2008.
20. Bamford SM, Holley-Moore G, Watons J. New perspectives and approaches to dementia and stigma. London: ILC; 2014. Date accessed: 30th June 2015. file:///Users/KeeleUni/Downloads/Compendium_Dementia_1%20(1).pdf.
21. Dowds L, McParland P, Devine P, Gray AM. Attitudes to and knowledge of dementia in Northern Ireland, University of Ulser, ARK. 2012. http://www.ark.ac.uk/publications/occasional/Dementia.pdf. Accessed 12 Feb 2015.

22. Daily Mail. I have a death pact with my sister. London: Daily Mail; 2011.
23. Barltett R, O'Connor D. Broadening the dementia debate: towards social citizenship. Bristol: Policy Press; 2010.
24. Thomas C, Milligan C. How can and should UK society adjust to dementia? York: Joseph Rowntree Foundation; 2015. Accessed 20th June 2015. http://www.jrf.org.uk/publications/how-can-and-should-uk-society-adjust-dementia.

Identification and Primary Care Management

19

Eugene Yee Hing Tang and Louise Robinson

19.1 Introduction

Owing to a global change in age demographic, dementia remains a major public health concern and a socioeconomic priority. In 2010, 35.6 million people were estimated to be living with dementia worldwide [1]. This number is expected to increase to 65.7 million by 2030 and 115.4 million by 2050 [1]. In the UK, there are currently around 700,000 people with dementia; this is estimated to rise to 1 million by 2020 and 1.7 million by 2050 [2]. The annual societal cost of dementia worldwide is estimated to be around US$604 billion [3] and in the UK £20 billion [4]. Amongst chronic disease, dementia remains one of the most important contributors to dependence, disability and nursing home placement [5]. Increasing prevalence has driven government responses. In the UK this has included the National Dementia Strategy, which sets out a number of key national commitments in dementia care, emphasising on good-quality earlier diagnosis, easy access to care and focus on better quality research into dementia [6].

It is recognised that dementia in general is underdiagnosed and undertreated by primary care physicians [7]. This is probably a reflection on case complexity and time pressures associated with primary care. Research has shown that "watchful waiting" is adopted for people presenting with symptoms suspicious of cognitive impairment rather than immediate referral to specialist services [7, 8]. Although we should not underestimate the obstacles that primary care physicians face when dealing with these

E.Y.H. Tang, MBChB, BSc, MRCSEd, MSc, PGDip (✉)
L. Robinson, MBBS, MRCGP, MD
Newcastle University Institute for Ageing and Institute of Health and Society,
Newcastle University, Newcastle upon Tyne, UK
e-mail: e.y.h.tang@newcastle.ac.uk; a.l.robinson@ncl.ac.uk

© Springer International Publishing Switzerland 2016
C.A. Chew-Graham, M. Ray (eds.), *Mental Health and Older People:
A Guide for Primary Care Practitioners*, DOI 10.1007/978-3-319-29492-6_19

complex individuals, timely diagnosis remains key if we are to provide timely intervention and support to enable these patients to live well in the community.

19.2 Mild Cognitive Impairment

People with dementia may exhibit an early preclinical phase of cognitive impairment. Mild cognitive impairment (MCI) was introduced as a "clinical entity" over 20 years ago to represent a stage of cognitive impairment where the individual does not have any impairment of activities of daily living. However, MCI may or may not represent a transition to dementia. The annual conversion rate of MCI to dementia varies from 5 % to 10 % according to the definition of MCI used [9]. Although the incidence of dementia in MCI individuals is higher than the general population (4.4 %), it is the minority that progress to dementia in the MCI population [9].

MCI is felt to be a distinct entity from the cognitive changes that will occur with normal ageing. The concept of MCI provides an intermediate clinical diagnosis, often for watchful waiting, and may facilitate preventative interventions to delay cognitive loss. Various classifications/definitions exist [10]. A change in cognitive abilities is required for a diagnosis of MCI, and this information is usually obtained from either the person with suspected cognitive impairment or from their next of kin. There is no gold standard to specify which neuropsychological test to use to assess cognitive impairment.

19.3 Screening for Dementia

To help improve diagnostic rates, calls for dementia screening have been advocated. However the UK National Screen Committee (in 2003, updated in 2006, 2009) concluded that there is no evidence base to introduce a routine population-screening programme [11]; committees outside the UK (e.g. US Preventive Services Task Force) have also reached similar conclusions [12].

However in the UK, a Direct Enhanced Service (DES) to encourage and reward general practitioner (GP) practices to facilitate earlier, more timely diagnosis of patients with dementia has recently been introduced. DESs are additional services outside the normal scope of primary care services to address the needs of the local population commissioned by local health boards. The emphasis of the DES is to identify patients at higher clinical risk of dementia as well as working with their local specialist services to offer assessment, referral and early intervention services to ensure the dementia diagnosis is made as close to the patient's home as possible [13].

19.3.1 Symptoms and Presentation

General practitioners (GPs) are well placed to recognise and diagnose symptoms of dementia. There may be a number of factors that may delay a diagnosis of dementia. Recognised difficulties encountered in primary care when diagnosing dementia include atypical or non-specific presentations and the presence of co-morbid features [14]. For the patient and their families, there can be a misinterpretation or denial of their symptoms (for fear of stigmatism) and also a fear of institutionalisation once a diagnosis has been made [15]. GPs are also impeded by a perceived lack of skills, knowledge and training with individuals having varying levels of experience [16, 17]. Individuals will have varying levels of experience in diagnosing and managing dementia, which can be supplemented by educational programmes tailored for primary care.

Dementia is a progressive, insidious and chronic disorder, and the initial clinical picture can be diverse ranging to what may be interpreted as normal ageing memory loss to difficulty in finding words or making decisions. The individual may present with a change in personality or mood with features similar to depression (see Sect. 19.3.3). Signs and symptoms may be subtle. They can present with memory problems, difficulties in communication and changes in behaviour and/or personality noticed by a concerned carer [8]. Suspicions tend to arise on a background of sudden changes of environment, e.g. hospitalisation, change in medications or the absence of his/her main carer [18]. There may also be subsequent problems in everyday tasks in work or at home [19]. This may be dependent on the individuals previous levels of education and baseline functioning.

19.3.2 Initial Assessment

Diagnosing dementia is still largely a clinical assessment [18] but is helped by increasingly accurate scanning techniques. Assessment of the patient in primary care requires careful history and examination, supplemented with a collateral history from their family and/or main carer(s) and brief cognitive assessment tests. The initial aim for the GP is to detect potentially reversible causes of cognitive impairment.

Discussion should be sensitively centred around any disturbance to daily living such as problems with finances, self-care, decision-making, missing appointments and behaviour that is new and not normally associated with the individual. The general practitioner, who may know the individual and family well, is in an ideal position to identify such problems. Assessment of past medical and educational history will also be important. Medication may also be an important factor; a review of the medication, the dosages and interactions between them is essential to ensure that they are not a trigger for cognitive impairment. This should also include over the counter and herbal remedies. An assessment of mood may also be relevant followed by a trial of antidepressants if "pseudodementia" is suspected.

19.3.3 Case Study 1: Memory Loss Following Bereavement

The daughter of an 86-year-old lady has requested a house call; she is present at this review of her mother. The lady lives alone and according to the daughter has been going "downhill" for around 6 months. She is refusing to look after herself properly and her daughter organised daily social care support in order to allow her to continue to live in the community independently. Her memory is "not as good as it used to be", and when questioned by her family, she is often unable to give an account of the previous days or weeks of events. The patient has a background of hypertension and non-insulin-dependent diabetes but is rarely seen at the practice except at annual reviews. She is well known in the community for having organised numerous charitable and social events in the past. On further questioning, the daughter is worried that her mother is developing dementia like her father who sadly passed away around 8 months ago. When questioning her mother, she reports that she has little interest in doing things she enjoys anymore, has felt down and "just wanted to be with her husband". Her General Practitioner Assessment of Cognition (GPCOG) score was 5. Six months later, following bereavement counselling and a course of antidepressant medication, although not back to herself completely, she feels much better and the social care package has been reduced. Her repeated GPCOG score was now 9.

Collateral history from the family or carer(s) can clarify what the symptoms are as well as the timescale involved in relation to their baseline premorbid mental function. Although not commonly used, informant-based questionnaires such as "Ascertain Dementia 8 (AD8)" can be used to structure the consultation [20] and can be done either face to face or via a telephone consult.

Examination should also include any uncorrected audiovisual disturbances as well as nutritional status (as evidence of self-neglect) [21]. Examination should also assess for any signs of either new illness such as cardiorespiratory disease, anaemia, thyroid disorder or deterioration in existing comorbidities. These are typically responsible for precipitating and prolonging dementia. Although a full-neurological examination may not always be possible in primary care, some abnormalities in the pyramidal and extrapyramidal pathways can be assessed for. Brisk reflexes and extensor plantar responses could indicate vascular dementia, whereas an expressionless face coupled with bradykinesia and cogwheel rigidity could indicate dementia with Lewy bodies [21].

The aim of initial investigations for possible dementia is to exclude potentially reversible causes. Routine blood tests and possibly also including chest radiography and electrocardiography to rule out cardiorespiratory disease are recommended. A midstream urine sample should also be routinely performed. Metabolic derangements such as hypercalcaemia and hypothyroidism are rarely the causes of dementia in clinical practice, but it is important to identify such causes.

Routine Blood Tests in Primary Care

Routine investigations should include full blood count, erythrocyte sedimentation rate, urea and electrolytes, thyroid function tests, serum B12 and folate. Syphilis serology and HIV testing are not recommended routinely but are justified if an atypical presentation is apparent [22].

19.3.4 Cognitive Assessment in Primary Care

Brief assessment tools are available to objectively assess cognition but they are not diagnostic of dementia. The most commonly used cognitive assessment tool is the

Mini-Mental State Examination (MMSE), with a score of ≤24 out of 30 suggestive of dementia [23]. However, adequate performance depends on cultural and educational influences as well as on intact language. In addition, legal copyright issues have limited the use of the MMSE in clinical practice. The test can also be time consuming and therefore less suitable for primary care consultations. Other brief cognitive assessment tools are available. The General Practitioner Assessment of Cognition (GPCOG) test (which is also available electronically) [24], the Mini-Cog Assessment Instrument [25] and the Memory Impairment Screen [26] are clinically robust tools that are more appropriate in primary care [27]. A six-item Cognitive Impairment Test (6-CIT) can also be used and has been found to be more reliable than the Mini-Mental State Examination [28].

19.3.5 Specialist Referral

Memory assessment services, e.g. community mental health teams, memory clinics or geriatric day centres, provide a single access point to multidisciplinary care for individuals suspected of dementia. They will have expertise in diagnosis of dementia subtypes and therefore be able to assess the practicalities and suitability for anti-dementia drugs. These services also have the capacity to assist in early identification and ideally should have a range of assessment, diagnostic, therapeutic and rehabilitation services. Social assessments will also be carried in order to assist families and other carers to help these individuals to live well in the community and support their carers. Multidisciplinary input will also be available for families and carers post-diagnosis and provide monitoring of any intervention started. It is important that memory clinics have the capacity to operate effectively and network with other components of the healthcare system within its locality. Effective communication with the general practitioner is therefore extremely important to assist these individuals post-diagnosis.

19.3.6 Case Study 2: Dementia

A concerned daughter has brought her father in for review in your morning clinic. He had been seen on a number of occasions over the last year for several issues including recurrent falls, low mood and reported fluctuations in cognition. However on each occasion he was able to provide an accurate history of what has been happening, had capacity to consent to investigations and remained very compliant throughout. His daughter however reiterates that he has "bad days" when his memory is poor; he is often drowsy and unable to make decisions about his personal or financial well-being. Given that he was a former head teacher who had always been very disciplined and organised, this was a significant shift in behaviour from his normal self. On further questioning, the patient reports that his sleep has been disturbed by extremely distressing dreams and this was why he was drowsy and lacked focus. Given this history he is referred to the old age psychiatry team where he is diagnosed as having Lewy body dementia. He is referred for physiotherapy and occupational therapy assessments, joins a local dementia support group to access more information and is referred to the psychology team for further cognitive rehabilitation.

19.4 Long-Term Management in the Community

Following the emergence of symptoms, individuals with dementia live an average of a further 5 years [29]. As no single healthcare team has the expertise to manage the issues associated with dementia care in the community, an integrated multidisciplinary approach needs to be adopted in order to assist these individuals to live well in the community and to ensure their family carers are well supported.

19.5 Information Provision

There are benefits and disadvantages to receiving a diagnosis of dementia; the key issue is for the diagnosis to be timely for the patient and their family. Some will be reassured that the difficulties they have encountered have been given a name. It may encourage them to plan ahead before they lose the capacity to make decisions in the future. Similarly families and carers may find that a diagnosis offers a full and proper explanation for the troubling observations they have witnessed.

For people diagnosed with dementia, accurate information provision to them and their families is key. If required this should be available on local support services and can be obtained from either primary or secondary care services. Unfortunately there is evidence that people with dementia and their families/carers do not receive either sufficient information or receive information in an acceptable format [30]. Voluntary organisations can provide support for patients and their families but their resources are often limited. The Alzheimer's Society (www.alzheimers.org.uk) provides local points of contacts for people with dementia and their carers. They also have a number of publications for patients and clinicians. "The Dementia Guide" is a free, comprehensive publication available to order for anyone who has recently been told they have dementia.

Peer support in dementia has the potential to be of great benefit to people with dementia and their families as they may be able to provide access to information that may not be readily available from their normal points of healthcare access. This could be in relation to, e.g. financial problems where individuals may benefit from signposting to financial or debt service agencies [31].

Providing carer support in the early stages of a patient's cognitive impairment can reduce future problems with depression and enable the carers to better cope with the behavioural problems associated with dementia [32].

19.6 Pharmacological Management

In the UK, following national guidance, pharmacological treatment of dementia is generally started by specialists in the care of people with dementia. Given the potential interactions associated with polypharmacy in a potentially frail older person, these should only be continued when it is considered to have worthwhile cognitive, global, functional or behavioural effect. There are currently two classes of drugs used in symptomatic (Alzheimer's and mixed) dementia. These include acetylcholinesterase inhibitors (AChEI) and N-methyl-D-aspartic acid (NMDA) receptor antagonists. Such medications do not alter the pathogenesis of dementia but do slow the rate of cognitive decline. The emphasis is to improve or maintain function following neuronal damage [33]. Severity of dementia is frequently defined by the Mini-Mental State Examination score (mild 21–26, moderate 10–20, moderately severe 10–14, severe less than 10).

The three AChEI (donepezil, galantamine and rivastigmine) are recommended as options to manage mild-to-moderate AD. If patients are intolerant of AChEI or have moderate or severe dementia, memantine can be started. However only specialists in the care of people with dementia should initiate treatment and only continued when there are perceived benefits to cognitive, global, functional or behavioural symptoms. A shared care protocol is normally locally agreed to ensure patients are reviewed appropriately.

Donepezil is initially given at 5 mg once daily at bedtime. Assessment of treatment should be carried out at 1 month with the dose increased to a maximum of 10 mg once a day if necessary and tolerated. Galantamine is given initially at 8 mg once a day for 4 weeks and then increased to 16 mg once a day for at least 4 weeks. The usual maintenance dose is 16–24 mg once a day depending on clinical benefit and tolerance. Rivastigmine is dosed initially at 1.5 mg twice a day increasing in steps of 1.5 mg twice a day at 2-week intervals. The maximum dose is 6 mg twice a day. Nausea and vomiting tend to be the main side effects of AChEI with donepezil also causing muscle cramps, fatigue and insomnia [34]. The NMDA receptor antagonist memantine is initially given as 5 mg once daily and increased in steps of 5 mg at weekly intervals to a maximum of 20 mg once a day. Common side effects include dizziness, headache and hypertension [34].

The key elements of managing dementia in primary care often lie out with conventional pharmacological treatments.

19.7 Non-pharmacological Interventions

The evidence base for non-pharmacological treatment of dementia is steadily increasing. These include psychosocial therapies, cognitive-based therapies and physical and sensorial therapies, which can be carried out at the patient's home or in their institutional care home [33]. Further advantages of non-pharmacological management include the avoidance of side effects, interaction and limited efficacy associated with conventional drug therapies [35]. For example, cognitive behavioural therapy can be used in those with mild-to-moderate dementia to overcome "catastrophic thinking" and reduce depressive withdrawal [27].

Cognitive training and rehabilitation are two of the most commonly used non-pharmacological treatments in the earliest stages of dementia. Emphasis is on training specific domains such as memory, attention and executive functions [36]. Cognitive rehabilitation offers a more individualised approach and can enhance functioning in everyday life. Cognitive stimulation therapies (CSTs) offer activities involving cognitive processing often as a group-based activity in a social context [36]. CSTs have been shown to be an effective secondary prevention therapy for older people with mild-to-moderate dementia [35]. CST has also been found to be as cost-effective as dementia drugs. CST comprises cognitive and social skills training, delivered in twice weekly sessions usually over 7 weeks. Information about training including course and information manuals can be found at www.cstdementia.com. Unfortunately due to a shortage of specialist services, psychological therapies may not be as accessible to people with dementia through primary care.

Other non-pharmacological interventions include physical therapies and occupational therapy. Like in other conditions, physical exercise programmes have been shown to be effective particularly as secondary prevention for people with mild-to-moderate dementia [37]. They have the potential to delay onset or slow dementia progression and are currently recommended as part of a care plan to assist people with dementia in maintaining their independence [38]. Occupational therapy (OT) assessment typically involves an evaluation of the severity of the individual's disability and the effects on daily living. This is usually followed by the modification of the individual's home and environment and educating the individual on compensatory strategies. A study looking at OT as a potential non-pharmacological therapy in home-based individuals found it to be both cost-effective and cost saving when compared to usual care for people with mild-to-moderate dementia living at home [43].

19.8 Driving and Dementia

A diagnosis of dementia can affect the individual in numerous ways and having a direct impact on their independence, for example, driving. If the patient wishes to continue to drive, they must, by law, inform the Driver and Vehicle Licensing Agency (DVLA). However it must be noted that a diagnosis of dementia does not automatically mean the person with dementia has to stop driving; however they must fulfil certain requirements which may include annual assessments by their GP [39]. It is also important to remember that the stage at which an individual loses the ability to drive safely varies.

Driving is a complex process as the individuals must make sense and then respond to their surroundings appropriately without causing accidents. They must also be able to plan their routes and remember their destination, something that can be difficult for the person with advanced dementia. A driving assessment can be offered if someone with dementia is unsure of his or her ability to continue to drive. Persons who feel as though they need to stop driving will need understanding and support from their family and carers [39]. Driving may be their only mode of acceptable transportation and the removal of this from their lives could mean a loss of independence.

19.9 Caring for the Carer

Some carers do not formally acknowledge the fact that they are carers as their input is seen as part of their family duties. However carers of people with dementia are more likely to experience depressed mood, to report a higher burden and to have worse physical health, compared with carers of people with other long-term conditions [40]. In dementia, carers may grieve as their relative loses their cognitive abilities and the tangible benefits of companionship, affection and intimacy; this experience has been likened to "coping with a living death". GPs are often the first point of access and are in prime position to detect those with physical or mental problems because of their caring responsibilities. GPs should therefore endeavour to provide proactive carer support and to monitor their health and well-being, in addition to caring for the person with dementia [41]. If the family carer is a patient on the GP's list, the GP should record them as a carer and assess their physical, psychological and practical needs.

In England, the 2006 General Practitioner Contract has encouraged such a proactive approach. Practices are rewarded for implementing a management system that includes a protocol for the identification of carers and a mechanism for the referral of carers for social services assessment in accordance with the Carers (Equal Opportunities) Act 2004. Carers expect realistic information about dementia, the implications of diagnosis and its prognosis, and how to make best use of available facilities. Respite care can also be provided regularly or sporadically. This can be in the person's home, in a centre or in institutional care [41] in response to the needs of the carer. Information about key voluntary organisations such as Dementia UK, with its special Admiral Nursing Services for carers of people with dementia, the Alzheimer's Society and Carers UK will be helpful. This has been supplemented by the Royal College of General Practitioners (http://www.rcgp.org.uk/carers).

The mental and physical health of carers is paramount if community care is to be a realistic, long-term possibility. A meta-analysis of psychosocial interventions for carers of people with dementia revealed that such interventions can reduce psychological morbidity for carers and help their relatives stay at home longer; interventions that were intensive, were individualised and also included people with dementia, as well as their carers, were the most successful [42]; however in terms of actual practice, it is difficult to know what sort of intervention works best for whom and when. Caregiver situations and characteristics need to be considered when individually tailoring flexible interventions in collaboration with the carer. Depression in the carer is one of the factors that influences their ability to keep on caring and should be periodically checked for and appropriately treated.

19.10 Supporting Patients to Live Independently in the Community

In the UK, two-thirds of people with dementia live independently in the community. This can pose significant challenges to primary and social care services. The ability of the individual to continue to live independently in the community may only be achieved through the support offered by neighbours, friends and social support. Medications can be provided through weekly dispensed Dosette boxes through the pharmacist, with any potential interactions and changes to medication readily flagged up as necessary. This can be facilitated through prompts and reminders to help them to remember to take the tablets. Assistive technologies such as tracking devices can be used in coordination with neighbours and friends to assist those who may be found wandering on an infrequent basis. Alarms and pendants can also be used to the same effect particularly if the individual requires prompt assistance. This can help the patient to remain safe at home, reduce the need for hospitalisation and delay institutionalisation which has its own financial implications. Further information on assistive technologies can be found at http://www.atdementia.org.uk/.

19.11 Suggested Activities

How do you support the family carers of people with dementia?

Discuss in your team how you raise subjects such as driving, financial planning and care planning with patients with dementia: Could you do it better?

Clinical audit of the physical health care of people with dementia.

Key Points
- Dementia remains a global health concern.
- Governmental strategies are focused on more timely diagnosis and enabling the patients to live in the community for as long as possible.
- Diagnosis can often be difficult; there is still considerable stigma associated with the illness and people may assume their symptoms are due to normal ageing.
- It is important to undertake an examination and investigations to rule out reversible causes of cognitive impairment; prompt referral to specialist services will allow access to earlier treatment and support.
- Pharmacological and non-pharmacological treatments are available but unacceptable variations in service provision exist.
- Factors such as driving and promoting independent living at home through assistive technology, social care packages and carer support need to be maximised.

References

1. Alzheimer's Disease International. World Alzheimer's report: the Global prevalence of dementia. 2009.
2. Alzheimer's Society. Dementia UK: the full report. 2007.
3. Alzheimer's Disease International. World Alzheimer's report: the Global economic impact of dementia. 2010.
4. All-Party Parliamentary Group on Dementia. The £20 Billion Question – an inquiry into improving lives through cost effective dementia services from the All-Party Parliamentary Group on Dementia. 2011.
5. Alzheimer's Disease International. World Alzheimer's report 2013: an analysis of long-term care for dementia. 2013.
6. Banerjee S. Living well with dementia—development of the national dementia strategy for England. Int J Geriatr Psychiatry. 2010;25:917–22.
7. Iliffe S, Robinson L, Brayne C, Goodman C, Rait G, Manthorpe J, Ashley P, DeNDRoN Primary Care Clinical Studies Group. Primary care and dementia: 1. Diagnosis, screening and disclosure. Int J Geriatr Psychiatry. 2009;24(9):895–901.
8. Bamford C, Eccles M, Steen N, Robinson L. Can primary care record review facilitate earlier diagnosis of dementia? Fam Pract. 2007;24(2):108–16.
9. Stephan BCM, Brayne C. Dementia: assessing the risk of dementia in the aging population. Nat Rev Neurol. 2009;5(8):417–8.
10. Petersen RC, Caracciolo B, Brayne C, Gauthier S, Jelic V, Fratiglioni L. Mild cognitive impairment: a concept in evolution. J Intern Med. 2014;275(3):214–28.
11. UK Screening Portal UK National Screening Committee. http://www.screening.nhs.uk/alzheimers.
12. Boustani M, Peterson B, Hanson L, Harris R, Lohr KN, Force UPT. Screening for dementia in primary care: a summary of the evidence for the U.S. Preventive Services Task Force. Ann Intern Med. 2003;138(11):927–37.
13. NHS Commissioning Board. Facilitating timely diagnosis and support for people with dementia. 2013. Retrieved from http://www.england.nhs.uk/wp-content/uploads/2013/03/ess-dementia.pdf.
14. Kostopoulou O, Delaney BC, Munro CW. Diagnostic difficulty and error in primary care – a systematic review. Fam Pract. 2008;6:400–13.
15. van den Dungen P, van Marwijk HW, van der Horst HE, Moll van Charante EP, Macneil Vroomen J, van de Ven PM, et al. The accuracy of family physicians' dementia diagnoses at different stages of dementia: a systematic review. Int J Geriatr Psychiatry. 2012;27(4):342–54.
16. De Lepeleire J, Wind AW, Iliffe S, Moniz-Cook ED, Wilcock J, Gonzalez VM, et al. The primary care diagnosis of dementia in Europe: an analysis using multidisciplinary, multinational expert groups. Aging Ment Health. 2008;12(5):568–76.
17. Turner S, Iliffe S, Downs M, Wilcock J, Bryans M, Levin E, et al. General practitioners' knowledge, confidence and attitudes in the diagnosis and management of dementia. Age Ageing. 2004;33(5):461–7.
18. Buntinx F, De Lepeleire J, Paquay L, Iliffe S, Schoenmakers B. Diagnosing dementia: no easy job. 2011. BMC Fam Pract. 27;12:60. doi: 10.1186/1471-2296-12-60.
19. De Lepeleire J, Heyman J, Buntinx F. The early diagnosis of dementia: triggers, early signs and luxating events. Fam Pract. 1998;15(5):431–6.
20. Galvin JE, Roe CM, Xiong C, Morris JC. Validity and reliability of the AD8 Informant interview in dementia. Neurology. 2006;67:1942–8.
21. Young J, Meagher D, MacLullich A. Cognitive assessment of older people. BMJ. 2011;343(d5042). doi: 10.1136/bmj.d5042.
22. National Institute for Health and Clinical Excellence. Dementia: supporting people with dementia and their carers in health and social care. 2006.
23. Folstein MF, Folstein SE, McHugh PR. Mini-mental state@ a practical method for grading the cognitive state of patients for the clinicians. J Psychiatr Res. 1975;12:189–98.

24. Brodaty H, Pond D, Kemp NM, Luscombe G, Harding L, Berman K, Huppert FA. The GPCOG: a new screening test for dementia designed for general practice. J Am Geriatr Soc. 2002;50(3):530–4.
25. Borson S, Scanlan J, Brush M, Vitaliano P, Dokmak A. The mini-cog: a cognitive 'vital signs' measure for dementia screening in multi-lingual elderly. Int J Geriatr Psychiatry. 2000;15:1021–7.
26. Buschke H, Kuslansky G, Katz M, Stewart WF, Sliwinski MJ, Eckholdt HM, Lipton RB. Screening for dementia with the memory impairment screen. Neurology. 1999;52:231–8.
27. Burns A, Iliffe S. Dementia. BMJ. 2009;338:b75.
28. Brooke P, Bullock R. Validation of the 6 item cognitive impairment test. Int J Geriatr Psychiatry. 1999;14(8):936–40.
29. Xie J, Brayne C, Matthews FE. Survival times in people with dementia: analysis from population based cohort study with 14 year follow-up. Br Med J. 2008;336:258–62.
30. van der Roest HG, Meiland FJM, Comijis HC, Derksen E, Jansen APD, van Hout HPJ, Jonker C, Droes RM. What do community-dwelling people with dementia need? A survey of those who are known to care and welfare services. Int Psychogeriatr. 2009;21(5):949–65.
31. Schneider J, Murray J, Banerjee S, Mann A. Eurocare: a cross-national study of co-resident spouse caters for people with Alzheimer's disease: i – factors associated with carer burden. Int J Geriatr Psychiatry. 1999;14(8):651–61.
32. Robinson L, Iliffe S, Brayne C, Goodman C, Rait G, Manthorpe J, Ashley P, Moniz-Cook E, DeNDRoN Primary Care Clinical Studies Group. Primary care and dementia: 2. Long-term care at home: psychosocial interventions, information provision, carer support and case management. Int J Geriatr Psychiatry. 2010;25(7):657–64.
33. Grand JHG, Caspar S, McacDonald S. Clinical features and multidisciplinary approaches to dementia care. J Multidiscplinary Healthc. 2011;4:125–47.
34. National Institute for Health and Clinical Excellence. Donepezil, galantamine, rivastigmine and memantine for the treatment of Alzheimer's disease Review of NICE technology appraisal guidance 111. NICE technology appraisal guidance 217. 2011.
35. Sadowsky CH, Galvin JE. Guidelines for the management of cognitive and behavioral problems in dementia. JABFM. 2012;25(3):350–66.
36. Knapp M, Iemmi V, Romeo R. Dementia care costs and outcomes: a systematic review. Int J Geriatr Psychiatry. 2013;28(6):551–61.
37. Medical Advisory Secretariat. Caregiver- and patient-directed interventions for dementia: an evidence-based analysis. Ont Health Technol Assess Ser. 2008;8(4):1–98.
38. NICE-SCIE. Dementia: supporting people with dementia and their carers in health and social care. Care guideline (amended March 2011). Clinical Guideline National Institute for Health and Clinical Excellence (NICE) and Social Care Institute for Excellence. 2011.
39. Alzheimer's Society. Driving and dementia. 2013. http://www.alzheimers.org.uk/site/scripts/documents_info.php?documentID=144.
40. Brodaty H, Green A. Who cares for the carer? The often forgotten patient. Aust Fam Physician. 2002;31(9):833–6.
41. Cameron ID, Aggar C, Robinson AL, Kurrle SE. Assessing and helping carers of older people. BMJ. 2011;343:d5202.
42. Brodaty H, Green A, Koschera A. Meta-analysis of psychosocial interventions for caregivers of people with dementia. J Am Geriatr Soc. 2003;51(5):657–64.
43. Graff MJ, Adang EM, Vernooij-Dassen MJ, Dekker J, Jönsson L, Thijssen M, Hoefnagels WH, Rikkert MG. Community occupational therapy for older patients with dementia and their care givers: cost effectiveness study. BMJ. 2008;336(7636):134–8. doi: 10.1136/bmj.39408.481898. BE. Epub 2008 Jan 2.

Psychotherapy Interventions with People Affected by Dementia

20

Richard Cheston

20.1 Post-diagnostic Interventions for People Affected by Dementia: Adapting the Living Well with Dementia Model of Group Therapy for Use Within Primary Care

20.1.1 Background

UK government policy makes it clear that people who are affected by dementia should not only receive a timely, ideally early diagnosis but that they should also be provided with support to help them to adapt to the illness. In part, this is based around a belief that early diagnosis and support will facilitate people who receive a diagnosis being able to plan ahead and to take control over their illness. Thus, the recent *"Dementia – State of the Nation"* report [1] set as a goal that by March 2015, two third of people diagnosed with dementia in the UK should *"be supported after diagnosis, to exercise control and choice over their lives and helped to manage their condition so they can live independently for longer"*.

While the State of the Nation report mentions the importance of peer support, it provides no guidance as to how this support can be provided effectively. Across the UK, the provision of post-diagnostic support within memory clinics is, at best, variable, with some services providing little or none, while others have structured forms of individual and group therapy. However, the research evidence suggests that effective support needs to involve at least two areas:

1. *The emotional impact of dementia.* There is strong evidence that receiving a diagnosis of dementia has a significant psychosocial impact which may not always be recognised [2]. Thus, initially after receiving a diagnosis, people with

---

R. Cheston, MA, PhD, Dip C Psychol
Department of Health and Social Sciences, University of the West of England, Bristol, UK
e-mail: Richard.cheston@uwe.ac.uk

dementia often describe moving from frustration and embarrassment through feelings of shock, grief and a wish to withdraw [3]. At the same time, research consistently shows that if given the choice most people would still want to know if they had dementia [4–6]. Thus, whilst many people affected by dementia want to know more about their illness, this process of learning needs to be done within a supportive and emotionally containing context.
2. *Advice and strategies for managing the impact of dementia.* There is a growing body of evidence both that people affected by dementia can learn to use more effective ways of remembering information and that use of these strategies reduces distress and improves quality of life. However, for these rehabilitative strategies to be successful, they need to be based around those psychological principles that underpin learning.

Given the combination of powerful emotional responses to dementia and the potential of rehabilitative approaches, it is perhaps unsurprising that there has been a consistent growth in reports of psychological therapy with people affected by dementia and in particular group therapy interventions [7]. This includes small-scale evaluations of group interventions from a wide range of countries including the USA [8], Denmark [9], Australia [10], Italy [11], Japan [12] and Germany [13, 14].

Previous research has provided preliminary evidence that a 10-week group intervention has clinical efficacy when delivered by a clinical psychologist. Thus, the Dementia Voice study group therapy study reported that for 19 people who attended six separate groups, a 10-week group therapy intervention significantly lowered average levels of depression compared to baseline with the gains being maintained at 10-week follow-up [15]. However, although data was collected independently of the clinical intervention, the study did not include a control group. A feasibility RCT with participants attending either a 10-week psychotherapy group or an educational group [16] showed a reduction in depression during the intervention amongst the intervention group compared to the educational group. However, the study only reported on eight participants in each arm, and allocation to the two conditions was not randomised. Moreover, the increase in depression levels amongst the educational group highlighted the dangers of providing information without also attending to the emotional needs of participants.

Analyses of the process of change within these groups have suggested that different aspects of group therapy might be associated with beneficial changes. First a qualitative, process analysis of transcripts from the Dementia Voice study identified the importance of sharing of experiences around potentially shameful, or taboo, areas [17]. Thus, after the group had been able to acknowledge their feelings of embarrassment, at least one participant moved from a position in which he denied having dementia to being able to talk openly not only about having Alzheimer's disease but also about how he had initially been unable to accept what was happening, because he was so frightened. This therapeutically important shift seems to have been facilitated by listening to others in the group talk about their embarrassment about the illness and their fears for the future. Other studies of the process of change occurring within therapy groups for people with dementia have suggested an important role for storytelling as an indirect or metaphorical process of exploration [15, 18]. The model developed from this work proposes that successful psychological adjustment to dementia involves three steps or tasks [19]. The first task is for people to be able to name their problems as being dementia – something that is only possible if people are supported so that they are not emotionally overwhelmed. Once people are able to talk about the dementia, then they have to find some emotional distance from the illness. Finally, they are able to see dementia as only one part of their lives, develop strategies (including those from memory rehabilitation) and make appropriate plans for the future.

As few memory clinics have substantial access to either a clinical psychologist or a psychotherapist, it was important for the LivDem programme to be delivered by clinical staff working within a memory service. This was achieved by incorporating the research evidence gained from previous research into the structure of the "*Memory matters*" developed by clinicians in Hampshire [20–22]. Memory clinic nurses receiving training and supervision by local clinical psychologists delivered the 8-week long Memory Matters group. Service evaluations of these groups suggested that participants reported both feeling more relaxed about their memory problems and especially valued the chance to meet others who shared their diagnosis.

The LivDem groups incorporate both the underlying structure of Memory Matters groups, but are also based around the model developed from psychotherapy process research of how people with dementia are able to adjust to their diagnosis and of how this process can be facilitated and obstructed. It was designed to be used by memory clinic staff who might have little, or no, prior experience of providing group therapy. Thus, staff attended a 2-day training course (and subsequently received supervision from a clinical psychologist) and then delivered a manualised therapy that included standardised supporting materials such as participant handouts and DVD.

While emotionally difficult aspects of dementia are addressed directly during the LivDem intervention, the content of sessions is paced, so that participants are not faced with material that is too threatening at too early a point in the group process. Participants are also provided with education about dementia and appropriate coping strategies while also being encouraged to talk more openly about dementia. The intervention is thus consistent with the recovery model of mental health, which places an emphasis on helping participants to find meaning in life, achieving acceptance of their illness and through this to renew hope. Central to this approach to well-being is the importance of redefining identity, challenging stigma and helping people with dementia to work with their family to take responsibility for living well with their illness [23].

The "*Living well with Dementia*" (LivDem) group therapy project was an NIHR-funded pilot randomised trial of a short-term group intervention delivered within memory clinics. Seven groups were established across Wiltshire and Hampshire with between five and eight people attending each group. Sixty participants were randomly allocated to receive either the 10-week LivDem group therapy led by memory clinic staff, or placed on a waiting list control. The acceptability of the intervention and research methods was studied through a series of semi-structured interviews that were carried out with a purposive sample of 18 participants and their families (including people identified as *"improvers"*, *"non-improvers"* and those participants who had dropped out) and all of the 17 group therapists who delivered the groups. Finally, sessions from one group were recorded, transcribed and subsequently analysed to explore whether the way in which people talked about their illness changed over the course of the group.

As a pilot study, this trial was not powered to find statistically significant results. However, there was a statistically significant improvement in levels of self-esteem and quality of life in the intervention group, although this effect was reduced to a non-significant level once baseline differences between the intervention and the control group were taken into account [24]. Qualitative analysis of the transcripts from one group suggested that all of the participants showed evidence of having assimilated awareness about their dementia [25]. Moreover, participants and their families as well as the staff running the groups were largely enthusiastic and supportive of the intervention. Feedback from all three stakeholder groups has been incorporated into a modified and enlarged manual.

However, for the LivDem intervention to be accessible, then it is important that it is delivered within a range of settings, rather than being restricted to memory clinics situated in secondary care. Consequently, we carried out a small-scale study to explore whether a LivDem group could be established within a Primary Care IAPT service [26].

20.2 Anna and Bill: A Case Study

Anna was a 75-year-old woman who had been diagnosed with a mixed form of Alzheimer's disease and vascular dementia the year before the group started. She was married to Bill, who described how before the groups Anna would occasionally deny that she could be forgetful, but that after the groups he noticed that she had become more accepting of her condition. This, in turn, made it easier for her to accept assistance for his help. After the group had finished, Bill said:

> Probably the most important thing, is that it encouraged you in front of other people to stand up and say "I have dementia". . . I think up until that hospital session Anna was in denial that she had it but after that she wasn't in denial and that helped a hell of a lot I think … although [this] seems small it is very, very big. I mean once you've accepted you've got a problem then you will accept people trying to help you more. But if you're in denial that you have this problem then of course you're not prepared to accept help from anybody.

For Anna, a key element in this change cane from being in an environment where others spoke openly about their dementia:

> And I'm not ashamed to say that I've got it whereas I think I might have been if it hadn't been, you know, for everybody else being so honest.

This change, too, had been apparent to the group leaders who noticed that in the sessions Anna moved from blaming any problems on her hearing to acknowledging openly that she

> She kept saying "Oh my hearing is bad" We got that she seemed to think it was about her hearing that was the issue. And as we went on through the groups it was kind of like the penny dropped a little bit and then she came to realise and accept that "My memory isn't as good as it once was but I can still do x, y and z. I can still lead a life" you know "A happy and productive life" So seeing that change, that acceptance in her, was really quite positive, it was really good … it kind of took her a while or a session or two to get to "Actually we're here for your memory". But then she kind of took it on board and would talk about her memory and how it isn't as good and how she doesn't remember what her partner says. So it was that realisation and acceptance

For the therapists, as for Anna herself, the key element within the group was *"just being quite open and honest …. talking about kind of the emotions, the feelings intertwined with a diagnosis, certainly helped move towards that change, that acceptance"*. Many therapeutic skills go into achieving an atmosphere which allows participants to explore their feelings about dementia. For Bill, the key was the way in which the therapists *"approached it [the group] from an extremely human way. It wasn't a question of nurse/patient, it was a question of human to human. And they had sort of empathy with the problems as they could see them from their point of view"*.

However, if the openness and honest discussion of feelings about dementia within the group helped Anna, then other elements of the group seemed to be less useful. In particular Bill felt that the handouts were of limited use: *"For people that haven't got memories the handouts almost become irrelevant because they forget to read them"*. However, although Anna recognised that her memory may have meant that the handouts were of limited use (*"every time I went I thought 'Oh that's good, you know, that's useful' but I'm blowed if I can remember them now"*), she nevertheless felt that she had incorporated some of the ideas from the group that related to memory aids and techniques into her daily life. Thus, Anna described how she now wrote out lists, bought birthday cards in advance and write on her calendar – *"probably the things that were useful I do automatically now without realising it was from that meeting that, you know, I'd learnt to use them [laughing]"*. Overall, Anna felt the groups had been useful:

> Well because it helped me so I'm sure it would help … it should help most people who go to them. I mean you always get the odd one or two who think 'I'm not doing that' or 'That's no good to me' But I mean if you go there with the right mind it is helpful.

20.3 Translating the Living Well with Dementia Group into a Primary Care

The participants for the group were recruited from primary care teams, and the local memory clinic. Eight referrals to the project were made, and five people affected by dementia were ultimately recruited to the study, although one man was forced to withdraw due to illness before the first session. All participants had received a diagnosis of dementia within the previous 18 months and acknowledged, at least occasionally, that they had a memory problem. They were all assessed as having capacity to give informed consent to taking part in the research. All of the four participants who subsequently attended were women. Of the carers, two were sons, one was a daughter-in-law and there was one husband.

Low-intensity therapists working within primary care as part of an Improving Access to Psychological Therapy (IAPT) service delivered the LivDem intervention. As IAPT therapists are experienced in group work, the training package was delivered in 1 rather than 2 days. Regular supervision was provided to therapists. Group participants and their carers attended the first and the final sessions together, with separate groups then being provided for participants and carers for the remaining eight sessions. Sessions for people affected by dementia involved a mixture of psycho-educational material (e.g. about the causes and treatment of dementia), skills training (e.g. in relaxation) and a psychotherapeutic focus on helping participants to discuss their experiences of dementia – and in particular the emotional impact of the illness. The parallel support group for carers shadowed the content of the participant sessions. At the end of every session, participants were provided with a handout describing the main issues that had been covered, and carers and participants with dementia were encouraged to discuss topics between sessions. A DVD of people affected by dementia talking about different aspects of their illness which paralleled the content of the sessions could also be played during sessions at the discretion of the group facilitators.

Participants completed the Quality of Life in Alzheimer's disease scale or QoL-AD [27] during the first and the final sessions, while carers completed a proxy rating of their perception of the quality of life of their partner. The ratings made by all of the carers suggested that the Quality of Life of participants was improved, while two of the three people affected by dementia also indicated improvement. The qualitative interviews largely confirmed this picture of change: all three carers described the groups as being helpful, while of the three people affected by dementia only Elsie (whose Qol-AD score increased) felt that they had not been helpful.

Therapists described important changes for participants, especially in the way in which participants spoke about their illness. One therapist (K) said:

> I found it really powerful in terms of change, how they think about dementia, and how that changes. To go from being unable to talk about dementia … there was stigma in how they viewed it, and we were taking away the fear.

For one couple (Ruby and Ron) in particular, the group seems to have been important in helping them to understand and empathise more with each other and to adjust to the difficulties they were facing. K described how *"at the start they were very polarised, and at the end session they held hands"*. Ruby and Ron also described changes:

> **Ruby**: What has been said and done has been very helpful, he did begin to understand what I've been trying to tell him, but he doesn't take it all in
> **Ron**: I think it helped her (Ruby) to come to terms with her own illness … She is more willing to talk about her illness and the problems it causes. The memory loss

None of the three psychologists who delivered the LivDem intervention to participants, or the two who worked with carers, had ever worked with people affected by dementia before. Although the therapists felt that the amount of training was adequate, the main difficulty that encountered in working with people affected by dementia was around managing the group process when people repeated themselves, for instance, when the same story was told over and over again.

The main problems identified by carers were around practical difficulties (e.g. taking time off work). One participant couple dropped out of the group due to illness with the caregiver. None of the participants felt that the lack of previous experience of the therapists with people affected by dementia impacted on the group.

20.4 Challenges Around Translating the LivDem Study into a Primary Care Setting

IAPT's initial mandate was to provide support for adults with depression and anxiety using a stepped-care module [28, 29]. In the IAPT service that took part in this project, the LivDem groups were located within Step Two of a stepped model of engagement. The aim of therapy at this level is to provide guided self-help, for instance, by therapists suggesting strategies that may be helpful, but not intervening more actively to ensure that these ideas are acted upon. Although the LivDem model fits within this ethos, this model of work presents a number of challenges when applied to people affected by dementia.

20.4.1 Recruitment

Of the eight people referred to the project, only three referrals were from a primary care setting, with the other five being referred from a local Memory clinic. IAPT services typically rely on self-referral, often using on-line processes, and may need to take a more active approach to initiating referrals when working with people affected by dementia, for instance, by drawing on local memory services and third-sector agencies.

20.4.2 Minimum Data Set

All IAPT services are required to administer the Minimum Data Set (MDS) to clients at the end of every session as a way of monitoring change. This involves standardised self-report questionnaires designed largely for use by adults of working age. However, very quickly it became apparent that all of the participants struggled to complete these questionnaires, and this form of data collection was abandoned.

20.4.3 Engaging with Therapeutic Material

In this study, I provided not only training but also visited the IAPT service regularly, providing informal support and supervision for therapists. Anecdotal feedback from a second LivDem group which has subsequently been run but which did not have the on-going support was that clients had quite complex needs, which therapists lacking a background in dementia struggled to meet. Thus, although the lack of familiarity of therapists with the needs of people with dementia did not seem to be an issue in this study, there is a danger that the expectations of step-two therapists for clients with dementia will be unrealistic – for instance, over-estimating the ability of participants to remember session material or to initiate the use of new self-help strategies. Similarly, if therapists are unused to working with older people, especially those who have a cognitive impairment, then as a consequence participants may struggle with even the basics of therapy such as hearing, understanding or retaining information that they are given.

20.4.4 Support for Carers

In this study, a parallel group for carers was run in which topics and ideas from the participant group were explained to carers, as a way of encouraging them to support the take-up of these strategies. The group for carers also provided peer support and stress management. Although labour intensive, this form of joint working is invaluable, particularly given therapists' lack of experience with people affected by dementia and the otherwise passive nature of IAPT services compared to more traditional secondary care and memory services.

In conclusion, providing post-diagnostic support to people affected by dementia is frequently cited as a gap in current services, regardless of whether a diagnosis is made in primary or in secondary care [30, 31]. More generally, access to primary care psychological therapies by older people has been disappointing in recent years, with many IAPT services now recognising a need to improve the training of therapists and to meet the shortfall in service delivery by providing new services. Providing therapeutic support groups to both people affected by dementia and to their carers using the LivDem model is thus one potential way to make up for this service deficit. Although the LivDem group was well received, and seems to have been beneficial for both the people affected by dementia and their carers, concerns remain about the fit between the LivDem intervention and the way in which primary care psychology is structured particularly if the intervention is seen as a step-two intervention, if therapists are not more actively supported by a dementia specialist and if a parallel carers' group is not run.

20.5 Follow-Up Work

The *"Dementia – State of the Nation"* report set as a goal that by 2015, two thirds of people diagnosed with dementia in the UK should *"be supported after diagnosis, to exercise control and choice over their lives and helped to manage their condition so* they can live independently for longer". In order for this to become a reality, people who receive a diagnosis of dementia and their families need to have access to a range of information, delivered sensitively and in a timely fashion. For many people, this will include access to facilitated peer support groups, although for others, this support will need to be provided directly to individuals and their families. It is, perhaps, good practice to carry out an audit into the types of support that is available, to establish the uptake of that support and to identify any gaps within the service.

20.6 Questions for Reflection

- If you, or someone that you love, has dementia, then what would be the hardest part of this illness for you to bear?
- If one of the main symptoms of dementia is a difficulty in learning new information, then what is the point of talking to people about their diagnosis?
- If you were to spend time talking to someone about their dementia, then what sorts of issues might be difficult to talk to them about?
- Are there occasions when talking to people about a diagnosis of dementia might not be the right course of action?

Acknowledgements I would like to thank all the participants for their involvement in the study and additionally the psychologists based at the LIFT psychology service in Swindon: Liz Howells OBE, Marianne Evans, Rosa Hoshi, Kim Jackson-Blott, Brian O'Cealliagh and Karen Wiltshire.

References

1. Department of Health. Dementia – a state of the nation report on dementia care and support in England. 2013. Retrieved from https://www.gov.uk/government/uploads/system/uploads/attachment_data/file/262139/Dementia.pdf.
2. Connell CM, Boise L, Stuckey JC, Holmes SB, Hudson ML. Attitudes toward the diagnosis and disclosure of dementia among family caregivers and primary care physicians. Gerontologist. 2004;44(4):500–7.
3. Aminzadeh F, Byszewski A, Molnar FJ, Eisner M. Emotional impact of dementia diagnosis: exploring persons with dementia and caregivers' perspectives. Aging Ment Health. 2007;11(3):281–90.
4. Ouimet MA, Dion D, Élie M, Dendukuri N, Belzile E. Disclosure of Alzheimer's disease Senior citizens' opinions. Can Fam Physician. 2004;50(12):1671–7.
5. Elson P. Do older adults presenting with memory complaints wish to be told if later diagnosed with Alzheimer's disease? Int J Geriatr Psychiatry. 2006;21:419–25.
6. Jha A, Tabet N, Orrell M. To tell or not to tell – comparison of older patients' reaction to their diagnosis of dementia and depression. Int J Geriatr Psychiatry. 2001;16(9):879–85.
7. Cheston R. Psychotherapy and dementia: a review of the literature. Br J Med Psychol. 1998;71:211–31.
8. Logsdon R, Pike KC, McCurry SM, Hunter P, Maher J, Snyder L, Teri L. Early-stage memory loss support groups: outcomes from a randomized controlled clinical trial. J Gerontol: B Psychol Sci Soc Sci. 2010;65B(6):691–7.

9. Sørensen LV, Waldorf FB, Waldemar G. Early counselling and support for patients with mild Alzheimer's disease and their caregivers: a qualitative study on outcome. Aging Ment Health. 2008;12(4):444–50.
10. Aarons S. Living with memory loss: a program for people with early stage dementia and their carers: a case study. Clin Psychol. 2003;7(1):63–6.
11. Fabris G. Psychotherapeutic groups for elderly people suffering from Alzheimer's disease or dementia. Gruppi. 2006;8(1):75–85.
12. Ishizaki J, Meguro K, Ishii H, Yamaguchi S, Shimada M, Yamadori A, Yambe Y, Yamazaki H. The effects of group work therapy in patients with Alzheimer's disease. Int J Geriatr Psychiatry. 2000;15(6):532–5.
13. Scheurich A, Schanz B, Muller MJ, Fellgiebel A. Early interventional group therapy for patients with incipient Alzheimer disease and their relatives. Psychother Psychosom Med Psychol. 2008;58(6):246–52.
14. Scheurich A, Fellgiebel A. Group therapy for patients with early Alzheimer disease. Z Neuropsychol. 2009;20(1):21–9.
15. Cheston R, Jones K, Gilliard J. Group psychotherapy and people with dementia. Aging Ment Health. 2003;7(6):452–61.
16. Cheston R, Jones R. A small-scale study comparing the impact of psycho-education and exploratory psychotherapy groups on newcomers to a group for people with dementia. Aging Ment Health. 2009;13(3):410–25.
17. Watkins B, Cheston R, Jones K, Gilliard J. "Coming out with Alzheimer's disease": changes in insight during a psychotherapy group for people with dementia. Aging Ment Health. 2006;10(2):1–11.
18. Cheston R. Stories and metaphors: talking about the past in a psychotherapy group for people with dementia. Ageing Soc. 1996;16:579–602.
19. Cheston R. Dementia as a problematic experience: using the Assimilation Model as a framework for psychotherapeutic work with people with dementia. Neurodisabil Psychother. 2013;1(1):70–95.
20. Marshall A. Coping in early dementia: findings of a new type of support group. In: Miesen B, Jones G, editors. Care-giving in dementia: research and applications, vol. 3. London: Routledge; 2004.
21. Preston L, Bucks RS, Marshall A. Investigating the ways that older people cope with dementia: the role of identity. BPS Spec Interes Group Elder Newsl. 2005;90:8–14.
22. Preston L, Marshall A, Bucks R. Investigating the ways that older people cope with dementia: a qualitative study. Aging Ment Health. 2007;11(2):131–43.
23. Hill L, Roberts G, Wildgoose J, Perkins R, Hahn S. Recovery and person-centred care in dementia: common purpose, common practice? Adv Psychiatr Treat. 2010;16:288–98.
24. Marshall A, Spreadbury J, Cheston R, Coleman P, Ballinger C, Mullee M, Pritchard J, Russell C, Bartlett E. A Pilot Randomised Control trial to compare changes in quality of life for participants with early diagnosis dementia who attend a "Living Well with Dementia" group compared to waiting list control. Aging Ment Health. 2014. doi:10.1080/13607863.2014.954527.
25. Cheston R, Gatting L, Marshall A, Spreadbury J and Coleman P. Markers of Assimilation of Problematic Experiences in Dementia within the LIVDEM project, Dementia: the International Journal of Social Research and Policy. 2015. doi:10.1177/1471301215602473. Published on-line September 2, 2015,
26. Cheston R, Howells L. A feasibility study of translating "Living Well with Dementia" groups into a Primary care IAPT service (innovative practice), Dementia: the International Journal of Social Research and Policy. 2015. doi:10.1177/1471301215582104. Published on-line April 17, 2015.
27. Logsdon RG, et al. Quality of life in Alzheimer's disease: patient and caregiver reports. J Ment Health Aging. 1999;5:21–32.

28. Department of Health. Improving Access to Psychological Therapies (IAPT) commissioning toolkit. London: Department of Health: The Stationery Office; 2008.
29. Turpin G, Richards D, Hope R, Duffy R. Delivering the IAPT programme. Healthc Couns Psychother J. 2008;8(2):2–7.
30. Dodd E, Cheston R, Fear T, Brown E, Fox C, Morley C, Jefferies R, Gray R. An evaluation of primary care led dementia diagnostic services in Bristol. BMC Health Serv Res. 2014;14:592. doi:10.1186/s12913-014-0592-3.
31. Dodd E, Cheston R, Ismail S, Cullum S, Gatting L, Jefferies R, Fear T, Gray R. Primary care led dementia services: themes from families, patients and health professionals. Dement: Int J Soc Res Policy. 2015. doi:10.1177/1471301214566476. First published on January 22, 2015.

'They Are Still the Same as You on the Outside Just a Bit Different on the Inside': Raising Awareness of Dementia Through the School Curriculum

21

Teresa Atkinson and Jennifer Bray

21.1 Introduction

Whilst memory loss is a significant feature of dementia, it is important to remember that people experience dementia in very unique and individual ways. In addition to physical symptoms, people living with dementia can be impacted upon by a range of behavioural and psychological symptoms which are debilitating for the person experiencing them and challenging for those around them, whether in a familial or caring capacity. Behaviour is often misunderstood when it is not considered within the context of a person's individual life history. Following a person-centred approach is therefore an essential part of appreciating someone's identity and identifying the underlying reason for the behaviour.

Maintaining 'personhood' [1] in dementia is key to supporting a person to 'live well'. Whilst this will not alter the physical progression of the disease, it will greatly enhance the quality of life and experiences of a person living with dementia. Warmth, empathy, respect and inclusion of people with dementia all help to maintain personhood and reduce the impact of the secondary symptoms of dementia. Raising awareness of dementia and helping people feel included and connected within their communities has been made a priority in developing dementia-friendly communities [2]. Creating dementia-friendly environments is embodied within current policy [3, 4] and is underpinned by good quality education which dispels myths, challenges stigma and builds confidence, understanding and knowledge.

The Prime Minister's Challenge on Dementia, Intergenerational Schools Project [5] provided an opportunity to explore the impact of introducing dementia awareness into the curriculum. A Pioneer Group of 22 schools across the country was

T. Atkinson, BSc Psy, MSc C.Neuropsychiatry (✉) • J. Bray, BSc French and Mathematics
Association for Dementia Studies, University of Worcester, Worcester, UK
e-mail: t.atkinson@worc.ac.uk; j.bray@worc.ac.uk

invited to take part in the project, with 13 engaging with an evaluation carried out by the Association for Dementia Studies, University of Worcester. In total over 250 primary school pupils aged between 7 and 11, together with over 1,600 secondary/college pupils aged 12–19, provided feedback on the impact of the dementia awareness curriculum.

Each school developed their own bespoke curriculum, resulting in a wide array of different approaches. In primary schools, common approaches included school assemblies, inviting professionals to come and talk to pupils and forming links with local care homes and activity groups. Secondary schools and colleges tended to explore the topic in greater detail by embedding dementia within key subjects such as science, personal social and health education and health and social care. The duration of the interventions varied, with some schools condensing their learning into a series of three to five lessons and others devoting a whole term to the subject.

Evidence from the evaluation demonstrated that regardless of the approach taken, improvements in dementia awareness were seen within every school. Prior to the project, 27 % of primary school pupils and 79 % of secondary/college pupils had heard of dementia. These figures rose to 100 % and 97 %, respectively. Similarly, at the start of the project, only 25 % of primary school pupils felt confident about meeting someone with dementia which rose to 76 % by the end of the interventions. A demonstrable increase in confidence was also seen for secondary/college pupils, with the impact being greater when they were able to meet a person with dementia.

The opportunity to meet someone living with dementia was found to be the most consistent factor impacting upon a young person's confidence, knowledge and understanding of dementia. Through local networking, schools were able to offer opportunities for pupils to meet a person living with dementia and/or their carers and engage in a range of activities. Sometimes these intergenerational activities were one-off opportunities such as visiting a local care home to sing for people with dementia or inviting people with dementia into schools to talk to pupils about their experiences. Other activities offered a deeper and more sustained learning experience where considerable benefits were experienced by all those involved, as illustrated by the following case study.

21.2 Case Study

Sixth form students at a large secondary school in the South of England chose the intergenerational aspect as the primary focus of their dementia awareness curriculum. Working in pairs and supported by a social care professional, students visited a person with dementia over a number of weeks to compile a life story book using personal photographs and pictures from the Internet. Life story work has long been valued as a therapeutic intervention for people with dementia [6].

Over a number of weeks, students were able to become involved in the lives of the people they visited, learning more about their childhood, their occupation as an adult, their wider family, their interests and their hobbies. A celebration tea party was hosted by the school at the end of the project which provided an opportunity for friends and family to come together to see the students present the life story books to the people they had worked with.

Learning from an older generation and working alongside people with dementia had a significant effect on the young people involved. Students were amazed to find that the people with dementia had '*had really interesting lives*' and began to understand the power of helping a person with dementia to recall events:

> Seeing his face when he remembered something he obviously hadn't remembered in quite a while, and when he told us about his late wife, 'cause he got quite worked up about that, […] and that was sad to see, but I was happy he could remember his wife
>
> I think the best thing for me was talking to him and he said […] 'the more I look back, the more I can remember' and he seemed very happy and he looked forward to seeing us every week

Students shared their initial apprehension at the thought of engaging in activities with people with dementia, but were able to reflect on the process and consider how this had helped them to alleviate their 'fear of the unknown':

> [I] was quite scared to meet them in case next time you go they've forgotten who you was (sic), but now that you know how to act with a dementia person it makes it easier

Family carers had also seen the impact of the project on the person with dementia. The son of a lady involved with students in making a life story book shared these thoughts about his experiences:

> Mum had a lovely smile when relating these events and issues. She seemed so much more animated […] whenever Mum looks at the life story book (which is often), she is always absorbed and interested. For my part, as a carer, it helped me to re-engage with Mum as a person, and not just somebody with a disease that needed looking after. It helped me remember the precious memories that can so easily be lost in the day to day routine of caring. It helped me offer a greater dignity and respect to her for all the richness that there is in her life, and to realise that the person hadn't disappeared, but was still there

21.3 Conclusion

Dementia is often shrouded in misconception and ignorance, which can result in people with dementia becoming lonely and isolated. Educating children from an early age about dementia and giving them the opportunity to interact with older adults was found to be key in helping children to engage with the introduction of dementia into their curriculum. Many children spoke of the lesson where they met someone with dementia as 'the best lesson they had ever had'.

There are many ways in which this type of intergenerational activity could be introduced into the curriculum, and there are indications that this would be well received in communities. During the course of the evaluation, it was evident that schools had formed partnerships with willing local care homes in close proximity to their schools. Many housing with care schemes and care homes operate as community hubs, providing a venue to bring together older and younger generations around a shared activity. Holistically, this keeps communities connected, supports informal caregivers, addresses issues of loneliness and helps to develop communities of understanding. Building dementia-friendly communities is reliant upon ensuring we prepare future generations to understand the issues that society faces and to value and respect people of all ages and all abilities. Helping children to overcome their fears of the unknown through good quality education and interactions helps communities to develop, sustain and stay connected.

21.4 Time to Reflect

- Can you think of ways to create links between your local schools and local services for people with dementia?
- Do you know of anyone in your community who would be willing to be involved in helping you to develop a dementia curriculum at your local school?
- What types of interventions could help to improve dementia awareness amongst the younger generations?
- Can you think of opportunities where older and younger generations could come together in a shared activity?
- How could you ensure that links are sustainable?

References

1. Brooker D. Person centred dementia care: making services better. London: Jessica Kingsley Publications; 2007.
2. Alzheimer's Society. Building dementia friendly communities: a priority for everyone. London: Alzheimer's Society; 2013.
3. Department of Health. Living well with dementia: a national dementia strategy. London: The Stationery Office; 2009.
4. Department of Health. The prime minister's challenge on dementia. London: The Stationery Office; 2012.
5. Atkinson T., Bray J. Dementia awareness & intergenerational exchange in schools: final report. 2013. Retrieved from: http://www.worcester.ac.uk/discover/dementia-prime-ministers-challenge-intergenerational-schools-project.html. Accessed 12th Feb 2015.
6. Thompson R. Using life story work to enhance care. Nurs Older People. 2011;23(8):16–21.

Mum and Me, a Journey with Dementia: A Personal Reflection

Jackie Jones and Mo Ray

As I reflect on and write something about our journey, Mum is safe and comfortable and now lives in a nursing home, which works very hard to provide high-quality, person-centred care. She is frail and has complex physical needs and is now deep in dementia. But despite Mum's physical and cognitive frailty, she is still able to express her wish to 'go home'. This is something that causes me great distress and the one thing that I wish I could achieve for her. But at the time of writing, it remains almost impossible to provide the level of care my Mum needs in her own home.

My aims in contributing this chapter are twofold: first, to increase awareness of the experience of living with and caring for someone with dementia and second, to highlight the need for integrated, coordinated dementia care throughout a person's journey in dementia.

When Mum was formally diagnosed with vascular dementia and Alzheimer's in 2008, I had a long-standing successful career as a Senior Manager in a large financial institution. My professional life was hectic and demanding, and I had a busy and enjoyable social life, hobbies and a wide circle of friends. I had always been and remain very close to my mother. She is simply my best friend.

Mum has always been a 'glass-half-full' kind of person – full of energy and zest for life. Her family was central to her life, and she relished being a wife, mother and grandmother. She worked as a school secretary and 'Avon lady' and was a member of various local clubs and groups. She is a loving and caring woman with a natural charisma with people, especially children. Always elegant, she loves to look good and to wear beautiful clothes.

J. Jones (✉)
Stoke-on-Trent, Staffordshire, UK
e-mail: jackiejones280@gmail.com

M. Ray, PhD
Gerontological Social Work and Programme, School of Social Science and Public Policy,
Keele University, Keele, Staffordshire, UK
e-mail: m.g.ray@keele.ac.uk

22.1 Diagnosis

Mum was 74 when she was formally diagnosed with dementia, but in common with many people, I noticed signs that suggested all was not well at least 12 months prior to her diagnosis. She stopped cooking for herself, and looking after the house became unimportant (but Mum still maintained that she did these activities); her finances became muddled, and she persistently lost or misplaced items about the house. I think the difficulties that she was having made her feel different and isolated, and she often commented about how lonely she felt.

The GP recommended referral to a memory clinic which Mum initially refused to consider. In common with many older people, she argued that being a 'bit forgetful' was just part of getting old and was understandably reluctant to talk about her difficulties or have them assessed by a medical team. We were grateful for a supportive and knowledgeable GP who believed that it was important for Mum to be referred and took the time to reassure and encourage her to go for the appointment.

Mum's appointment at the memory clinic was with a clinical psychiatric nurse who involved her in taking a 'Mini-Mental' examination and taking Mum's history. Mum was very alarmed by the referral for a brain scan and needed a lot of reassurance about the process. A few weeks after the appointment, we returned to see the consultant who informed Mum that she had 'mixed dementia', a combination of vascular dementia and Alzheimer's disease. He told us that Mum qualified for Aricept which had the potential – but no guarantees – to slow the halt of the disease. And he told us that there was no cure. We left the consulting room dazed and confused and in tears as we tried to process what we had been told, and Mum tried to comprehend what was wrong with her. What was worse was that we were left in a 'black hole'. The consultant had given Mum a prescription and told us that he would contact her GP and see Mum again in 6 months. That was it. We did not understand what the diagnosis meant, what we should do next or where to go for help or support. So we went home and waited – but of course, we had no idea what it was we were waiting for. Conversation about the diagnosis was difficult, as we did not know what we were facing, and Mum was very frightened.

With the benefit of hindsight and if I could rewrite my mother's experience, being given a diagnosis of dementia would look more like this:

> After the Consultant had explained a little bit about the diagnosis, we were put in touch with a Dementia Care Nurse and given more information about Mum's diagnosis and an opportunity to ask questions. We were given accessible information about where we might go for support (e.g. help lines, information centres) and an initial plan of support or signposts for information for mum was developed and agreed. We were given information about social care and how to make a referral for a social work assessment. The social work assessment would as part of the process, give us information about what kinds of resources were available – for example, day care opportunities, lunch clubs, domiciliary care services, carer support and education and personal budgets. With mum's permission, care plans and key biographical information was kept by the link nurse so that as mum's journey in dementia progressed, important information was known about her and we did not have to spend hours of our lives repeating information and mum did not have to cope with the indignity of not always being able to answer questions about key information. I was given help by the social worker and/or link nurse about caring for mum and what I might expect.

In my experience, many – but not all – of the professionals who were involved with us focused on their area of expertise and either could not or would not acknowledge a wider, complex picture that was emerging as Mum's symptoms became more complex. There was so much to do as a carer of someone whose cognitive capacities were declining and who was also in poor physical health. Figure 22.1 shows how many agencies and people were involved in Mum's care and support – and who we had to relate to during Mum's dementia journey. Medical appointments, changing care needs and financial and legal issues – the list seemed endless and I rarely felt that I knew what I was doing, what I should do first or where I should go for help. Most of the time, especially in the months following Mum's diagnosis, I was trying to work it out alone. Unfortunately Mum and I learnt the hard way, and the coordination and integration of Mum's care was one of the greatest personal challenges I have ever faced. Mum was rapidly losing capacity, and I felt and, indeed was, responsible for her future.

From my perspective and experience, the emotional consequences of a diagnosis of dementia are also critically important and can be easily overlooked. For Mum the emotional consequences of living with uncertainty, growing communication difficulties, declining memory and challenges with everyday tasks that had once been commonplace were all too evident. For me, it was hard to accept that the roles between Mum and her daughter were reversing. And I had no idea in the months following Mum's diagnosis what a tough, life-changing experience this was going to be.

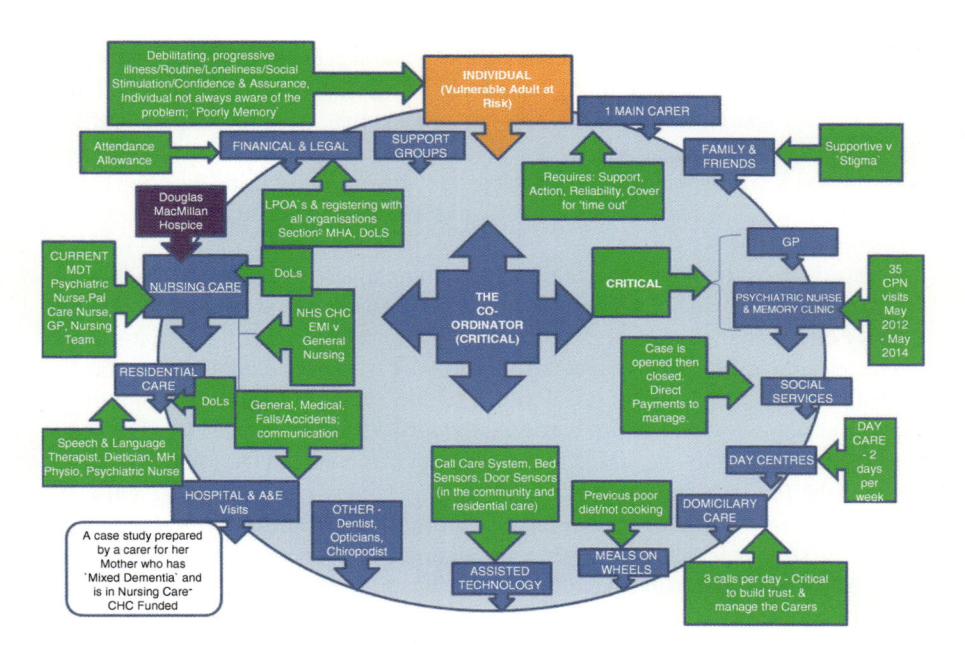

Fig. 22.1 The team and interventions required for J's care

22.2 Supporting Mum at Home

Following her diagnosis, Mum lived at home for 3.5 years. In common with many people living with dementia, her major struggles initially focused on coping with everyday activities such as cooking, maintaining a decent diet and taking medicine. Socially and emotionally, loneliness and her sense of intense isolation was a very serious worry and impacted on her mood and well-being.

In response to Mum feeling lonely and isolated, I managed to find out about day centres. I applied for her to attend although at the time, I was very unsure whether she would even consider going. In common with most things that I tried to put in place at the time, the application process seemed impenetrably mysterious and lengthy. I applied and Mum was being put on a waiting list. When a place was eventually offered, I was delighted and relieved that Mum immediately enjoyed going to the Centre. In fact, she blossomed and her sense of well-being and motivation improved. It seemed to reignite and keep her spirit alive – I think largely because she had a purpose and some structure to her week and she felt valued too. Prior to going to the day Centre and after diagnosis, it was as if she was in limbo – at home and waiting – for what we were unsure about. At the Centre she was able to engage again with going out on trips, playing social games, singing and dancing, baking and enjoying the company of others. The Centre developed a communication book, which summarised what Mum had done during the day. This excellent practice meant that we were able to participate in conversations to support, reinforce and extend the sense of well-being and achievement she experienced after being at the Centre. It provided a valuable and important opportunity for conversation that Mum led and actively participated in.

At about the same time, I was advised to make a referral to social services to request an assessment to see if any help could be offered to support Mum with personal care, preparing food and taking her medication. Our first experience of a social work visit was not positive. It seemed that the social worker's main purpose was to fill in a pile of forms which she set about achieving by firing questions at me while Mum was left out the conversation and was effectively separated from what was going on.

I was dismayed by our experience and so complained about the approach of the social worker. The social service team did send a new social worker that had an entirely different approach. She spoke directly with Mum and showed that she was interested in who she was – especially her love of gardening and about her family. Over time, the social worker developed a relationship with Mum and introduced support at home – which Mum was initially very reluctant to consider. The social worker had the skill to encourage Mum to accept help while at the same time ensuring that she felt involved. I realise that it is increasingly rare to have a continuous relationship with a social worker, but we did for 4 years until Mum moved into a care home. It was invaluable in terms of continuity of support from someone who knew Mum and could understand therefore when there were changes in Mum's condition and how best to respond. Her presence over 3 years was an important lifeline.

Even with the assistance of a capable and committed social worker, nothing seemed straightforward. Undertaking a financial assessment meant that I had to be present as the assessor needed information about Mum's income, savings and bank accounts – which she could not have managed on her own. A personal budget was allocated which I had to manage and necessitated opening a separate bank account and keeping records of all transactions and receipts. I was also responsible for paying the carers and for Mum's meals service and day care, which was another significant task to add to my growing list. While in many ways the skills I needed were second nature to me, awareness of the challenge of managing new roles and responsibilities was rarely acknowledged by health and social care professionals.

It took a good while to establish support at home. Mum hated having strangers in her house and disliked the implication that she could no longer cope alone. To try and support Mum and make things work, I took a week off work when care started. I found carers coming into Mum's house several times a day strange, uncomfortable and not what I really wanted for her. But there was no choice, and if my aim was to support Mum to remain in her own home, then we had to give it a go.

Establishing routines that reflected Mum's preferences and the way she preferred to do things was crucial for success. This helped her to feel that what she wanted was still important, and the more familiar care support felt to her, the more comfortable she was with it. Eventually, we developed routines for everything. It helped Mum to feel safe and secure about where she was in the day and what was happening at specific times of the day. Initially, when Mum could process written information, we used 'Post It' notes as reminders. We had a family organiser diary with everything that Mum needed to know prominently displayed on the wall. If Mum forgot anything, she would telephone me, and I could direct her over the telephone as to where something was or where a reminder was written down. I was conscious that I wanted her to be able to do what she could for herself, and I did not want to take any part in taking her independence away.

Mum has always taken great pride in her appearance and is an elegant and stylish lady. It was difficult to see therefore when she put on odd shoes or her clothes did not match. The carers played a huge role in supporting her to achieve and maintain her presentation and to manage everyday tasks. Changes in routine though could cause considerable stress and extra effort to sort out. If, for example, Mum was prescribed antibiotics, this threw the medication routine. Antibiotics were not in the pre-prepared medication pack, so this meant trying to get authorisation for a carer to supervise Mum taking from the pack or a neighbour calling, or it meant me driving over to give Mum her medication. Managing Mum's medication felt almost impossible at times and, as her needs became more complex, continued to be a significant challenge in the journey of Mum's care.

Care at home was vitally important in supporting Mum with basic activities of daily living. But there was a lot to do besides to ensure that Mum's life ran smoothly. Tasks such as gardening, changing bed linen, washing and ironing are rarely provided by care services. As a lifelong gardener, it caused Mum distress if her garden was not tidy. These issues might not appear of importance to health and social care that tend to focus on 'life and limb' but to someone's sense of identity, or to preserve their well-being – they are often centrally important. It cannot be acceptable for a person living with dementia to have to accept that gardens become overgrown, clothing is not washed and homes are not cleaned. I managed to find a gardener to cut lawns and a friend who provided some housework and laundry every Friday. This visit became an important part of Mum's week, and a warm and positive relationship was established. I would visit and go on outings with Mum at the weekend. Overall, the routine of day care, meals on wheels, carers, my input provided a structure which supported Mum to remain at home and I believe that overall, Mum had a good quality of life and managed well for the best part of almost 4 years.

22.3 Change and Uncertainty

By autumn 2011, I could see a profound change in Mum's health, and at a routine appointment at the Memory Clinic, I was warned of changes in her condition. The clinical psychiatric nurse felt that Mum's condition was progressing, and a few months later, she experienced a significant stepped change. A multidisciplinary meeting was held, and it was agreed that we should proactively increase the support that Mum was given. The domiciliary care service was increased to four calls a day, and bed and door sensors were put in place to minimise the risk of leaving the house during the night (although this never happened).

Within 6 weeks of the increase in support and as a result of vascular change, Mum went to her neighbours and reported concerns that people were trying to harm her. There followed months of Mum experiencing delusions and hallucinations which was distressing for her and for us all. The social worker and psychiatric nurse debated at length what should happen to Mum – was it a 'health issue' or a 'care issue'? Eventually, it was agreed that Mum would be admitted to respite care.

In the 4 weeks that Mum spent in respite care, her condition declined beyond what I thought was possible. She did not know where she was and what had happened to her and so was afraid and fearful. She stopped eating, lost weight, wandered around the building and was highly emotional and anxious. She frequently attempted to leave the building and was very fearful and angry. After 4 weeks, Mum was admitted to the hospital under Section Two of the Mental Health Act. It was unplanned and happened suddenly with no coordination or liaison and was a very traumatic experience for Mum and for her family. But it was also a relief that she might be somewhere which was safe and where she could be properly assessed.

After 7 weeks in the hospital, the 'Care at Home' team assessed Mum to establish if she could return home. Mum begged to go home, and all viable options were explored to see if it could be achieved. With great sadness, I had to accept that there were no viable ways that this could be achieved with current care and support arrangements and in light of Mum's cognitive impairments. It was agreed that she needed to move to a residential care home. Once again I faced the prospect of finding care for someone I love very much, with very little help or assistance – other than a booklet with a list of registered care homes. How would I know what counted as a 'good' care home and how could I know whether a care home would be able to provide the care and support my mother needed? I soon found as I started visiting countless homes that there are vast variations in the standards of care homes.

In the absence of any other help, I applied the principle that if I was to consider a care home suitable for Mum, then it had to be somewhere that I would stay myself. I also tried to get beyond the 'look' of the place to understand how care was provided. I struggled to find an appropriate setting in the time we had available, but eventually, I found a somewhere close to my own home and Mum moved there from hospital. But, she longed for her home and did not settle. She often felt agitated and worried and responded aggressively to carers – largely I think because she was afraid of what was happening to her and the difficulties in coping with the huge changes she had experienced. Life became punctuated by visits from the CPN (18 times in 10 months), uncertainty as Mum's medical needs became more complex including seizures, a low heart rate, infections and falling. Medical care became more complex and involved more people. Mum lost her mobility following a severe infection and was unable to eat and drink adequately resulting in yet more weight loss. It was evident that the care home was not sufficiently trained or resourced to cope with Mum's needs, and it was confirmed that she needed to move to a nursing home.

A multidisciplinary meeting was convened to discuss my mother's care, and it was agreed that an application could be considered for continuing health care. I made a call to social services to request a social worker to be present as Mum was not self-funding. It took over a week of increasingly desperate calls to get any kind of response. Subsequently, I was faced with trying to find a suitable nursing home for Mum, but had no idea if she was likely to be funded under continuing health care or not. It felt as if the clock was ticking as Mum was very poorly and her needs were not being met in the care home – but nor was it considered to be in her best interests to go to hospital.

I experienced applying for continuing healthcare funding as a difficult, challenging and lengthy process. Apart from the intellectual challenge of preparing evidence against 12 assessment domains, at a personal and emotional level, it forced me to face the changes in my Mum's condition over the past year. It took 2 days to produce our contribution, and it feels to me, that for many people, the process is too difficult both practically and emotionally. Mum was awarded continuing healthcare funding, and I eventually found a nursing home that I thought would give good care. But we hit an obstacle because I had found a general nursing home rather than a so-called, 'EMI' registered home. As a result, two further psychiatric assessments were required in order to confirm that Mum's physical needs had superseded her mental health needs. I managed to achieve this alongside being deeply concerned about my mother's deteriorating health. The level of coordination and commitment that seemed to be required personally from me escalated to unmanageable levels.

Mum was transferred to a nursing setting in February 2013. My Mum currently remains at this nursing setting, and at the time of writing, a continuing healthcare review is imminent. This is another stressful date in the care calendar that continues to shape my life. Mum is now in the late stages of her illness; she needs care and support in all aspects of her day-to-day life. She has severe cognitive decline; her behaviour remains unpredictable and at times challenges those around her. She has multiple complex needs, including swallowing difficulties, and her nutritional needs remain compromised. A multidisciplinary team consisting of me, the GP, the nurses at the home, the psychiatric nurse, speech and language specialist and the palliative care nurse work to try to ensure the best quality of life for Mum that is possible under difficult circumstances.

I spend as much time as I can with her and try to keep life as normal as possible in a situation that is heart breaking to witness. Occasionally there is a good day; Mum may have more lucid moments, and there is sometimes an opportunity to get her up for a few hours. I read to her, talk to her and spend time helping her eat, and we both sing to endless songs she loves.

22.4 Summary

As you read this, you may be thinking that overall, my Mum has received good care. You would be right. But it is also the case that I have had to fight to get what is needed for Mum. I have had to use all of my negotiation, communication and facilitation skills. I have had to challenge at times, to complain when it has been necessary and to use my advocacy skills to ensure as best as I can that my Mum remains central and that decisions about her care are more about her than they are about what might be convenient or expedient. My role became project manager, relationship manager, influencer, challenger, and decision maker of all care issues, but I remain – above all – her daughter. While I believe that I know my Mum very well and have done my best to advocate for her, at the time of her diagnosis, I knew nothing about health and social care services or mental health services. Of course, I have learned a lot over the past years. But it would be a mistake to think that my exposure to complex and, at times, impenetrable care pathways increased my resilience to the personal pain and the emotional consequences of witnessing Mum's despair and fear as her health and cognition declined.

The key question I have continued to ask myself throughout the journey is as follows: 'was the care and support Mum received person centred, integrated and coordinated to the best it could be? And what would have happened to Mum if she hadn't got me?' The answer is that the care was not coordinated. The system is complex, and navigating a pathway is difficult; there isn't a roadmap with clear signposting at present. Figure 23.1 illustrates every intervention Mum received on her journey. We lived through endless assessments, visits and interventions from various sources and endless repetitions of the same information but to different people – who often did not seem to know anything about my mother.

The care Mum receives is good, but it is what everyone living with dementia should receive – but in a more seamless, effective and integrated way. There should not be the need for 'a me' to coordinate everything. I remain troubled by the people living with complex dementia who do not have anyone who are able to negotiate 'the system' or to advocate for their best interests to be upheld. We must make it easier for people who lose their capacity and their carers and supporters to experience the care in a way that everyone deserves to have in a way which preserves identity and dignity.

If you are a carer or you have cared for someone in the past with dementia, then you will probably recognise much of what I have said. Some people, unfamiliar with dementia, say to me 'it's not your Mum'; well, my response is 'yes it is'. There is something left. Mum is still Mum, and when I turn up to visit, I believe she still knows who I am. On days where she is lucid and alert, she gives me a look as if to say 'I know you, you're my daughter', and if I say, 'I love you Mum', she will say 'you too'.

22.5 Reflection

How can primary care services contribute to providing timely and integrated support to people diagnosed with dementia and their families?

How can health and social care services demonstrate that they take proper account of the best interests of people living with dementia in care decisions when they do not have supporters or carers available?

How might services work together better to avoid people with dementia and their carers repeating information to separate agencies and workers over lengthy periods of time?

What would appropriate support after diagnosis look like to you?

Role of Specialist Care in Dementia

Chris Fox, Andrea Hilton, Ken Laidlaw,
Jochen René Thyrian, Ian Maidment,
and David G. Smithard

There are 835,000 people in the UK who have dementia [1] at an annual cost to the UK economy of £26 billion. Most people with dementia live in the community with one in three living alone at home [2] with much of the care being met by unpaid carers [3]. Seventy percent of care home residents have dementia [1].

Dementia is an umbrella term that covers a multitude of diagnoses and problems from vascular dementia through to Alzheimer's disease via the fronto-temporal dementia and Lewy body disease.

Specialist care has a critical role in supporting primary care's role in management. Specialist care includes old age psychiatry, geriatric medicine and neurology.

C. Fox, MB, BS, Mmedsci, MRCPsych MD (✉)
Department of Clinical Psychology, Norwich Medical School, Norwich, Norfolk, UK
e-mail: Chris.Fox@uea.ac.uk

A. Hilton, BPharm (Hons), MSc, PhD
Faculty of Health and Social Care, University of Hull, Hull, UK
e-mail: a.hilton@hull.ac.uk

K. Laidlaw, MA (Hons), MPhil., PhD, C.Psychol.
Department of Clinical Psychology, Faculty of Medicine and Health Sciences,
Norwich Medical School, University of East Anglia, Norwich, UK

J.R. Thyrian, PhD, Dipl-Psych
Site Rostock/Greifswald, German Center for Neurodegenerative Diseases (DZNE),
Greifswald, Germany
e-mail: rene.thyrian@dzne.de

I. Maidment, PhD
School of Life and Health Sciences, Aston University, Birmingham, UK
e-mail: i.maidment@aston.ac.uk

D.G. Smithard, BSc, MBBS, MD, FRCP
Department of Clinical Gerontology, King's College Hospital NHS Foundation Trust,
Princess Royal University Hospital, Farnborough, Kent, UK
e-mail: david.smithard@nhs.net

In addition non-medical specialties have a significant role. These include community psychiatric nurses, occupational therapists, psychologists and pharmacists. Physiotherapy and speech and language therapists can be a part of management and assessment. In this chapter we will describe the role of specialist care in dementia. There is no one model that fits the care pathways in dementia, and some of the collaborative models will be described.

23.1 Mental Health Care in Dementia

In the last 20 years, there have been changes in mental health services in dementia with expansion of multidisciplinary teams. Typical services for dementia in mental health are organised around a memory service, which functions to diagnose and treat patients and then signpost to other services.

Memory services do vary in structure and there is a national accreditation scheme in the UK (http://www.rcpsych.ac.uk/workinpsychiatry/qualityimprovement/qualityandaccreditation/memoryservices/memoryservicesaccreditation/msnapstandards.aspx).

Typically, patients are referred by primary care, less commonly by cross referral and in some centres can self-refer.

The changes in care have been brought about by the development of cognitive enhancer medications (of which there are 4 – donepezil, rivastigmine, galantamine and memantine) and innovation in psychological approaches. With the availability of generic medications in dementia, the role of primary care has been expanding [4]. In addition, there have been restrictions levied on psychotropic medications due to adverse effects in people with dementia, for example, stroke risk with antipsychotic usage.

Mental health services in dementia include old age psychiatry, community and inpatient psychiatric nurses, occupational therapists, psychology, support workers and social workers.

Specialist mental health services in dementia are primarily delivered in the community. In addition, there are day centres/hospitals in some services. For the more severe cases, there are inpatient services.

Diagnostic services are usually delivered by some form of memory assessment service so-called memory clinic [5]. However, these are sometimes delivered by neurologists and geriatrician more commonly in some healthcare systems, for example, the USA.

23.1.1 Psychological Approaches to Dementia Care

Mental health professionals have many contributions to the assessment, care and management of people with dementia and also to the support provided to dementia caregivers. Psychologists have an important role in neuropsychological assessment of dementia, and this is a highly specialised skill. The different dementias

(Alzheimer's, vascular, Lewy body, frontotemporal, etc.) may have a different neuropsychological profile [6–9]. It may be useful to take account of potential differences when working with people with dementia, but this is a very complex and challenging area for non-specialists.

Any dementia is likely to have a number of different consequences for the person with dementia and for those who care for them. There are obviously different dementias with different consequences for each individual and at different stages in the person's journey with dementia.

23.1.2 BPSD

In terms of behavioural and psychological symptoms of dementia (BPSD), mental health has a key role to play in working with informal and formal carers when dealing with behaviours that challenge in dementia. Behaviours that challenge cause significant distress to carers and can often result in a breakdown in care arrangements [10]. The first-line approach to treatment is recommended as nonpharmacological, because the potential benefits of antipsychotics are outweighed by the adverse effects evident from general use [11].

Understanding behaviour as having different functions for every individual psychologists, a key part of mental health services for dementia, has developed different ways of helping carers understand and respond appropriately to behaviour. Cohen-Mansfield and colleagues understand challenging behaviour in dementia as indicating an unmet need [12]. In the case of understanding a person with behaviour considered to be challenging in dementia, a psychological formulation-led individualised approach augments standard functional analytic approaches [10] by focusing on the person and the range of factors impacting upon them. As people with dementia may not be able to directly communicate their stress and distress in environments in many cases that are not under the direct control of an individual with dementia, individualised formulation-led interventions are going to be essential in order to meet the needs of the person with dementia [13].

Distress in Dementia Caregivers

Most care for people with dementia is provided within the family [14]. Strong evidence for psychological approaches (e.g. cognitive behaviour therapy, CBT) for dementia caregivers exists with a number of systematic reviews demonstrating that CBT is an efficacious approach [15–17].

Overall, the evidence for dementia caregiving suggests interventions are more effective when they are active rather than passive. While psychoeducation improves subjective wellbeing, it is effective in reducing distress *only* if it is active. CBT works best when used for more focal targets such as reducing caregiver depression and burden. As dementia is a deteriorating condition, interventions focused on one target may be less effective overall, and this is reflected in findings that only structured multicomponent interventions are effective in reducing and delaying institutionalisation [18].

Psychological Approaches for People with Dementia

Psychological therapists have often shied away from working with older people with dementia as they assume that such clients will be unable to engage in the process of therapy; however, this is disempowering of individuals and is contrary to the ethos of CBT. Many people diagnosed with dementia in the early stages will retain enough insight and capacity to engage in therapy as long as simple adjustments are made by the therapists to accommodate to any mild memory or communication difficulties [18].

At the post-diagnosis stage in the experience of dementia, there may be lot that an individual can benefit from psychological therapy as they come to terms with the implications of their diagnosis. CBT is especially appropriate with older people diagnosed with dementia because it is a structured problem-focused, present-oriented, evidence-based treatment making it straightforward to use, as well as effective in building coping strategies and skills that are empowering for individuals who are faced with challenges of living well with dementia.

Inspiration for tailoring CBT interventions for those with dementia can be drawn from CBT for chronic physical health conditions. Central to CBT for people with chronic health conditions is the concept that it is the individual's appraisal of their experience rather than the experience itself that is important in understanding how well they cope with an event. This is a standard concept in CBT. It is not the situation per se that causes an individual's problems; it is the personal meaning attached to the situation that determines its impact. In this way, two individuals may experience similar situations and report markedly different emotional responses. An individual's illness-related beliefs and illness-related behaviours are also likely to be important. How one views dementia will influence one's behaviour in response. Depressive attributions about how an individual with dementia characterises their problems may also be a useful focus for CBT interventions [19]. Thus, if an individual attributes all memory, reasoning or communication failures to the onset of dementia symptoms, this may be an overgeneralisation that may undermine an individual's self-confidence. Although people living with dementia have to deal with realistic challenges, nonetheless, individuals can endorse many unhelpful or erroneous cognitions that may make living with dementia much more difficult.

When working with people with dementia, there may be important data to be derived from understanding how an individual reacts in response to actual or real memory failings. A disproportionate reaction may leave an individual feeling more diminished as a competent person, and this may have an adverse approach on a person's cognition, affect and behaviour.

Evidence for the efficacy of CBT in anxiety and depression in dementia comes mainly from a range of small intriguing clinical trials and case studies. Mohlman and Gorman [20] note that treatment outcome for CBT for anxiety disorder can be compromised when clients have executive dysfunction (i.e. specific cognitive deficits in planning organising and reasoning abilities). If attention-training and enhanced self-monitoring in therapy are used to augment CBT, deficits can be overcome and enhanced treatment outcome achieved [20]. The evidence base for CBT interventions for people with anxiety or depression in dementia is summarised in Table 23.1.

Table 23.1 Table of psychological therapy for depression and anxiety in dementia, executive dysfunction and varying levels of cognitive impairment

Author(s)	Primary focus	Design	Intervention	Results
Teri et al. [21]	Depression in dementia	Open trial of 'Seattle Protocols'	22 BT and 19 control (this is intern report for Teri et al. 1997)	Treatment took place over 9 weekly sessions of BT (including carers in the intervention). 68 % of carers reported as clinically depressed at start. 20/22 PwD improved and carers' wellbeing also shows improvement. No change evident in W/L control group
Teri et al. [21]	Depression in dementia	Controlled trial	72 dyads: BT-PE, BT-PS, TAU and W/L. CGs involved actively	Both active treatments more effective in reducing depression than TAU or W/L. 60 % of participants in active BT conditions improved, whereas 70 % in TAU and W/L show no improvement. Carer's depression also improved significantly even though this was not directly targeted. Changes in depression in carers and PwD maintained at 6 months follow-up
Koder [23]	Anxiety disorder in dementia	Single cases CBT	2 cases	Two single cases of 82-year-old males with depression and anxiety. Treatment involved carers and positive effects were reported in both cases. Treatment was structured and time-limited in both cases
Scholey and Woods [24]	Depression in dementia	Single cases CBT	7 single cases	All participants met diagnostic criteria for depression and dementia. Individualised CBT protocol used without apparent difficulty. Overall significant difference in outcome in mood over treatment. 2/7 participants evidencing clinically significant improvement in mood using standardised mood scales (e.g. Beck Depression Inventory; BDI, Geriatric Depression Scale; GDS)
Walker [25]	Depression in dementia	Single case CBT	1 single case	71-year-old male living with spousal carer, both demoralised at intake. Treatment nonresponsive to ADM. Couple seen together for 16 sessions of CBT. At end of Tx and 12-month follow-up, cognition improved (MMSE) and anxiety improved (GHQ 32 at b/l, reduced to 5 at follow-up)

(continued)

Table 23.1 (continued)

Author(s)	Primary focus	Design	Intervention	Results
Burns et al. [26]	Depression in dementia	RCT	20 psychodynamic interpersonal therapy vs 20 TAU	While participants reported positive attitudes towards psychotherapy, there were no positive outcomes on any of the main domains of interest. Psychodynamic psychotherapy does not appear efficacious although treatment length (6 sessions) in this study is very short for this type of intervention
Carreira et al. [27]	Depression in varying levels of CI	Subgroup analysis of large RCT	52 participants with CI randomly compared IPT (35) to supportive clinical management (18)	The cognitively impaired participants receiving monthly IPT sessions fared better than participants receiving support clinical management. This surprising finding was contrasted with non-CI participants receiving the same interventions, and there was no difference. IPT seems to have potential as an efficacious psychotherapy with people with depression and cognitive impairment
Kraus et al. [28]	Anxiety in dementia	Single cases	7 cases	Treatment emphasises active self-monitoring by the clients (i.e. keeping a notebook handy to remember and monitor homework tasks, use of checklists to remain oriented to task and time). Emphasis on behavioural rather than cognitive change. Specific strategies used to enhance recall such as use of cues and other retrieval-based strategies
Kiosses et al. [29]	Depression in dementia	RCT (interim data)	15 PATH vs 15 ST	12-week home-delivered PATH (problem adaptation therapy); a behavioural problem-solving treatment was compared to 12 weeks of supportive therapy (ST) for people with depression in dementia. Carers actively involved in treatment. PATH participants reported 51 % greater improvement in depression compared to those allocated to ST

Table 23.1 (continued)

Author(s)	Primary focus	Design	Intervention	Results
Paukert et al. [30]	Anxiety in dementia	Open trial	9 intervention, 7 complete Tx	Six-month treatment with weekly session for first 12 weeks followed by telephone sessions. Carers active participants in treatment. Most participants reduced anxiety and depression, and carers concerns about PwD reduced over treatment
Arean et al. [31]; Alexopolous et al. [32]	Depression in executive dysfunction	RCT	110 problem-solving therapy (PST), 111 ST	Participants recorded moderately severe levels of depression and mild-to-moderate levels of ED. Randomly allocated to 12 weekly sessions of either ST or PST (a version of CBT focussing on problem-solving). Participants reported reduction in depression symptoms for both treatments. At week 12 (end of Tx), PST > ST (46 % vs 28 %) in terms of remission and response. No follow-up at end of Tx
Spector et al. [33]	Anxiety in dementia	RCT	25 CBT, 25 TAU	Randomly allocated to receive either CBT or treatment as usual (TAU). CBT participants reported reduction in anxiety and depression symptoms not experienced by participants in receipt of TAU. Gains maintained at 6 months after follow-up with CBT participants alone in reporting improvement in their relationships

From Laidlaw [18] with permission
ADM antidepressant medication, *BT* behaviour therapy, *BT-PE* behaviour therapy with psychoeducation, *BT-PS* behaviour therapy with problem solving, *CBT* cognitive behavioural therapy, *CI* cognitive impairment, *ED* executive dysfunction, *GAD* generalised anxiety disorder, *IPT* interpersonal psychotherapy, *PST* problem-solving therapy, *RCT* randomised-controlled trial, *ST* supportive therapy (counselling), *TAU* treatment as usual

23.2 Geriatrician

There is a considerable overlap between the geriatrician and the old age psychiatrist. As many as 50 % of older people with physical illness will have issues with recall and memory. For some, this will be little more than an irritation for others; it will indicate a more serious and underlying problem. Dementia or cognitive problems have been recognised as one of the geriatric giants for many years.

Older people with dementia may present to the geriatrician in a number of ways. These include an outpatient referral for diagnosis, a referral where the dementia is a comorbidity or a delirium or other acute or elective medical problem complicated by the presence of dementia. The role of the geriatrician is to exclude possible organic disease that may be the underlying aetiological factor and help the old age psychiatrist or general practitioner identify pseudodementia (hypothyroidism, metabolic disorders or depression).

Acute medical services are, at times, used as a service of last resort in an emergency to provide a place of safety. This is usual in the situation where there has been an exacerbation of the dementia by delirium or deterioration in behaviour due to disease progression or stress resulting in behavioural problems.

Delirium is increasingly common in older people with 60 % of those in post acute settings (including care homes) and 53 % of those in hospital, and failure to recognise delirium or consider the diagnosis can be fatal. People with dementia are 6–11 times more likely to develop delirium. It is the role of the geriatrician to recognise the presence of delirium and then to seek its cause. Increasing frailty, medication changes, constipation, urinary retention and a previous episode of dementia are some of the predisposing factors [34].

In this situation the geriatrician has to be able to recognise the underlying problem and work with the multidisciplinary team (including liaison psychiatry). Once the problem has been identified, not only must the aetiological factors need to be managed, but consequences also need to be recognised and managed. People may not have eaten or drunk for many hours or days, medication may not have been taken and the agitation and risk of harm need to be managed [24–36].

Behavioural and psychological symptoms of dementia (BPSD) or disturbed behaviour in the context of dementia will occur in over 90 % of people with dementia at some stage. The important role of the geriatrician is to recognise the underlying cause of the change in behaviour. The problem may again range from constipation and pain to a silent organic medical problem such as a myocardial infarction.

People with dementia are not only found on the acute medical wards, but are frequently occupying surgical beds, either due to the bed situation or because they have undergone surgery. The geriatrician is required to provide a liaison service to support the surgeons in the appropriate management of people with dementia.

Geriatric services also provide a liaison service to work with old age psychiatry to provide a medical input into the inpatient service to provide holistic care to review and manage any comorbid medical conditions [35].

Many older people live in care homes. Staffs in residential homes, in particular, are often poorly trained in dementia care, even if the primary focus of the home is dementia care. The geriatrician with the old age psychiatrist and the general practitioner need to work together to ensure appropriate management plans are in place to prevent inappropriate transfers of care.

People with dementia face repeated episodes of transfer of care to hospital from their care home or own home as the dementia deteriorates. There is a need to make an assessment of the appropriate treatment/management so as not to increase suffering unnecessarily. Close working with primary care, psychiatry and care homes are required to ensure that appropriate anticipatory care plans are agreed and put into place. The PEACE documentation [37] and Gold Standards Framework [38] are examples of good practice. There needs to be a clinical recognition that a refusal to eat and drink may be part of the terminal decline and may be complicated by dysphagia. When dysphagia occurs resorting to enteral feeding is an inappropriate response. Carers need to be supported and encouraged to use oral feeding, recognising that this is a risk, but will provide comfort to the person with dementia.

Geriatricians access community nurses, physiotherapists, occupational therapists and speech and language therapists across the care pathway. They should also have links to old age psychiatry and neurology.

23.3 Collaborative Care as a Bridge Between Primary and Secondary Care

Optimising medical treatment in primary care for people with dementia needs integrative approach with specialists.

The underlying challenges in providing good medical care to people with dementia are similar across nations. The complexity of treatment and care needs cooperation between different professions and stakeholders. Amongst the tasks to be considered, medication management and drug safety plays an important role. For example, it has been reported that the incidence of hospitalisation in Germany due to potentially inadequate medication is 3,25 % with 205 of these being avoidable [39]. The action plan to improve drug safety in Germany (www.ap-amts.de) highlights interdisciplinarity and the knowledge of the entire medication are the key components of successful pharmaceutical treatment. However, in reality, each patient gets prescriptions from a variety of different physician specialists and is provided these medications by different pharmacies. There is no structural interface between those, so that potentially inadequate medication (Pim) and drug-related problems (DRP) are common. There has been the call for cooperation, for example, in the guideline 'multimedication' (www.pmvforschungsgruppe.de). In Germany, the general physician (GP) can serve as a gatekeeper for patients in primary care and the local pharmacies are well prepared to deliver their share in medication management. Since 2012, in Germany, medication management is part of the pharmacy rules of operation.

An innovative concept to overcome these interface problems is currently evaluated in the DelpHi trial following a successful US trial [40, 41], a cluster-randomised, population-based intervention trial. A dementia care manager (DCM), a specifically qualified nurse, is the function that is integrated into the healthcare system. The DCM works GP-based, with the GP screening patients for cognitive impairments and upon identification providing the DCM. The DCM visits the patient at home and amongst other topics conducts an extensive medication analysis. Using a computer system, the DCM scans the barcodes of all medication present in the patients' household. The DCM notes medication plans, dosage, frequency, storage and adherence problems, according to a systematic assessment tool [42]. This information is summarised and given to the local pharmacist for evaluation, when the pharmacist participates in the study. For all other patients, the role of the pharmacist is provided by study pharmacists. They evaluate the medication plan, check for potentially inappropriate medication, drug-related problems and drug-drug interactions and provide pharmaceutical recommendations. This is done in a standardised way, and the DCM summarises the pharmacist's evaluation into a recommendation letter to the GP. The recommendation letter to the GP is basis for planning further treatment and care for the patient and is discussed between GP and DCM with the GP being able to delegate tasks to the DCM. Thus the GP is able to base his decision on systematically assessed and evaluated information and modifies pharmacotherapy and/or drug administration. The DCM, however, monitors the changes and is able to give feedback to the GP frequently. Results so far indicate that the structured and computer-supported assessment improves the identification of needs [43], however, not restricted or limited to medication. The interaction between GP and pharmacist has improved without adding too much on the work load on either profession. The function of a DCM is perceived as support and preliminary analysis shows an effect on medication as well.

The NHS has recently been piloted and was found unsustainable, and there was a need to redefine the role of case managers and better targeting of which people with dementia could benefit from collaborative care [44].

23.4 Role of Pharmacy in Dementia Care

23.4.1 Role of Community Pharmacists

Community pharmacists are amongst the most accessible healthcare professionals, on high-streets countrywide, and therefore could play a key role in supporting people with dementia and their family carers. It is acknowledged that community pharmacists are an underutilised resource; according to the NHS confederation, the 'NHS has historically undervalued the role that community pharmacists can play in improving and maintaining the public's health' [45]. However, as highlighted by Gidman et al. in a research conducted in Scotland, awareness of community pharmacists' extended roles is low [46]. The NHS is promoting community pharmacy with campaigns such as 'feeling under the weather' and in the report 'urgent and emergency care review' – 'we can capitalise on the untapped potential, and convenience, that greater utilisation of the skills and expertise of the pharmacy workforce can offer' [47].

Family carers are commonly housebound and home delivery services offered by community pharmacists can be valuable. Community pharmacists have a key role in supporting appropriate self-medication by people with dementia. Many over-the-counter (OTC) medicines possess anticholinergic activity and should therefore be avoided in people with dementia [48]. There are a number of OTC medicines including Souvenaid and ginkgo products, which may improve memory, and community pharmacists are in an ideal position to advise people with dementia and older people, more generally, on the use of such products. The community pharmacist may be the healthcare professional that the family carer and person with dementia have most regular contact with. Community pharmacists can provide medicines use reviews (MURs). MURs are structured reviews for patients on multiple medications especially those patients who have a long-term condition [49].

Comorbidity is common in people with dementia, and community pharmacists can have a key role in supporting safe and effective management of medication both for the dementia and for any comorbidities [50]. However, preliminary evidence suggests that family carers, who commonly take on responsibility for medication management as the dementia progresses, lack appropriate support and find medication management challenging [51]. More research is needed on how community pharmacists can support family carers, including the usefulness of domiciliary visits that could include a medication review.

23.4.2 Medication Management Dementia Care Pathways

Pharmacists (community, secondary care, interface and prescribing support) all have roles to play in producing organisational and trust guidelines. Pharmacists are involved in drug and therapeutic committees (DTC). These committees are responsible amongst other things for improving drug use and evaluating drugs for the formulary list. Interface pharmacists provide the link between secondary and primary care, particularly around medication which may have a shared care protocol. These may be medications which started in secondary care and continue to be prescribed by general practitioners, for example, acetylcholinesterase inhibitors. The role of the clinical commissioning groups (CCG) pharmacists can involve, for example, cost-effective prescribing, medicines optimisation and many other aspects.

23.4.3 Specialist Pharmacy Services

Specialist pharmacy services are generally provided by pharmacy staff employed by mental health organisations and include both pharmacists and pharmacy technicians. Specialist pharmacists have diverse roles and responsibilities including:

- Developing secondary or cross sector guidelines, for example, the treatment of the behavioural and psychological symptoms of dementia (BPSD) [52].
- Attending ward rounds, case conferences and multidisciplinary team meetings to advise clinicians on the most appropriate medication regimen.
- Conducting individual one-to-one medication reviews.
- A supplementary or independent prescribing role.

- Counselling patients and carers on their medication regimen including potential adverse events and how to manage them. This may be one-to-one or in a group setting and include the supply of written information.
- Providing a medical information service and answering frequently complex queries from both health and social care professionals and members of the public.

Historically, pharmacy technicians have tended to have a mainly supply function and their roles have included dispensing. However, increasingly pharmacy technicians are developing a clinical function; a good example of such a role is medication reconciliation – when patients move between primary and secondary care. The Mid Staffordshire NHS Foundation Trust Public Inquiry highlighted the need for safe systems within healthcare, and recent research has identified the importance of this clinical role, delivered by pharmacy technicians, in improving patient safety [53, 54].

The Sainsbury Centre identified in 2007 the need for more investment in specialist pharmacy services [55], and such pharmacy practitioners need to receive appropriate training and support for this specialist, complex role. Specialist pharmacists can study for appropriate postgraduate qualifications at Aston University [56]; however, currently there is no such specialist qualification for pharmacy technicians. The College of Mental Health Pharmacy also provides support and runs training courses for both pharmacists and pharmacy technicians.

23.5 Conclusions

In the future, particularly with the contraction of bed numbers, specialists will need to work more within a community setting rather than in hospital services. One particularly innovative approach could involve joint working between primary care pharmacists and specialists to support GPs, for example, in the management of BPSD [57]. However, more research is required on the impact of such an outreach role for specialist dementia care pharmacists and potential for collaborative care between specialists and primary care [44].

> **Key Points**
> - Old age psychiatrists have a key role in making the diagnosis of dementia but will need to liaise with a geriatrician, the primary care team and social services.
> - A number of models of care for the management of people with dementia have been proposed, including a collaborative care framework.
> - Liaison between primary and specialist care should enable rapid access to support if a patient develops BPSD.
> - Specialist pharmacists have a potentially important role in supporting medication concordance in patients with dementia.

23.6 Suggested Activities

- What is the role of mental health specialists in dementia in your healthcare system?
  - Is there a need?
  - Where do you fit into this system?
- What is the role of the geriatrician in managing people with dementia in your healthcare system?
  - Where do you fit in with the working of geriatric care in dementia?
- If a case management model was adopted, who could be a case manager in your healthcare system?
  - Could you be a case manager?
  - Where would you fit in with the working of a case manager?
- What is the role of the community pharmacist in supporting the management of people with dementia in your healthcare system?
  - How do you work with the community pharmacist in supporting the management of people with dementia?

References

1. Alzheimer's Society. Dementia UK: 2014 edition. London: Alzheimer's Society; 2014.
2. Mirando-Costillo C, et al. People with dementia living alone: what are their needs and what kind of support are they receiving? Int Psychogeriatr. 2010;22(4):607–17.
3. Luengo-Fernandez R, Leal J, Gray A. Dementia 2010: the economic burden of dementia and associated research funding in the United Kingdom. Cambridge: Alzheimer's Research Trust; 2010.
4. Fox C, Maidment I, Moniz-Cooke E, White J, Thyrian JR, Young J, Katona C, Chew-Graham C. Optimising primary care for people with dementia. Ment Health Fam Med. 2013;10:143–51. ISSM 1756-8358.
5. Fox GC, Moniz-Cooke M, Boustani M. The treatment of dementia where is it going? Br J Hosp Med. 2009;70(8):450–5.
6. Caputo M, Monastero R, Mariani E, Santucci A, Mangialasche F, Camarda R, Senin U, Mecocci P. Neuropsychiatric symptoms in 921 elderly subjects with dementia: a comparison between vascular and neurodegenerative types. Acta Psychiatr Scand. 2008;117(6):455–64. doi:10.1111/j.1600-0447.2008.01175.x.
7. Hodges JR, Miller B. The neuropsychology of frontal variant frontotemporal dementia and semantic dementia. Introduction to the special topic papers: part II. Neurocase. 2001;7(2):113–21. Review.
8. Hodges JR, Miller B. The classification, genetics and neuropathology of frontotemporal dementia. Introduction to the special topic papers: part I. Neurocase. 2001;7(1):31–5. Review.
9. Palmqvist S, Hansson O, Minthon L, Londos E. Practical suggestions on how to differentiate dementia with Lewy bodies from Alzheimer's disease with common cognitive tests. Int J Geriatr Psychiatry. 2009;24(12):1405–12. doi:10.1002/gps.2277.
10. Bird M, Llewellyn-Jones R, Smithers H, et al. Psychosocial approaches to challenging behaviour in dementia: a controlled trial. Report to the Commonwealth Department of Health and Ageing. Canberra: CDHA; 2002.

11. Bannerjee S. The use of antipsychotic medication for people with dementia: time for action. Independent report commissioned and funded by the Department of Health. 2009.
12. Cohen-Mansfield J. Nonpharmacologic interventions for inappropriate behaviors in dementia: a review, summary, and critique. Am J Geriatr Psychiatry. 2001;9:361–81.
13. James IA. Understanding behaviour in dementia that challenges: a guide to assessment and treatment. London: Jessica Kingsley Publishers; 2011.
14. World Health Organization and Alzheimer's Disease International. Dementia: a public health priority. Geneva: World Health Organization; 2012. p. 92–3. http://www.who.int/mental_health/publications/dementia_report_2012/en/.
15. Brodaty H, Arasaratnam C. Meta-analysis of nonpharmacological symptoms of dementia. Am J Psychiatry. 2012;169:946–53.
16. Goy E, Freeman M, Kansagara D. A systematic evidence review of interventions for non-professional caregivers of individuals with dementia. VA-ESP Project #05-225. 2010.
17. Elvish R, Lever S-J, Johnstone J, Cawley R, Keady J. Psychological interventions for carers of people with dementia: a systematic review of quantitative and qualitative evidence. London: BACP UK; 2012.
18. Laidlaw K. Cognitive behaviour therapy for older people: an introduction. London: SAGE Publications; in press, 2015.
19. Walker DA. Cognitive behaviour therapy for depression in a person with Alzheimer's dementia. Behav Cogn Psychother. 2004;32(4):495–500.
20. Mohlman J, Gorman JM. The role of executive functioning in CBT: a pilot study with anxious older adults. Behav Res Ther. 2005;43(4):447–65.
21. Teri L. Behavioral treatment of depression in patients with dementia. Alzheimer Dis Assoc Disord. 1994;8 Suppl 3:66–74.
22. Teri L, Logsdon RG, Uomoto J, McCurry S. Behavioral treatment of depression in dementia patients: a controlled clinical trial. J Gerontol B Psychol Sci Soc Sci. 1997;52B(4):159–66.
23. Koder DA. Treatment of anxiety in the cognitively impaired elderly: can cognitive-behavior therapy help? Int Psychogeriatr. 1998;10:173–82.
24. Scholey KA, Woods BT. A series of brief cognitive therapy interventions with people experiencing both dementia and depression. Clin Psychol Psychother. 2003;10:175–85.
25. Walker DA. Cognitive behavioural therapy for depression in a person with Alzheimer's dementia. Behav Cogn Psychother. 2004;32:495–500.
26. Burns A, Guthrie E, Marino-Francis F, et al. Brief psychotherapy in Alzheimer's disease. Br J Psychiatry. 2005;187:143–7.
27. Carreira K, Miller MD, Frank E, Houck PR, Morse JQ, Dew MA, Butters MA, Reynolds CF. A controlled evaluation of monthly maintenance interpersonal psychotherapy in late-life depression with varying levels of cognitive function. Int J Geriatr Psychiatry. 2008;23:1110–3.
28. Kraus CA, et al. Cognitive-behavioral treatment for anxiety in patients with dementia: two case studies. J Psychiatr Pract. 2009;14:186–92.
29. Kiosses D, Teri L, Velligan DL, Alexopoulous G. A home-delivered intervention for depressed, cognitively impaired disabled elders. Int J Geriatr Psychiatry. 2011;26:256–62.
30. Paukert AL, Calleo J, Kraus-Schuman C, Snow L, Wilson N, Petersen NJ, Kunik ME, Stanley MA. Peaceful mind: an open trial of cognitive-behavioral therapy for anxiety in persons with dementia. Int Psychogeriatr. 2010;22:1012–21.
31. Arean PA, Raue PJ, Macklin RS, Kanellopoulos D, McCulloch C, Alexopolous GS. Problem-solving therapy and supportive therapy in older adults with major depression and executive dysfunction. Am J Psychiatry. 2010;167:1391–8.
32. Alexopolous GS, Raue PJ, Kiosses DN, Macklin RS, Kanellopoulos D, McCulloch C, Arean PA. Problem-solving therapy and supportive therapy in older adults with major depression and executive dysfunction: effect on disability. Arch Gen Psychiatry. 2011;68:33–41.
33. Spector A, Orrell M, Charlesworth G, Qazi S, Hoe J, Hardwood K, King M. I can't forget to worry: a pilot randomized controlled trial of CBT for anxiety in people with dementia. NIHR, Research for Patient Benefit (FrPB). Programme, Final Report Form. 2013.

34. Inouye SK. Delirium in older persons. NEJM. 2006;354:1157–65.
35. George J, Adamson J, Woodford H. Joint geriatric and psychiatric wards: a review of the literature. Age Ageing. 2011;40:543–8.
36. Cooke M, Oliver D, Burns A. Quality care for older people with urgent & emergency care needs ('Silver Book'). http://bgs.org.uk/campaigns/silverb/silver_book_complete.pdf.
37. Hayes N, Kalsi T, Steves C, Martin F, Evans J, Briant L. Advance care planning (PEACE) for care home residents in an acute hospital setting: impact of ongoing advance care planning and readmission. BMJ Support Palliat Care. 2011;1:99. doi:10.1136/bmjspcare-2011-000053.114.
38. Gold standards framework-http://www.goldstandardsframework.org.uk/dementia-care-training-programme.
39. Rottenkolber D, Schmiedl S, Rottenkolber M, Farker K, Saljé K, Mueller S, Hippius M, Thuermann PA, Hasford J, for the Net of Regional Pharmacovigilance Centers. Adverse drug reactions in Germany: direct costs of internal medicine hospitalizations. Pharmacoepidemiol Drug Saf. 2011;20:626–34.
40. Callahan CM, Boustani MA, Unverzagt FW, Austrom MG, Damush TM, Perkins AJ, Fultz BA, Hui SL, Counsell SR, Hendrie HC. Effectiveness of collaborative care for older adults with Alzheimer disease in primary care: a randomized controlled trial. JAMA. 2006;295(18):2148–57.
41. Thyrian JR, Fiß T, Dreier A, Böwing G, Angelow A, Lueke S, Teipel S, Fleßa S, Grabe HJ, Freyberger HJ, Hoffmann W. Life- and person-centred help in Mecklenburg-Western Pomerania, Germany (DelpHi): study protocol for a randomised controlled trial. Trials. 2012;13:56. doi:10.1186/1745-6215-13-56.
42. Fiß T, Thyrian JR, Wucherer D, Aßmann G, Kilimann I, Teipel SJ, Hoffmann W. Medication management for people with dementia in primary care: description of implementation in the DelpHi study. BMC Geriatr. 2013;13(1):121.
43. Eichler T, Thyrian JR, Fredrich D, Köhler L, Wucherer D, Michalowsky B, Dreier A, Hoffmann W. The benefits of implementing a computerized intervention-management-system (IMS) on delivering integrated dementia care in the primary care setting. Int Psychogeriatr. 2014;26(8):1377–85. doi:10.1017/S1041610214000830. Epub 2014 May 9.
44. Iliffe S, Waugh A, Poole M, Bamford C, Brittain K, Chew-Graham C, Fox C, Katona C, Livingston G, Manthorpe J, Steen N, Stephens B, Hogan V, Robinson L. The effectiveness of collaborative care for people with memory problems in primary care: results of the CAREDEM case management modelling and feasibility study. Health Technol Assess. 2014;18(52):1–148. doi:10.3310/hta18520.
45. NHS confederation. Health on the high street: rethinking the role of community pharmacy. Available from http://www.nhsconfed.org/resources/2013/10/health-on-the-high-street-rethinking-the-role-of-community-pharmacy. 2013. Accessed Aug 2014.
46. Gidman W, Ward P, McGregor L. Understanding public trust in services provided by community pharmacists relative to those provided by general practitioners: a qualitative study. BMJ Open. 2012. doi:10.1136/bmjopen-2012-000939.
47. Urgent and Emergency Care Review Team. Transforming urgent and emergency care services in England Urgent and Emergency Care Review End of Phase 1 Report (NHS England). 2013. Available from: http://www.nhs.uk/NHSEngland/keogh-review/Documents/UECR.Ph1Report.FV.pdf. Accessed Aug 2014.
48. Fox C, Richardson K, Maidment ID, Savva GM, Matthews FE, Smithard D, Coulton S, Katona C, Boustani MA, Brayne C. Anticholinergic medication use and cognitive impairment in the older population: the Medical Research Council Cognitive Function and Ageing Study (CFAS). J Am Geriatr Soc. First published online: 24 JUN 2011. doi:10.1111/j.1532-5415.2011.03491.x.
49. Pharmaceutical Services Negotiating Committee. Medicine use Review (MUR). Available from: http://psnc.org.uk/services-commissioning/advanced-services/murs/. 2014. Accessed Aug 2014.
50. Smith T, Maidment I, Hebding J, Madzima T, Cheater F, Cross J, Poland F, White J, Young J, Fox C. Systematic review investigating the reporting of comorbidities and medication in

randomized controlled trials of people with dementia. Age Ageing. 2014;19:2014. doi:10.1093/ageing/afu100.
51. Poland F, Mapes S, Pinnock H, Katona C, Sorensen S, Fox C, Maidment ID. Perspectives of carers on medication management in dementia: lessons from collaboratively developing a research proposal. BMC Res Notes. 2014;7:463. doi:10.1186/1756-0500-7-463.URL. http://www.biomedcentral.com/1756-0500/7/463.
52. NHS Kent. Treatment of behaviour in dementia that challenges. Available on http://www.easternandcoastalkent.nhs.uk/home/independent-contractors/medicines-management/drug-formulary-and-prescribing-policies/central-nervous-system/. 2011. Accessed 30th Sept 2014.
53. Francis Report (The Mid Staffordshire NHS Foundation Trust Public Inquiry). Report of the Mid Staffordshire NHS Foundation Trust Public Inquiry. Executive summary. London: The Stationery Office; 2013. http://www.midstaffspublicinquiry.com/sites/default/files/report/Executivesummary.pdf.
54. Brownlie K, Schneider C, Culliford R, Fox C, Boukouvalas A, Willan C, Maidment ID. Medication reconciliation by a pharmacy technician in a mental health assessment unit. Int J Clin Pharm. 2014;36:303–9.
55. Boardman J, Parsonage M. Delivering the government's mental health policies services, staffing and costs. London: The Sainsbury Centre; 2007. http://www.centreformentalhealth.org.uk/pdfs/scmh_delivering_govt_mental_health_policy.pdf.
56. Aston University. Life and Health Sciences. 2014. http://www.aston.ac.uk/study/postgraduate/taught-programmes/school/life-health-sciences/.
57. Child A, Clarke A, Fox C, Maidment ID. A pharmacy led program to review anti-psychotic prescribing for people with dementia. BMC Psychiatry. 2012;12:155. doi:10.1186/1471-244X-12-155. http://www.biomedcentral.com/1471-244X/12/155.

Living with Dementia in a Care Home: The Importance of Well-Being and Quality of Life on Physical and Mental Health

Lynne Phair

As a person travels the journey of dementia, the impact of the condition will affect their physical, emotional and intellectual abilities, and the risk of increased complications of frailty such as, chest infections, urine infections, falls, constipation and pressure damage increases. Frailty is now recognised as a distinctive health state related to the ageing process in which multiple body systems gradually lose their inbuilt reserves [1]. Older people who live with frailty will have multiple conditions which may cause the diagnosis or management of any particular condition to be masked or harder to identify. For people living with dementia in care homes, the opportunities for them to undertake normal life activities that can assist in staving off or reducing the risks of physical or mental health conditions occurring are reduced. The impact of institutional living coupled with the progressive nature of dementia can complicate opportunities for both diagnosis and the management of conditions.

Care homes should be a place where the person not only receives care to manage the physical or cognitive consequences of dementia, but where they are supported to flourish, within their capabilities, and where the speciality of long-term care encompasses the support of quality of life and well-being alongside any physical or mental health conditions.

This chapter will explore some essential aspects of care and suggest how the qualities of the staff, the environment and the milieu can be used to benefit people living with dementia. So often the value of the physical environment is not considered as essential, except in respect of orientation and reducing distress. Whether a primary care professional is assessing a person's needs, is responding to concerns regarding their health or is involved in commissioning or contract monitoring the service a resident receives, the impact of the environment and activity on the person's quality of life and well-being should be central.

L. Phair, MA, BSc (Hons), Nursing RMN, RGN
Lynne Phair Consulting Ltd, Heathfield, East Sussex, UK
e-mail: lynne@lynnephair.co.uk

There are increasing numbers of regulatory and commissioning organisations who are developing competencies for staff who work with people with dementia in care homes. However, the focus is too often on ensuring that care workers respond to physical needs in a competent and person-centred way. While responding to physical need is a vital component of care, the importance of meaningful activity on physical and mental health is often overlooked or seen as something that is only relevant to an overall need for occupation. There are scarce examples of standards which measure how staff can demonstrate competence that incorporates an understanding of the wider benefits of the environment, the milieu and meaningful activity on the health of older people who live in care homes.

The guidance produced by the National Institute for Health and Care Excellence (NICE) on the mental well-being of older people in care homes is an important source designed to drive measurable quality improvements within a particular service [2]. The guidance sets out a concise set of six statements reflecting standards on:

1. Maintaining personal identity
2. Recognising signs and symptoms of a mental condition
3. Support of sensory impairment
4. Support of physical problems
5. Participation in meaningful activity
6. Access a full range of healthcare service

NICE highlights research which evidences that many older people are dissatisfied, lonely and depressed and many are living with low levels of life satisfaction and well-being. They refer to additional research, for example, from the Alzheimer's Society which shows that many care homes do not have enough activity or ways of positively occupying residents' time, coupled with poor access to NHS primary and secondary care services. Lack of activity and limited access to essential healthcare services are shown to have a detrimental impact on a person's mental well-being.

Meaningful activity is described by the NICE as activities that include physical, social and leisure activities that are tailored to a person's needs and preferences. Activities can range from activities of daily living, leisure, gardening, reading, arts and crafts, conversation and singing. An activity can provide emotional, creative, intellectual and spiritual stimulation and should include using outdoor spaces.

The NICE further describes mental well-being to include areas that are key to optimum functioning and independence, such as life satisfaction, optimism, self-esteem, feeling in control, having a purpose in life and a sense of belonging and support.

24.1 Traditional Approaches to Well-Being and Quality of Life in a Care Home

Traditional approaches to activity and the expected norms of promoting quality of life in care homes may include group activities following a standard timetable and an activity that has, as its common denominator, something that everyone can do. In a traditional culture of care, little attention is paid to the desires, intellectual ability or interests of the resident. Activities are 'done to' a person rather than with a person. Musical entertainers who lead 'sing-alongs', group quizzes and the television playing daytime TV are examples of entertainment designed for everyone.

Gardens too may be accessible, but in more traditional care homes, they are not considered as 'a room without a roof'. Rather, they are more likely to be used when the sun is bright, and residents can be placed under a parasol rather than sit in the lounge.

The physical environment in the care home may have paid little attention to the impact of factors such as light, noise or age and culturally appropriate furnishings. Cultural diversity may be most likely to be understood in respect of black and minority ethnic people but fails to pay attention to ensuring that care staff understand the culture of local residents including local history, food, festivals and events. There are very few induction programmes, for example, where care staff from overseas are helped to learn about the culture and traditions of the place they will live and work or helped to understand information that may support them to converse with a local person living with dementia about their life, work and pastimes.

24.2 Changing Cultures of Care to Promote and Support Quality of Life and Well-Being

Changes in traditional cultures of dementia care have been developing since the 1990s and focus on the need to value the person as an individual. The importance of personhood as a central theme aims to ensure that person who lives with dementia is not undermined and lost within the disease and medical management [3, 4]. Supporting quality of life through meaningful activity and an enriched physical environment has also developed and, in progressive care homes, reflects the developed understanding of how meaningful activity and the environment impact on quality of life which in turn impacts on the physical and emotional well-being of the person and their families.

The need for physical activity is better understood and is now supported by national guidance identifying the need for older people to be moderately active for 150 min a week to improve balance, coordination and strength. The benefits of exercise offer opportunities for social contact, engagement and communication [5]. The therapeutic value of the garden can bring benefits to people with dementia in a variety of ways, not simply to obtain fresh air and natural sunlight. The design can provide passive or active space, sensory stimulation and opportunities to walk and assist with gardening activity according to interest and ability [6].

The use of technology is becoming popular in specialist care homes for people with dementia: supporting activity with game consoles which encourage communication, coordination and sociable fun. Tablets are used to access resources that are online to encourage conversation, reminiscence, films or music, family photos or even direct contact with families abroad via web-based visual communication [7]. For people with advanced dementia, programmes are being developed to enhance the senses and give compassionate care. For example, the Namaste care programme (the Hindu greeting meaning to honour the spirit within), focuses on meeting the needs of attachment, comfort, identity, occupation and inclusion [8].

The impact of the environment has also become better understood. It is now appreciated that a person with dementia may have a reduced stress threshold to environmental stimuli, such as the noise of call bells, machines, office chatter and equipment or the motion of people through a living area. Some research suggests that continuous exposure to noise can increase alterations in memory and increase agitation, reduce tolerance of pain and increase feelings of isolation [9]. The impact of light and lighting is also more fully appreciated. For example, the benefit of natural light enhancing a room while avoiding glare and the importance of having enough bright light and using task lighting in areas where residents are doing activities are grounded in evidence.

The need to balance risk and potential benefits of any activity should always be considered in collaboration between the individual, family carers and any other involved staff. The promotion of risk taking rather than being risk averse can enhance quality of life and improve well-being but requires positive understanding of the importance of quality of life, sometimes outweighing the importance of trying to achieve total safety [10].

24.3 Assessing Common Health Problems Where Poor Quality of Life and Well-Being May Be a Hidden Factor

Primary care professionals are regularly asked to attend a person in a care home who is experiencing problems such as continence difficulties, constipation, falls, poor nutrition, urinary tract or chest infections, sleep problems, the development of pressure ulcers, distressed behaviour or the management of pain. The traditional and usual assessment process will be to consider the presentation by assessing the physiological aspects of the presenting problem, with a review of medication, nutritional intake, weight and perhaps pain or other attributed factors.

But many of these common problems become exacerbated by lack of activity and psychological engagement. If the person is unable to initiate their own activity due to their cognitive impairment, the spiral of dependency can escalate, as a sedentary life leads to boredom, sleepiness, lowered self-esteem, loss of appetite and lowered nutritional intake. These initial factors can then lead to increased dependency as mobility becomes more impaired, which leads to increased risk of pain, continence difficulties, sleep difficulties, constipation, increased cognitive decline and risk of pressure damage [11]. While continuing to consider physiological factors, primary care professionals should consider how quality of life for the person in the care home may be impacting on their physical and mental health and should consider reviewing the psychosocial aspects of care before resorting to, or alongside, more orthodox approaches. Set out in Box 24.1 are some examples of factors that may affect a person health that could be considered when assessing and treating a person for some common concerns.

Box 24.1 Common causes for GP referral, quality of life factors that may be important

Problems of continence and constipation
Signage to the toilet should be clear and use both words and symbols
Malodours should be managed so that the person is not distressed by using a toilet that others have used
Staff should use language that the person is familiar with
Activities should be encouraged that support physical movement
Clothing, including any continence aids, should be easy for the person to manage themselves
Residents that cannot move about may benefit from abdominal massage on a regular basis
Fresh fruit and vegetables and fluids should be available in all public spaces and encouraged throughout the day
Falls
Lighting and floor contrasts should be audited in areas where falls occur
Rails should be fitted at hand height on corridors and walk ways and places to rest should be readily accessible
Floor covering should be considered along with foot wear and the use of mobility aids
Signage should be available (words and symbols) throughout the home (e.g. to the toilet, the dining area, bedrooms)
People who have difficulty locating their room should have easily identifiable room doors
People should have access to outdoors and opportunities for walking, outdoor activity, exploring, fresh air and sunlight
Opportunities for activity should be encouraged as an integral and normal part of the day for all residents; exercise should be encouraged to maintain balance, muscle strength and intellectual stimulation
Appetite and drinking
Inviting smells of food may assist in promoting an appetite and encouraging a natural biological awareness of the time to eat
Portion size and presentation should be appropriate and the texture of the food should be correct to encourage appetite
Snack and finger food may be a better alternative for a person who cannot manage a 'normal' meal
Full fat milky drinks and fortified meals could be tried before resorting to nutritional supplements
The lighting, noise levels, table settings, atmosphere and care culture of the dining room and mealtimes should be audited regularly against the well-being and nutritional intake of residents
Picture menus or showing food presented on plates can assist in understanding and making food choices
Eating and drinking can be encouraged through social events and cooking activities. For example, tea dances, party nights, peeling vegetables or making cakes
Monitoring snack foods given to the resident by families prior to meals, particularly if the person has abnormal blood glucose readings and there is no simple explanation

(continued)

Box 24.1 (continued)

Enabling residents to help with laying the tables or clearing away afterwards
Encouraging and supporting physical activity, including time outdoors, to promote appetite and hunger
Problems with sleep
Fresh air and activity during the day may help a person to become tired
Encourage activities where possible such as raking leaves, sweeping, dusting, pegging out laundry or helping to push trolleys
Ensure good sleep hygiene and, as far as possible, follow the preferred routine of the individual person; for example, does the person prefer a particular nighttime drink? Do they like a cool room? Music?
Noise, light, ventilation should be considered
Consider night time pain, joint stiffness or the need to go to the toilet that may cause disturbed sleep
Quiet music, talking books or gentle soothing sounds may help settle the person, after a cup of hot chocolate
Consideration of biographical continuity is important. For example, has the person worked night shifts? Have they typically been 'poor' sleepers or preferred to 'burn the midnight oil'?
Staff may need to consider enabling the person to be up at night and sleep during the day, ensuring the day is set around the person
Problems with distressed behaviour
Behaviours that cause distress should be carefully recorded and antecedents should be considered (e.g. time of the day, staff involved, their approach and responses to the person, how long it goes on for). Analysis of these factors will support any intervention
Physical factors such as pain, constipation and infection may be important
Is the person experiencing anxiety or depression?
What might the person be communicating by their behaviour? (refer also to Chapter 24: Communicating with People Living with Dementia)
Psychosocial care should include consideration of individual biography and factors which may cause distress, occupation and activity, comforting and reassuring care and support and social networks and support

In conclusion, this chapter has briefly reviewed the importance of the physical and care environment, including awareness of meaningful activity as a means of supporting and encouraging well-being and quality of life for people living with dementia in care homes. While considerable progress has been made in challenging traditional approaches to care, there is still work to be done. Primary care practitioners have an important role to play in asking questions about the care and psychosocial support that residents receive in the care home. A commitment, for example, to providing meaningful activities as part of the day rather than assuming that residents can be corralled into timetabled, group activities may play an important role in promoting well-being and ultimately reduce calls on the time of primary care practitioners.

24.4 Case Study

Senga Williams moved to a care home after repeated episodes of being found outdoors, often lost, and not dressed for cold weather. It was felt by her family that she would be safer in a care home environment. Senga has not settled well in the care home and appears agitated and restless and spends most of her time on her feet, walking about. Staff perceived Senga's behaviour as 'wandering' (i.e. walking without purpose) and asked the GP to visit as she had lost weight. The GP asked about Senga's biography, and it was evident that care staff had not asked about Senga's past life, her work and family history and her likes and dislikes. Further investigation revealed that Senga had been a postwoman and had walked a long postal round every day of her long working life. Moreover, she was a keen walker when not at work. The care staff worked to develop a care and support plan which included asking Senga to sort and deliver the post and newspapers in the care home each morning, going out with care staff when they went out for shopping or to run errands, encouraging Senga's family to walk with her and encouraging Senga to work in the garden whenever possible. These activities did not entirely resolve Senga's apparent restlessness, but she appeared more settled. This was evidenced by, for example, an increase in her ability to sit at meal times and eat; providing snacks and finger foods for Senga to take with her when she was walking, and some improvement in sleeping and some weight gain.

24.5 A Quick Audit for Busy Primary Care Practitioners

Box 24.2 is about quality of life – impact on health and well-being audit.

Box 24.2 Quality of life – impact on health and well-being audit

	Quality of life and well-being activity	Evidence in the care home
1	What can the staff tell you about the person, their character, their interests and their past life, not simply about their medical condition or physical care needs?	
2	What can the staff tell you about the person and what makes them laugh or smile?	
3	Can the staff tell you how involved the family are and how they like to share the persons care and meaningful activity?	
4	How does the atmosphere feel in the public areas of the home? Calm, positively engaging? Noisy and distressing? Soporific?	
5	As you look around, are any residents 'helping staff' in any way or engaged in meaningful activity?	
6	As you look around, are residents engaging in any activity that appears to be unique to them (rather than general group activity)?	

(continued)

Box 24.2 (continued)

	Quality of life and well-being activity	Evidence in the care home
7	Can the residents go outside to get fresh air, and be safe?	
8	When did the resident you are visiting last go out in the fresh air? Do you feel this is adequate considering the weather or health condition?	
9	How has the resident been engaged in activity/occupation over the past week that: (i) Encouraged physical activity (ii) Stimulated the senses (iii) Engaged in meaningful intellectual stimulation (appropriate to their cognitive ability) (iv) Engaged with the community or environment outside of the main living area (v) Supported positive engagement and communication with family/friends or people other than staff	
10	How have the staff been using psychosocial interventions to improve or support the physical or mental health concerns?	

24.6 Appendix 24.1 Additional Resources

Stirling University Dementia Development Centre

The Virtual Care Home is an online resource that demonstrates dementia-friendly design in care home settings or people's own homes: http://dementia.stir.ac.uk/design/virtual-environments/virtual-care-home.

My Home Life; a UK-wide initiative with the aim of developing care practice in care homes: http://myhomelife.org.uk.

The Kings Fund's Enhancing the Healing Environment is an initiative aimed to improve dementia design in NHS and collective care settings: http://www.kingsfund.org.uk/search/site/enhancing%20healing%20environment.

National Association for the Provision of Activity for Older People – promoting best practice in activity provision including in care home settings: http://www.napa-activities.com/how-we-work/.

References

1. British Geriatric Society. Fit for frailty. London: BGS; 2014.
2. NICE. Mental well-being of older people in care homes. London: National Institute of Health and Care Excellence; 2013.
3. Kitwood T. Dementia reconsidered: the person comes first. Maidenhead: Open University Press; 1997.

4. Brooker D. Person-centred dementia care making services better. London: Jessica Kingsley Publishers; 2007.
5. Wallace R. Effects of a 12 week community exercise programme on older people. Nurs Older People. 2014;26(1):20–6.
6. Chalfont G, Walker A. Dementia green care handbook of therapeutic design and practice. Mesa: Safehouse Books; Chelfont Design Sheffield England; 2013. http://www.housinglin.org.uk/_library/Resources/Housing/OtherOrganisation/Dementia_Green_Care_Handbook.pdf
7. Cutlet C, Hick B, Innes A. Technology, fun and games. J Dement Care. 2014;22(4):12–3.
8. Thompsell A, Stackpoole M, Hockley J. Namaste care: the benefits and the challenges. J Dement Care. 2014;22(2):28–30.
9. Dewing J. Caring for people with dementia: noise and light. Nurs Older People. 2009;2(5):34–8.
10. Department of Health. Nothing ventured, nothing gained: risk guidance for dementia. London: Department of Health; 2010.
11. Phair L, Good V. Dementia a positive approach. London: Whurr; 1998.

Communication with People with Dementia

25

Louise McCabe

This chapter considers communication with people with dementia while recognising the growing recognition of the need to include people in their own care and treatment. Dementia affects a person's ability to communicate and their comprehension of the world around them; however, the success or failure to communicate is related to a whole range of factors not least of which is the other person(s) involved in the communication. Current understandings of dementia reflect a condition that is as much to do with an individual's environment, both social and physical, as it is to do with specific neurological damage [1–3]. It is acknowledged that communication can be enhanced through some simple considerations and through a focus on the person with dementia as someone who has the same rights to information about their condition and care as anyone else. However, stigma often plays a significant role in the lives of people with dementia and affects how (and if) communication takes place [4]. This chapter reflects on the various challenges and facilitators to communicating with people with dementia, breaking down the impact of different factors within the personal, social and physical environment of the person with dementia. By thinking about dementia in a more holistic manner, we can then find ways to compensate for impairment, address challenges and improve communication. The chapter finishes with a discussion about diagnosis and the disclosure of a dementia diagnosis to the person and their family, perhaps one of the most important times for effective communication with a person with dementia.

L. McCabe, MA, MPhil, PhD
School of Social Sciences, University of Stirling, Stirling, UK
e-mail: louise.mccabe@stir.ac.uk

25.1 Barriers and Facilitators to Communication

Communication is a complex process with different components including the people, the message, the medium of communication, the code or language, the sound environment, the feedback from the receiver and the social and physical context [5]. Understanding this complexity illuminates why people with dementia face difficulties and suggests routes to improve communication.

25.1.1 The Person

Dementia can affect communication in a number of ways, but it is important to note that dementia affects individuals differently, and these symptoms will not be common to everyone. Specific difficulties will relate to the type of dementia and the length of time someone has had the condition. People with dementia may have difficulty thinking and using the right words (anomia) and may reply to a question with a repeat of an answer to a previous question (intrusion) or repeat one phrase twice or more in succession (perseveration). There may also be a high degree of circumlocution, where a subject is 'talked around'. People may experience difficulties in word finding (aphasia), and they may talk at length without seeming to make sense (confabulation). However, they may still retain an understanding of how words are combined in sentences to make grammatical sense (syntax) and may communicate more easily about topics that are relevant and familiar to them. Dementia also affects an individual's reasoning, concentration and memory, and all of these aspects can further impact on their ability to communicate.

25.1.2 Physical and Mental Health

Most people with dementia are older and, therefore, more likely to be affected by hearing loss and low vision. These impairments may not have been correctly identified or addressed perhaps due to problems with communication; so it is possible to see how a spiral effect is set up leading to a worse outcome for the person with dementia. It is also important to consider the individual's physical health; they may be experiencing symptoms such as pain or breathlessness which can impact on their ability to communicate. Low mood and low self-esteem will also affect an individual's ability to communicate as will more debilitating conditions such as depression and anxiety.

25.1.3 Physical Environment

People with dementia are sensitive to their physical environments, and aspects such as background noise, interruptions, echoes as well as poor lighting, unfamiliar settings and inadequate signage/wayfinding can cause greater confusion and impact negatively on communication.

25.1.4 The Other Person

People may speak with different accents or dialects, and they may mumble or talk too quickly. The other person may also forget to include the person with dementia or focus their attention on the carer rather than the person with dementia themselves.

25.1.5 The Social Environment

People with dementia face stigma, and this may result in them being ignored, patronised or misinterpreted as well as excluded from conversations that concern them [6]. Sabat [2] refers to this as malignant positioning, and it occurs when people with dementia are positioned within social interactions as incompetent due to a focus on their dementia. Low expectations can lead to loss of self-esteem and reduced opportunities for communication. For example, by addressing questions to a carer while the person with dementia is present only reinforces to them their lack of worth and further excludes them, leading to less communication and further withdrawal.

There are many reasons why a person with dementia may have difficulty communicating. Some of this will be related to the type and degree of cognitive impairment they experience, but most will be related to social or physical factors that can be readily addressed.

25.2 What Can Be Done?

The first step is to believe that communication with people with dementia is possible and valuable and to challenge the stigma and negative social positioning that people with dementia experience.

There are some simple things to consider such as body language; changes that can be made to speech such as tone, speed, and content of speech; as well as considerations of the physical and social environment. It is also important to think about the memory problems someone with dementia may face and provide opportunities for information to be communicated in different forms and at different times.

25.2.1 Body Language

It is important to be aware of the non-verbal aspects of communication and use gestures, touch and tone of voice appropriately. Words only constitute about 7 % of the information we pick up from someone in any one interaction with 93 % of information coming from what we see, hear or experience from a spatial or somatic level [7]. A person with dementia who has difficulty following the path of conversations will have an increased reliance on non-verbal information. People with dementia may also use behaviour as a way to communicate. Unusual, repetitive and perhaps difficult behaviours can all be ways in which people with dementia try to communicate. Be alert to any visual or behavioural cues from the person with dementia.

25.2.2 Speech Patterns, Speed and What You Say

Speaking slowly and clearly to people with dementia while maintaining eye contact will aid communication. Also consider cues and feedback from them to gauge how much of what is being said is being understood. Give them plenty of time to reply [8]. It may be helpful to stick to one idea or piece of information at a time to allow the person with dementia to keep up with the conversation.

25.2.3 Physical and Mental Health

Sensory impairment increases with age, and older people may need extra support to ensure they have the right glasses and/or hearing aid. Paying attention to these basic aspects of health care can make significant differences to a person's ability to communicate. Similarly, considerations should be given mental health problems and how addressing these may impact positively on communication.

25.2.4 Listening

Be an active listener, giving the person with dementia your full attention. People with dementia may not use verbal speech to directly convey their message, and as such it is important to be aware of any emotional message or need that is being conveyed, rather than the specific words spoken.

25.2.5 Physical Environment

Be conscious of the physical environment and try to minimise any possible distractions; keep noise levels down and light levels high, and ensure the person is comfortable.

25.2.6 Social Interactions

It is important to pay attention to the dynamics of communication, to avoid 'malignant positioning' and to ensure people with dementia are included in conversations about their care and support. Good communication can support decision making about care as well as supporting the person with dementia to feel valued, promoting self-esteem and contributing to well-being.

25.2.7 Memory Problems

One of the most impactful symptoms of dementia is memory impairment. Someone with dementia may communicate well in the moment, but it may not be clear whether they will remember information provided at a later date. Providing written information, a route for people to call back for more information or a follow-up appointment will help address this issue.

The task of improving communication with people with dementia is not difficult, but it does require a multidimensional approach that considers personal, environmental and social factors. Awareness of barriers to communication can suggest solutions to facilitate communication.

25.3 Disclosing a Diagnosis of Dementia and Talking About Dementia

One important aspect of a GP's role may be in talking to people with dementia and their families about the diagnosis of dementia and what they can expect following this. GPs are the gatekeepers to services because they are most likely to be the professional whom relatives of the person with dementia approach for help [9]. However, research suggests that GPs may be reluctant to disclose the diagnosis [10]. There is ongoing debate about the positives and negatives of disclosure. A recent review [11] highlights the main positives associated with disclosure: the person's right to know diagnosis; to facilitate planning; potential psychological benefit to person with dementia and/or carers; opportunities to maximise treatment possibilities; the possibility to obtain a second opinion; and to travel or go on holiday. The review suggested that majority of people with dementia wish to be told their diagnosis. However, risks associated with disclosure include emotional distress, inability of the person with dementia to understand and/or retain diagnosis, no clear benefits to diagnosis, lack of a cure or effective treatment and the stigma associated with dementia.

This review found that there is a dearth of empirical research observing how a diagnosis of dementia is disclosed. A small number of studies within the review examined the longer-term impact of disclosure and found that the majority of people do not develop significant psychological ill-health although people with dementia may experience short-term distress. One study [12] found that people who had received their diagnosis had significantly higher environmental and physical quality of life scores than those to whom the diagnosis had not been disclosed. There is consensus that disclosure should be an ongoing process with provision of information and support for people with dementia and their families.

A key aspect of disclosure is the manner in which it takes place and the quality of communication with the person with dementia. Good communication at this point is crucial, and compassion, sensitivity and good listening skills are considered important skills for professionals delivering a diagnosis [13]. Written information should also accompany the diagnosis to support recall of information about the diagnosis and any recommendations made at that time.

25.4 Conclusions

Good communication with people with dementia is a crucial part of providing good quality care and support, and there are simple routes to improving communication. Attention should be paid to all aspects of the communication process, taking account of an individual's dementia, their sensory impairments, their physical and mental health, their physical environment and perhaps most importantly their social environment. Understanding the complexity of communication helps to suggest solutions and promote better communication for people with dementia.

25.5 Case Study

John had been having memory difficulties for some time, and eventually his wife Eva encouraged him to go to the GP. John realised that day-to-day life was getting more difficult. He found it very difficult to do many of the things that until relatively recently he had taken for granted. He developed an interest in local history when he retired, and he noticed these days that he could not concentrate on reading, found it difficult to retain information and had lost his confidence to go to the group meetings. Even getting organised in the mornings and getting dressed was becoming a problem, and John often felt muddled, anxious and upset. The GP listened sensitively to John and Eva's worries. The GP wanted to spend a little more time making a preliminary assessment of John's symptoms and so asked the couple to return for a double appointment at the end of a surgery. Throughout both appointments and in a subsequent referral, John felt that the GP spoke to him directly and respected his views and concerns. She recognised that John needed time to share his worries and also that she needed to take account of the impact of memory difficulties on his ability to follow a conversation. John was subsequently referred to a memory clinic and was diagnosed with Alzheimer's disease. When John visited the surgery again, the GP was clearly aware of his diagnosis and was helpful in signposting Eva and John to places where they might get more help and support. The surgery had made an effort to be 'dementia friendly' and had paid attention to their signage and lighting and to the information they had available about local resources.

25.6 Audit

The following questions provide a quick audit of your current approach to communicating with people with dementia and involving them in making choices about their care. The resources that follow provide tools to improve communication with people with dementia.

1. Does your clinical/practice environment have a sufficient level of lighting, clear signage and low noise levels?
2. Do the staff have basic knowledge about communication with people with dementia? The resources below could be used to provide this.
3. Is there a culture of inclusion within your practice, for example, are people with dementia routinely involved in decisions about their care and treatment?
4. Do you have information leaflets about dementia for families and people with dementia?
5. Do you have information about local services and support for people with dementia and their families and someone who can signpost them to relevant support?
6. Do you provide opportunities for a follow-up visit or phone call with a practice nurse (or other staff member) to clarify information and answer questions? This would be especially important soon after a diagnosis has been disclosed.

25.7 Resources

Dem Talk – An evidence-based tool for improving communication with people with dementia with versions for health professionals, social care workers and family carers [14].
   http://www.demtalk.org.uk/
   Talking Mats© – A low-tech communication framework to help people with communication difficulties to think about issues and provide them with a way to effectively express their opinions. Talking Mats has been used successfully with people with dementia [15].
   http://www.talkingmats.com/
   Environmental design – The Dementia Services Development Centre website has two virtual environments where you can find out how to improve the physical environment.
   http://dementia.stir.ac.uk/design/virtual-environments
   Alzheimer's Society, England, fact sheet on communication:
   http://www.alzheimers.org.uk/site/scripts/documents_info.php?documentID=130

References

1. Kitwood T. Dementia reconsidered. Buckingham: Open University Press; 1997.
2. Sabat S. Surviving manifestations of selfhood in Alzheimer's disease. Dementia. 2002;1(1):25–36.
3. Bartlett R, O'Connor D. Broadening the dementia debate: towards social citizenship. Bristol: Policy Press; 2010.
4. Vernooij-Dassen M, Moniz-Cook E, Woods R, Lepeleire J, Leuschner A, Zanetti O, Rotrou J, Kenny G, Franco M, Peters V, Iliffe S. Factors affecting timely recognition and diagnosis of dementia across Europe: from awareness to stigma. Int J Geriatr Psychiatry. 2005;20:377–86.
5. Young T, Manthorpe C, Howells D. Communication and dementia. Madrid: Editorial Aresta; 2010.
6. Beard R, Fox P. Resisting social disenfranchisement: negotiating collective identities and everyday life with memory loss. Soc Sci Med. 2008;66(1):1509–20.
7. Robinson A, Spencer B, White L. Understanding difficult behaviours. Michigan: Eastern Michigan University; 2007.
8. Stevenson L. Hearing the voice: improving communication with people with dementia. Stirling: University of Stirling; 2008.
9. Bamford C, Eccles M, Steen N, Robinson L. Can primary care record review facilitate earlier diagnosis of dementia? Fam Pract. 2007;24(2):108–1165.
10. Moore V, Cahill S. Diagnosis and disclosure of dementia: a comparative qualitative study of Irish and Swedish General Practitioners. Aging Ment Health. 2013;17(1):77–84.
11. Robinson L, Gemski A, Abley C, Bond J, Keady J, Campbell S, Samsi K, Manthorpe J. The transition to dementia – individual and family experiences of receiving a diagnosis: a review. Int Psychogeriatr. 2011;23(7):1026–43.
12. Mate K, Pond C, Magin P, Goode S, McElduff P, Stocks N. Diagnosis and disclosure of a memory problem is associated with quality of life in community based older Australians with dementia. Int Psychogeriatr. 2012;24(12):1962–71.
13. Mastwyk M, Ames D, Ellis K, Chiu E, Dow B. Disclosing a dementia diagnosis: what do patients and family consider important? Int Psychogeratr. 2014;26(8):1263–72.
14. Young T, Manthorp C, Howells D, Tullo E. Developing a carer communication intervention to support personhood and quality of life in dementia. Ageing Soc. 2011;31(6):1003–25.
15. Murphy J, Oliver T. Talking mats and dementia. Speech Lang Ther Pract. 2011;6: p. 6 (Spring).

The Dementias: Risks to Self and Others

Steve Iliffe and Jill Manthorpe

Risk and danger are pervasive in dementia syndrome, from its cause through its course, to its care. When seen from a medical perspective, many people with dementia are the outcomes of risky behaviour, their neurodegeneration being the consequence of high alcohol consumption, obesity or smoking and other potentially modifiable 'lifestyle' behaviours.

The diagnostic label of dementia carries risks with it, one being that it can turn someone who is muddled and forgetful into the bearer of a stigmatised disease, propelling them onto an escalator to disability [1] or infantilism. The risk for the person with dementia is that they become 'uncivil', embarrassing and visibly lacking in self-control [2]. This risk appears along a spectrum from words lost and sentences not completed through messy eating to incontinence. Dementia is a condition well suited to an era of uncertainty and unease, in which risks clamour for attention and possible dangers crowd in from all sides. In this 'risk society', everyone is 'subject to political rules of recognition, compensation and avoidance' [3]. These political rules are made explicit in the National Dementia Strategy [4] and the Prime Minister's Challenge for Dementia [5].

Behavioural and psychological symptoms such as aggression, agitation, 'wandering' and disinhibition, which typify dementia, create additional risks for the person with dementia and those around them by causing distress, misunderstanding and inappropriate reactions. These symptoms occur in 40 % of those people who

---

S. Iliffe, MBBS, FRCGP (✉)
Research Department of Primary Care and Population Health, University College London, London, UK
e-mail: s.iliffe@ucl.ac.uk

J. Manthorpe, MA
Social Care Workforce Research Unit, Kings College London, London, UK
e-mail: jill.manthorpe@kcl.ac.uk

have 'mild cognitive impairment' and in 60 % of those in the early stage of dementia and often become more frequent and troublesome with advancing dementia. Carers spend much of their time supervising and controlling the care environment [6], and carers' health may be at risk of harm from the stress of caring [7].

Understanding the risks associated with dementia matters to the care assistant in a nursing home as much to the community nurse who visits the home. They matter too to the community-based physiotherapist providing rehabilitation, to the practice nurse managing long-term conditions or to the social worker arranging for a 'suitable person' (generally a relative) to manage the social care direct payment and support plan.

This chapter explores what is meant by risk for people with dementia, describes which 'risks' cause most concern and offers some ways of understanding risk for people with dementia and their carers. It proposes three types of response to risk: a 'safety-first' stance; seeing benefits in risk; and adopting a right-based approach to risk taking, emphasising 'risk enablement' and 'positive risk taking'. In practice cautious approaches to risk predominate, with risk seen as a danger more than liberation. 'Managing risk' is now as important than 'meeting needs', at least in social care [8].

26.1 Dementia and the (Dis)embodiment of Risk

The possibility that dementia could be prevented focusses attention on the 'risk of' developing dementia, with the cause of dementia being attributed to multiple 'risk factors'. The 'risk factor' approach reduces change to decontextualised and disembodied behaviours and exposures, with potential for blaming the individual's present condition on their past lifestyle choices [9] or sometimes their genes. The alternative is the embodiment of risk, which finds clues about current health in the dynamic social, material and ecological context into which we are born, develop, interact and endeavour to live meaningful lives [10]. The wide range of possible risk factors – from gum disease to sleep disturbance in midlife, not forgetting all cardiovascular risk factors and head injuries – suggests that the causes of dementia are multiple and as much environmental as behavioural. The embodiment view of dementia risks fits the evidence better, but it is harder to grasp, measure and manipulate, which may be why the epidemiological 'risk factor' view is more popular, at least in medicine. This epidemiological view only allows for safety-first approaches – we should not smoke, drink too much, eat too much and exercise too little, or we may get dementia. And we should keep our cholesterol levels and blood pressure low with medication, too.

26.2 The Hazards of Diagnosing Dementia

Incorrect categorisation of other forms of behaviour or cognitive change as dementia creates the potential for under-treatment of treatable conditions like depression and the misdirection of individuals and families to inappropriate services. The increased referral of individuals to specialist services or memory clinics may heighten patient and family anxiety during investigation and even reduce availability of such services by extending waiting times. A 'false-positive' diagnosis may jeopardise patient and family trust in practitioner judgements.

The desire to communicate honestly and directly with a patient may be at variance with an equally strong desire to accept a family's reluctance to disclose the diagnosis [11]. This problem exists for specialists as well as generalists, with 60 % of psychiatrists and geriatricians in one UK study over a decade ago regularly not telling patients their diagnosis because of concerns about the patient's insight or about possible detrimental effects [12]. In the United Kingdom (UK) with the pressure for early or timely diagnosis, this situation is likely to have changed [13]. However, practitioners have every reason to be anxious about risks and hazards in diagnosis, given the intense debate about the balance of benefits and harms of an early diagnosis in dementia and the suggestion even of a 'curse of diagnosis' [14]. Alzheimer's Disease International has pointed out that there is almost no research conducted into the effect of the timing of dementia diagnosis upon subsequent disease course and outcomes for the person with dementia and their carers [15].

Being at risk because of having dementia has consequences for everyday life – such as not being able to obtain travel insurance easily or at all or losing social roles and status – some of which can lead to conflicts. The older person with dementia can come into conflict with practitioners about a range of options facing them [16]:

- Living at home at risk or moving to a care home.
- Following advice on diet when swallowing difficulties begin or declining a pureed diet that will reduce the risk of aspiration pneumonia.
- Remaining active despite the risk of falling or restricting activity to reduce falls.
- Driving or losing the driving licence. Loss of the right to drive is becoming a major practical and psychological problem for many people with dementia in the developed world [17].

26.3 Challenging Behaviour in Dementia

Understanding behavioural and psychological symptoms in dementia is important to avoid risks of worsening functional impairment, overmedication (especially with antipsychotic medication), relocation to a care home and elder abuse. 'Risky' behaviour is especially associated with fronto-temporal and Lewy body dementias (as is loss of insight, but distinguishing poor insight and judgement from stoicism or even courage can be difficult) [11]. Agitation or aggression may indicate pain (which the individual cannot describe or localise), infection or misinterpretation of others' actions. 'Wandering' may have meaning for people with dementia [18], as a form of re-familiarisation with the environment, or of 'window shopping'. A high proportion of people with dementia who have behavioural and psychological symptoms experiences significant improvement over 4 weeks with no specific treatment. Thus, watchful waiting is the safest and most effective therapeutic approach unless there is severe risk or extreme distress [19]. A safety-first approach may lead to avoidable constraints being applied, like sedation. A pragmatic approach may see benefits in walking for mood and sleep and arrange the environment to make 'wandering' safer. A right-based stance will accept risks and work around them, as long as the individual has capacity to make decisions – including wrong ones. Such risk management needs to include support for family or other carers to reduce their risk of breakdown or crisis.

26.4 Carers and Risk

Professionals tend to look at risk in a generalised way [20], whilst people with dementia and family carers take a more personalised view and also engage in self-regulation of risky behaviours, for instance, giving up driving or working with hazardous tools. The risk themes which are currently debated are the 'big' topics of diagnosis, driving, money management and moves into long-term care. There is much less discussion about everyday issues like leaving a person with dementia alone in the house or what to do about their smoking. For example, sometimes problems arise for carers when eating out with the person with dementia, which they deal with pragmatically or by avoiding going out [21]. This emphasis is still on 'big decisions' rather than smaller everyday decisions and typifies wider debates about rights to take risks versus the 'safeguarding' of vulnerable groups. For practitioners a key resource is likely to be other 'experts by experience' such as carers' groups in the locality. While some of these are dementia focused, in some areas more generic groups potentially offer emotional as well as practical support with day-to-day dilemmas.

26.5 Putting Risk in Its Place

Both practitioners and family carers now have a clearer legal framework for action in England and Wales in the Mental Capacity Act 2005 (which we will discuss further in the next chapter). The Care Act 2014 provides a further set of principles to guide service commissioning of services to promote well-being and to support family carers. However, risk is situated in people's own experiences and expectations [22], so 'risk' assessment is context specific and necessarily person centred. We need to be aware that an emphasis on risk enablement rather than harm minimisation may not fit all professional assessment systems, even though national risk guidance is multi-professional [8]. Greater community awareness of dementia (and its risks) and the involvement of other family members, friends and neighbours in supporting an individual with dementia will widen the debate about risks. And in a super-diverse society, we cannot assume that dominant notions of risk are shared by people from different backgrounds who may have very different views on autonomy and independence.

26.6 A Risk 'Heat Map' for Primary Care

Figure 26.1 below, taken from the UK Department of Health's Risk Guidance for Dementia [17], sets out methods for conceptualising risk as a matter of assessment and of judgments about importance and likelihood. The 'heat map' shown in Fig. 26.1 provides a framework in which to consider each potentially hazardous behaviour or activity as a balance between quality of life and risk. There is no scoring system, but it can be used to trigger a discussion between the key parties involved. A strategy for mitigating risks can be worked out using the 'heat' map with a range of professionals or supporters as well as with the person with dementia (if this is possible) and with family carers. This may helpfully be used in collecting information (how often does the person with dementia leave a lighted cigarette unattended, when and where?) and making an assessment (the person may enjoy smoking and it may be calming) and in the sharing of different perspectives (the right to smoke may be fiercely contested and present risks of harm to others).

In primary care, there may be opportunities to influence such assessment and risk management through knowledge of the person with dementia and also of family carers' possibly different viewpoints. The role of the primary care practitioner may be to offer opportunities for discussion, forms of mediation and some clarity over the legality of decision making and sometimes to act as an expert opinion provider

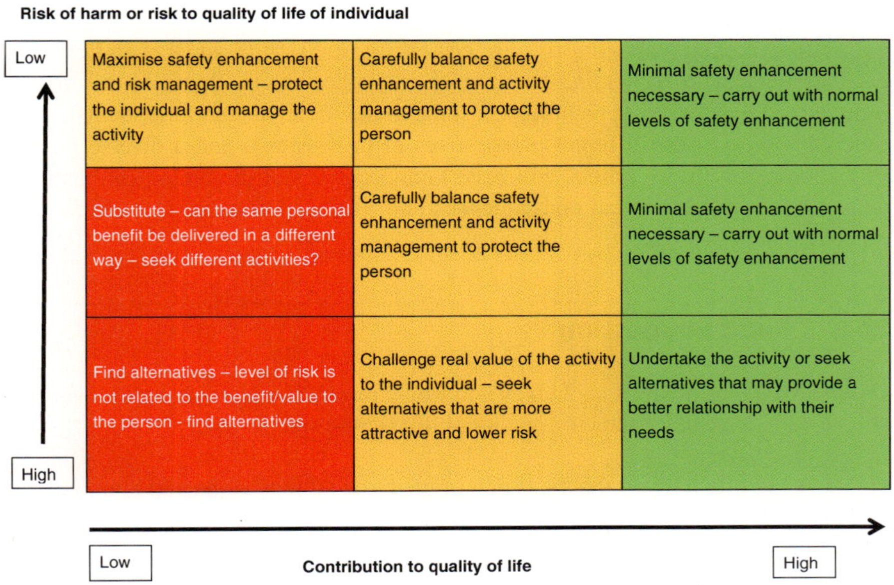

Risk of harm or risk to quality of life of individual

Low	Maximise safety enhancement and risk management – protect the individual and manage the activity	Carefully balance safety enhancement and activity management to protect the person	Minimal safety enhancement necessary – carry out with normal levels of safety enhancement
	Substitute – can the same personal benefit be delivered in a different way – seek different activities?	Carefully balance safety enhancement and activity management to protect the person	Minimal safety enhancement necessary – carry out with normal levels of safety enhancement
High	Find alternatives – level of risk is not related to the benefit/value to the person - find alternatives	Challenge real value of the activity to the individual – seek alternatives that are more attractive and lower risk	Undertake the activity or seek alternatives that may provide a better relationship with their needs

Low   **Contribution to quality of life**   High

Fig. 26.1 Risk 'heat map' (From Manthorpe and Moriarty [8]; contains public sector information licensed under the Open Government Licence v3.0 https://www.nationalarchives.gov.uk/doc/open-government-licence/version/3/)

when a patient is at the difficult stage of becoming less able to understand information and to act in their own best interests.

In the United Kingdom, the risks of exploitation of people with dementia are being increasingly recognised [23] and practitioners should be alert to signs of this and all other forms of elder abuse and familiar with local safeguarding policies and procedures. Interestingly the term 'adult at risk' is used in the Care Act 2014 (England) to replace 'vulnerable adult' suggesting a new emphasis on risk as a form of social classification. For primary care practitioners, the use of the word 'risk' therefore needs to be used with caution and applied to specific situations in which likelihood and severity of harm or gain are identified. For example, a family carer consulting her GP may talk in some distress of her relative's risky behaviour, but elucidation of this is warranted.

Close multi-professional working may assist in the analysis of the presenting risks but also in the negotiation of a support plan, its monitoring and review. As we have observed above, behavioural symptoms that are difficult to manage are often cast as presenting risks, and primary care practitioners may be the first professionals to be informed of these. Theirs is a key role in securing expert support, which may range from specialist interventions by secondary care practitioners to peer support for people with dementia and for family carers.

26.7 Conclusion

Understanding and managing risk are central to provision of support and care for the individual with dementia, their family and other carers. Some of this risk is intrinsic to the underlying pathologies, some to the social and cultural habits of our time and some to the different perspectives of professional and a diverse public. Practitioners of all disciplines will need knowledge about the biological basis for dementia, its psychological consequences and its social context, to provide adequate and tailored support.

26.8 Audit Suggestion

Use the 'heat map' to think about how you would respond to these scenarios involving people with dementia, balancing quality of life against risk:

- Mr. A's family tell you that he is determined to do things alone and often goes to Post Office, but frequently gets lost on the way and, because he does not dress appropriately for the weather, sometimes gets very cold.
- The children of Mrs. B – who lives alone – complain to social services that she likes meeting people when show goes round the town, but has invited a new 'friend' home, and they think she is being exploited.
- Mrs. C's spouse knows that she has paid someone who called at the house to clean their windows, but no cleaning has been done and he thinks she has been conned.

Key Points

- A 'false-positive' diagnosis of dementia will jeopardise patient and family trust in practitioner judgements.
- 'Risky' behaviour is especially associated with fronto-temporal and Lewy body dementias.
- The UK Department of Health's Risk Guidance for Dementia conceptualises risk as a matter of assessment and of judgments about importance and likelihood.
- Close multi-professional working may assist in the analysis of the presenting risks but also in the negotiation of a support plan, its monitoring and review.

References

1. Iliffe S, Manthorpe J. The hazards of early recognition of dementia: a risk assessment. Aging Ment Health. 2004;8(2):99–105.
2. Williams SJ, Gave J, Calman M. Health, medicine & society: key theories, future agendas. London: Routledge; 2000.
3. Beck U. From industrial society to risk society. In: Featherstone M, editor. Cultural theory and cultural change. London: Sage; 1992. p. 99.
4. Department of Health. National dementia strategy living well with dementia: a national dementia strategy. London: Department of Health; 2009.
5. Department of Health. Prime Minister's challenge on dementia delivering major improvements in dementia care and research by 2015. London: Department of Health; 2012.
6. Walker AE, Livingston G, Cooper CA, Katona CLE, Kitchen GL. Caregivers experience of risk in dementia: the LASER-AD study. Aging Ment Health. 2006;10(5):532–8.
7. Gordon DS, Carter H, Scott S. Profiling the care needs of the population with dementia: a survey in Central Scotland. Int J Geriatr Psychiatry. 1997;12:753–9. Carers value people to listen to them and respond personally.
8. Manthorpe J, Moriarty J. 'Nothing ventured, nothing gained': risk guidance for people with dementia. London: Department of Health; 2010.
9. Mythen G, Walklate S. Beyond the risk society: critical reflections on risk and human security. Buckingham: Open University Press; 2006.
10. Krieger N. Embodiment: a conceptual glossary for epidemiology. J Epidemiol Community Health. 2005;59:350–5.
11. Gordon M, Goldstein D. Alzheimer's disease – to tell or not to tell. Can Fam Physician. 2001;47:1803–8.
12. Johnson H, Bouman W, Pinner G. On telling the truth in Alzheimer's disease: a pilot study of current practice and attitudes. Int Psychogeriatr. 2000;12(2):221–9.
13. Burns A, Buckman L, on behalf of the Timely Diagnosis of Dementia Consensus Group. Timely diagnosis of dementia: integrating perspectives, achieving consensus. London: BMA/NHS England; 2013.
14. Le Couteur DG, Doust J, Creasey H, Brayne C. Political drive to screen for pre-dementia: not evidence based and ignores the harms of diagnosis. BMJ. 2013;347:f5125.
15. Prince M, Bryce R, Ferri C. World Alzheimer's report 2011. The benefits of early diagnosis and intervention. London: ADI; 2011.
16. Patterson C, Rosenthal C. Living a little more dangerously. Lancet. 1997;350:1164–5.
17. Mason A, Wilkinson H. Whose hands are on the wheel? Experiences of giving up driving. J Dement Care. 2001;9:33–6.

18. Dewing J. Screening for wandering among older people with dementia. Nurs Older People 2005;17(3):20–2, 24.
19. Alzheimer's Society. Optimising treatment and care for behavioural and psychological symptoms of dementia: a best practice guide. http://www.alzheimers.org.uk/site/scripts/download_info.php?downloadID=609.
20. Carr S. Enabling risk, ensuring safety: self-directed support and personal budgets enabling risk, ensuring safety. London: Social Care Institute for Excellence; 2010.
21. Manthorpe J. Eating out: dementia carers' views on the pleasures and pitfalls. J Dement Care. 2002;10:26–7.
22. Kemshall H. Risk rationalities in contemporary social work policy and practice. Br J Soc Work. 2010;40(4):1247–62.
23. Samsi K, Manthorpe J, Chandaria K. Risks of financial abuse of older people with dementia: findings from a survey of UK voluntary sector dementia community services staff. J Adult Prot. 2014;16(3):180–92.

The Dementias: Mental Capacity Act and Legal Aspects

27

Jill Manthorpe and Steve Iliffe

This chapter outlines the legal framework for the care and support of older people with dementia. There is no law specifically relating to older people's mental health, or dementia, per se, for the laws relating to adults in respect of mental healthcare and treatment apply regardless of age. Thus, a working knowledge of the Mental Health Act 1983 is important, and easy access to specialist advice is essential when patients appear to be a danger to themselves or others. However, practitioners working with older people may find that they are asked about decision-making and advance care planning more often than those working with other age groups and so need to understand the basics of the Mental Capacity Act 2005 (applicable in England and Wales). Given the likelihood that older patients will have multi-morbidity, the law relating to social care and support is also highly relevant, and this includes rights to support for family carers. In a wider context, both the Human Rights Act 1988 and the Equalities Act 2010 are important in ensuring that older people's rights are respected, especially as dementia is a disability. There is no space in this chapter to mention the laws related to social security benefits. Their complexity means that primary care professionals should ask whether people are getting all the help they are entitled to and recommend that they have a 'benefits check', most commonly available from Citizens Advice (commonly referred to as the CAB).

J. Manthorpe, MA (✉)
Social Care Workforce Research Unit, King's College London, London, UK
e-mail: jill.manthorpe@kcl.ac.uk

S. Iliffe, MBBS, FRCGP
Research Department of Primary Care and Population Health, University College London, London, UK
e-mail: s.iliffe@ucl.ac.uk

In this chapter, we outline some of the key legal frameworks relevant to primary care practice. It is by necessity only a brief summary and readers are advised to seek specific advice when uncertain. In most areas this will be available from professional colleagues in specialist mental health services, from local authorities in regard to social care and safeguarding and from their own professional bodies. We begin with the legal framework most relevant to those with cognitive impairment – the Mental Capacity Act 2005 – and move on to the Mental Health Act and the Care Act (readers in Scotland may wish to consult the British Medical Association's Mental Capacity Act toolkit [1] and the Adults with Incapacity Act (Scotland) 2000 and use the Alzheimer's Scotland resource [2]).

27.1 Mental Capacity Act (MCA) 2005

The MCA provides a statutory framework to protect and empower adults who may lack capacity (ability) to make all or some decisions about their lives [3]. It also governs the way decisions can be made for an individual who lacks decision-making capacity. On a proactive level, the MCA enables people to set out their wishes in advance and to appoint proxy decision-maker(s) in areas such as welfare, finance and healthcare (lasting power of attorney). 'Advance decisions' can also be made in respect of care and treatment (patients may refer to these as 'living wills'). While these are often suggested as important in early discussions around dementia diagnosis, they are applicable to other patients who may wish to set out their choices in the event that they become too ill to consent to or refuse treatment or to express their preferences.

Section 1 of the MCA sets out five principles to support decision-making, either by or on behalf of a person who may lack capacity. In brief:

1. There is a presumption of capacity – every adult has the right to make his or her own decisions and must be assumed to have capacity to do so unless it is proved otherwise.
2. Individuals should be supported to make their own decisions.
3. People have the right to make unwise decisions, and making an unwise decision does not mean they lack capacity to make that decision.
4. If someone lacks capacity, then an act done or a decision made for them under the Act must be done in their best interests.
5. Anything done for or on behalf of a person who lacks capacity should be the less restrictive option.

These principles promote the human rights of people who may lack capacity because they enshrine respect for individual autonomy but also set out principles for professional decision- making, including risk assessment and risk management (see preceding chapter). They make it clear that we should always presume that a person has capacity to make decisions unless it is established otherwise. They further make it clear that the decision needs to be specific. Particular difficulties may arise when a patient lacks capacity to consent to a particular intervention. The MCA helps resolve these difficulties, and as noted above, it is built upon human rights principles. It protects and empowers people who lack capacity to make decisions or to consent to care and treatment in a variety of ways. One of the most important of these is to ensure that practitioners or other care providers including relatives act in the best interests of the person who is not able to make specific decisions.

27.2 The MCA Code of Practice

The MCA Code of Practice [3] is a key document for practitioners and for other people, for example, family members who have been granted lasting power of attorney (LPA) or have been made court-appointed deputies for those who have not made LPAs and where major decisions need to be made. Other new roles were created under the MCA. These include Independent Mental Capacity Advocates (IMCAs), who have specific powers and responsibilities when certain decisions are being considered for people lacking capacity (e.g. about medical treatment, move to a care home) or represent the person lacking capacity when there is an investigation of suspected abuse or neglect.

Many primary care practitioners will be required at some point to act in the best interests of an individual who lacks capacity, to make a decision or to consent to aspects of their care and treatment. The MCA (Sections 1–4) supports the common law principle that any decision or action taken on behalf of a person who lacks capacity to make this decision or give consent must be in his or her best interests. What actually is in someone's best interests depends upon the circumstances of each individual case. Interventions, such as medical treatment, will be lawful where there is both a necessity to act and any action is in the best interests of the incapacitated adult as long as (a) any action is proportionate and (b) when the practitioner has a choice of actions, they must choose the alternative which is the less restrictive of the patient's freedom. If a person has been appointed a lawful proxy decision-maker, then this cannot generally be overridden. Primary care records should contain details of such documents and their status.

In order to establish whether a patient is able to make a particular decision, the person who would have to make this decision otherwise must ask two questions:

Stage 1. Is there an impairment of or disturbance in the functioning of a person's mind or brain?
Stage 2. Is the impairment or disturbance sufficient that the person lacks the capacity to make a particular decision?

A person is unable to make their own decision if they cannot do one or more of the following four things:

1. Understand the information given to them.

2. Retain that information long enough to be able to make the decision.
3. Weigh up the information available to make the decision.
4. Communicate their decision – this could be by talking, using sign language or simple movements such as blinking or squeezing a hand.

The results of the two-stage test should be contained in the patient's records. For people with dementia, their abilities to make decisions may fluctuate, and the two-stage test may need to be applied on several occasions.

Knowledge and confidence in applying and abiding by the MCA in practice are growing as practitioners gain experience. In a first round of interviews conducted in 2008–2009, Admiral Nurses (community nurses specialising in dementia) [4] reported receiving MCA training and estimated their knowledge as 'reasonable' but displayed limited confidence. In a second round of interviews in 2010 [5], their knowledge and confidence had grown especially in recognising when referrals should be made for specialist legal advice. They also noted that the MCA could be of benefit to family carers as well as people with dementia, because it could prove their authority to act behalf of their relative (e.g. to bank officials) and could give them an important voice in discussions with professionals.

The MCA was designed to empower those who feared dementia (amongst others), citing the opportunity to appoint an LPA as a prime example of being able to exercise choice and having the right to have such choices respected. Advance planning amongst older people is not always undertaken or seen as acceptable. Personal preferences, for example, may mean people do not want to think about the future, while others may plan for some areas and not others. For example, LPAs can be made about some types of decisions and not others – financial LPAs are currently more common than health and welfare LPAs.

However, the usefulness of the MCA is evident in that over 300,000 lasting powers of attorney applications were registered with the Office of the Public Guardian in 2014 indicating that many members of the public find this useful and relevant to their lives.

Primary care professionals may find that they are asked about the processes of drawing up an LPA – it is now possible to do this online. They may also need to let patients' families know if this is 'too late' (e.g. the person with dementia cannot understand what they are signing) but then should inform them about the processes of becoming a deputy appointed by the Court of Protection. This facility may also be of use to patients who have no one to appoint as LPA or whose family appear to be in conflict.

27.3 Difficult Decisions

Family carers of people often have to make difficult decisions throughout the course of dementia. Livingston and her colleagues asked a large, purposively sampled, diverse range of people caring for someone with dementia to identify their most difficult decisions and what were the barriers and solutions to these dilemmas. Participants consistently described particular problems but also emphasised their need to overcome the resistance of the person with dementia as well as changes to their family roles. Even with the legal authority to make decisions for the person without capacity (such as LPA), in practice families nearly always needed to gain agreement or cooperation to ensure that the person with dementia retained their dignity [6].

Some research has commented on the lack of awareness of the MCA amongst the public, especially amongst black and minority ethnic (BME) groups [7]. One earlier study found that awareness-raising events amongst a BME community was successful in increasing their knowledge and awareness of the Act and suggested that such events should be encouraged by health and social care professionals [8].

The findings from several studies of MCA practice are emerging. A study of IMCA use in practice revealed the importance of raising awareness and training staff around legal requirements to seek IMCA involvement [9]. A recent House of Lords 2014 review [10] criticised variations in understanding of the MCA amongst different professional groups and called for more scrutiny of records about advice, decision-making and practice by the Care Quality Commission.

The EVIDEM MCA study focused on dementia services in community settings [11]. A particular feature of this research was its investigation of the interface of the MCA with the safeguarding of people with dementia from abuse and neglect. It found that local authority safeguarding specialists were generally well informed about the MCA and were increasingly called upon by other professionals to provide guidance and advice. Prosecutions of the new offences under the Act (ill treatment and wilful neglect) were providing case examples of the criminalisation of poor practice and potentially upheld the rights to justice of people with dementia [12]. Some of these related to incidents in care homes, but others covered incidents where a person lacking capacity was living at home. Money management and concerns about the risk of financial abuse were of growing concern to dementia and safeguarding practitioners – highlighting the need for stronger communication between professionals to reduce risks and expose hazardous situations [13].

27.4 Mental Health Powers

In addition to being mindful of the MCA in practice, primary care services support many older people for whom elements of other mental health legislation are relevant. The Mental Health Act 1983 provides a framework for assessment and treatment, and within that, there are community-based powers such as Community Treatment Orders and the use of Guardianship under Sections 7 and 37 of the Mental Health Act 1983. The purpose of such orders is to enable patients to receive care in the community where it cannot be provided without the use of compulsory powers. Expert advice on these provisions is available from local secondary mental health services, while information useful to older people and their carers explaining the law is to be found on sites such as those run by the Mental Health Foundation, MIND and for carers the Carers Trust and Carers UK.

Table 27.1 Care Act 2014: summary of carers' provisions

The Act consolidates and extends public services' duties to carers (to be met by themselves or others) including:
Extending the duty to promote well-being to include carers (clause 1)
Adding a duty for local authorities to prevent and reduce needs for care and support for carers (clause 2)
Adding duties for local authorities to integrate services and provide information and advice (clauses 3 and 4)
Mandating local authorities to provide sufficient provision to enable carers to participate in work, education and training (clause 5)
Establishing a new single duty for carers' assessments based on appearance of need and a duty to meet carers' needs for support (clause 20)
Ensuring that carers should be consulted on care and support plans; giving carers the right to a support plan to decide how their needs should be met; entitling carers to request a copy of the care and support plan (clause 25)
Giving carers new entitlements to personal budgets and new rights to request direct payments payable to the carer or the adult needing care (clause 26 and 31)
Data from Care Act 2014, London, The Stationary Office, http://www.legislation.gov.uk/ukpga/2014/23/pdfs/ukpga_20140023_en.pdf (accessed 6 June 2015)

27.5 The Care Act 2014

The Care Act has recently become statute, but practice and implementation guidance are in the course of construction. The Act has potential implications for primary care support of older people with dementia, particularly its emphasis on direct payments and on carers' rights to assessments (see Table 27.1 for a summary of carers' provisions). There is increased emphasis on prevention and the duty of public bodies to promote well-being.

For carers of older people with dementia, these provisions are important and aim to address the long-standing criticism that they receive too little and too late, whether that is legal information and advice, access to advocacy and rights to short-break care. For carers and older people with mental health problems, the increased emphasis on and legal entitlements to direct payments (cash for care) in both social care and personal health budgets holds out the promise of greater choice and control – particularly being able to use these flexibly and also to ensure greater continuity of care. However, the mosaic of local services is changing. For example, specialist voluntary services are less often supported by funding contracts, and day care centres are losing funding – both leading to closures or increased charges. Links with local safeguarding services will be increasingly important when there are suspicions that such public money is not being used appropriately. The Care Act 2014 contains specific sections on financial abuse, and its guidance will be an important resource for many professionals.

For primary care practitioners, there is a need to keep up to date with the evolution of local services to inform patients about personal budgets. There is much evidence of high unmet need for advice, social networks and community and peer support amongst people with dementia and their carers [14]. Information from voluntary or third sector organisations is also valued. The Dementia Roadmap, recently developed in the UK by the Royal College of General Practitioners [15], is an example of a website designed to assist primary care staff to support people with dementia and their families. It includes local information that professionals are advised to consult when telling patients or carers about local services, support groups and networks. The expectation is for the Roadmap to bring together practitioners, people with dementia and carers and provide a resource for "understanding dementia, memory worries, the diagnostic process, post-diagnosis support, living well with dementia, carer health and planning for the future". At the time of writing, four English regions have registered Roadmaps on this site and cited several potential advantages to the process.

27.6 Conclusion

The law relating to dementia (and indeed social care) has been remarkably unchanged during the lifetime of many older people, but the past 10 years have seen major changes. All primary care professionals working with older people need to be more 'legally literate'. Many now have greater responsibilities for commissioning accessible and accurate advice services together with the local authority and for drawing attention to matters that now contravene the law or regulations. Many older people themselves and their carers are also better aware of their legal rights; and they may wish for primary care professionals to assist them in thinking through their applicability to them and their family. Primary care practitioners may be asked to provide expert opinion when complex, disputed or major decisions are under discussion; however, patients and carers are also likely to need advice about sources of help and basic information locally. Knowledge of how to contact local agencies and their remit should be at the primary care professionals' disposal.

> **Key Points**
> - All practitioners supporting older people with dementia need a working knowledge of the Mental Health Act 1983 and Mental Capacity Act 2005[1].
> - Current policies emphasise the importance of the health and well-being of carers of people with dementia.

---

[1] This applies in England and Wales.

27.7 Learning Exercise

Think about how you would respond to these scenarios involving people with dementia:

- Miss C tells you she has power of attorney for her mother and does not want her mother to have a flu injection or any more antibiotics.
- The children of Mrs B – who lives alone with dementia – think you should tell social services that Mrs B needs to be in a care home.
- Mrs C's spouse is increasingly reluctant to let the community nurse in to the house to dress his wife's leg ulcers.
- Mr Z wants to know if his father can make a will even though he has early dementia
- Mrs Y is tearful in a consultation and says caring is getting too much. She says that many people are worse off than her and that her mum doesn't want anyone but her in the house.

References

1. BMA Mental Capacity Act Toolkit. http://bma.org.uk/practical-support-at-work/ethics/mental-capacity.
2. Killeen J. Research summary and recommendations for policy and practice dementia: autonomy and decision-making: putting principles into practice, Edinburgh, Alzheimer's Scotland 2012. http://www.alzscot.org/assets/0000/5332/dementia-autonomy-decision-making-ResearchReport.pdf.
3. Mental Capacity Act 2005 Code of Practice, London, Ministry of Justice. https://www.justice.gov.uk/downloads/protecting-the-vulnerable/mca/mca-code-practice-0509.pdf.
4. Samsi K, Manthorpe J, Nagendaran T, Heath H. Challenges and expectations of the Mental Capacity Act 2005: the perspectives of community-based specialist nurses working in dementia care. J Clin Nurs. 2011;21:1697–705.
5. Manthorpe J, Samsi K. Care homes and the Mental Capacity Act 2005: changes in understanding and practice over time. Dementia. 2014. doi:10.1177/1471301214542623.
6. Livingston G, Leavey G, Manela M, Livingston D, Rait G, Sampson E, et al. Making decisions for people with dementia who lack capacity: qualitative study of family carers in UK. Br Med J. 2010;341:4184.
7. Mental Health Foundation. Engaging with black and minority ethnic communities about the mental capacity act. London: Mental Health Foundation; 2012. http://www.mentalhealth.org.uk/publications/engaging-black-minority-ethnic/.
8. Shah A, Heginbotham C, Fulford B, Buffin J, Newbigging K. The effectiveness of events to raise awareness of the Mental Capacity Act 2005 among representatives of ethnic minority communities. Ethn Inequalities Health Soc Care. 2010;3(3):44–8.
9. Redley M, Clare ICH, Dunn MC, Platten P, Holland AJ. Introducing the Mental Capacity Advocate (IMCA) service and the reform of adult safeguarding procedures. Br J Soc Work. 2011;41(6):1058–69.
10. House of Lords. Mental Capacity Act 2005: post-legislative scrutiny, Parliament, London; 2014. http://www.publications.parliament.uk/pa/ld201314/ldselect/ldmentalcap/139/139.pdf.
11. Iliffe S, Wilcock J, Drennan V, Goodman C, et al. Changing practice in dementia care in the community: developing and testing evidence-based interventions (EVIDEM), Programmes for Applied Research, by 2015, http://www.journalslibrary.nihr.ac.uk/__data/assets/pdf_file/0019/142093/FullReport-pgfar03030.pdf.

12. Manthorpe J, Samsi K. Care professional' understanding of the new criminal offences created by the Mental Capacity Act 2005. Int J Geriatr Psychiatry. by 2015;30(4):384–92. doi:10.1002/gps.4147.
13. Samsi K, Manthorpe J, Chandaria K. Risks of financial abuse of older people with dementia: findings from a survey of UK voluntary sector dementia community services staff. J Adult Protect. 2014;16(3):180–92.
14. Moriarty J. Carers and the role of the family. In: Sinclair AJ, Morley JE, Vellas B, editors. Pathy's principles and practice of geriatric medicine. 5th ed. Chichester: Wiley; 2012. p. 2838–55.
15. Royal College of General Practitioners Dementia Roadmap. 2014. http://dementiaroadmap.info/.

Caring for People with Dementia Towards, and at, the End of Life

28

Louise Robinson and Eugene Yee Hing Tang

28.1 Introduction: Evidence to Date

Due to our ageing societies, more older people will experience a slower, more unpredictable dying pathway from a combination of age-related cognitive impairment, multi-morbidity and frailty. In the UK, one in three people aged over 60 years die with dementia [1]. Costs of dementia care in England are currently estimated at £20 billion, with community care costs accounting for almost half of this [2]; a significant proportion of these are accounted for by care in the last year of life [3]. In the UK, few people with dementia die at home, with the majority dying in care homes, and around a third dying in hospital [4]. Despite being considered a palliative illness, very few people with a primary diagnosis of dementia access specialist hospice care.

Research reveals many staff find prognostication in dementia difficult and both medical and nursing home staff consistently overestimate prognosis [5]. People with advanced dementia suffer a range of symptoms comparable to those dying with cancer: 64 % of people dying with dementia experience pain and 57 % loss of appetite, [6]. Evidence has consistently shown that people with advanced dementia experience suboptimal care compared to those dying with cancer, with increased hospitalisation, worse pain control and fewer palliative care interventions [7, 8]. Many of these physical symptoms are poorly detected and often remain untreated;

L. Robinson, MBBS, MRCGP, MD (✉)
E.Y.H. Tang, MBChB, BSc, MRCSEd, MSc, PGDip
Newcastle University Institute for Ageing and Institute of Health and Society,
Newcastle University, Newcastle upon Tyne, UK
e-mail: a.l.robinson@ncl.ac.uk; e.y.h.tang@newcastle.ac.uk

assessment and management of pain is particularly difficult as patients cannot verbalise their symptoms and there is currently no single pain/distress assessment tool deemed useful for widespread use in practice [9].

In addition, family carers of people with advanced dementia may require more emotional support prior to the person's death than afterwards; they experience symptoms of grief even though their loved one is still alive (*living bereavement*). They have limited knowledge about the symptoms and prognosis of advanced dementia and may not consider their relative to have a terminal illness. There is some evidence that advance care planning may improve the 'quality of dying' in people with dementia, largely through reducing unnecessary hospital admissions [10]; however, few people with dementia complete formal care planning documents compared to those with cancer [11]. The key to providing good quality end of life care in dementia is to start at the beginning with open and sensitive discussions, whilst the person with dementia has the capacity to discuss their future preferences for care, a process called advance care planning.

28.2 Future Care Planning

Advance care planning is a term used to refer to a series of discussions between a patient, their family and the professionals involved in their care about their future wishes should they lose capacity; a person's GP is well placed to undertake such discussions. Following these discussions, patients can formally record their wishes in a number of ways including the completion of an advance directive, or living will as it was previously known. A summary of the different types of documents that can be produced from such discussions is shown in Table 28.1. In the UK, the National End of Life Care Programme website provides both advice for patients and professionals about ACP and also examples of documentation (http://www.endoflifecareforadults.nhs.uk/).

In England, the introduction of the Mental Capacity Act in 2005 provided a statutory framework for making decisions on behalf of adults who lack the mental capacity to do so for themselves. The Act's 'code of practice' affords guidance on good practice for professionals. It contains (i) a staged approach to the assessment of capacity (see Table 28.2), (ii) a statutory framework for an advance directive and (iii) advice on how to manage patient decisions, once the advance directive is applied. The Act also established a new role, the Independent Mental Capacity Advocate (IMCA) Service, to represent individuals who lack capacity, but who have no one to support them when major decisions need to be made about their lives.

The Act has also seen the introduction of a new formal power of attorney, Lasting Power of Attorney (LPA), which has replaced the existing Enduring Powers of Attorney (EPA), although an EPA will remain valid if executed before the implementation of the new Act. LPAs are particularly useful in dementia care and extend

Table 28.1 Outcomes of ACP discussions: international and national terminology

Statement of wishes and preferences: Documents an individual's wishes for future care and is not a legally binding document. In the UK, this is known as an advance statement
An advance directive for refusal of treatment (or 'living will'): This is a statement of an individual's refusal to receive specific medical treatment in a pre-defined future situation. It is legally binding and comes into effect when a person loses mental capacity. In the UK, this is known as an advance decision to refuse treatment (ADRT)
A proxy decision maker or Power of Attorney (POA): This is a legally binding document whereby the person ('donor') nominates another ('attorney') to make decisions on their behalf should they lose capacity. In England, following the Mental Capacity Act, this is now known as a Lasting Power of Attorney (LPA); there are two separate aspects to LPA, first relating to a person's health and welfare and second in relation to property and affairs

Table 28.2 Assessment of mental capacity

Two stage test:
1. Does the patient have an impairment or disturbance of function of the brain?
2. Regarding a specific decision, can the patient:
Understand the decision to be made
Retain sufficient information to make an informed decision
Use information appropriately
Communicate their decision
Practical tips for assessment of capacity:
Information may need to be provided in different forms
The GP may need to assess on several occasions, i.e. if morning is best time for them
Record information and two stages accurately in patient notes
Refer to expert (old age psychiatry) if in doubt

the areas in which patients can authorise others to make decisions on their behalf to include personal care and medical treatment, in addition to property and finance. Families need to be advised that these are separate documents and may carry two separate fees if they seek legal advice to complete the appropriate LPA.

Advance care planning is particularly important for people with dementia in care homes and can be helpful in reducing inappropriate hospital admissions, especially towards, and at, the end of life. The number of care home residents admitted to hospital is concerning as many of these admissions are avoidable [12]. Hospitals are less than ideal environments for people with dementia and can lead to disorientation and deterioration in their physical health, through falls and acquired infection as well as being costly. Through discussing patients and their families' wishes, and completing a Do Not Attempt Resuscitation or Do Not Admit to Hospital form, unnecessary admissions can be avoided.

28.3 Preferred Place of Care

One of the outcomes of care planning discussions is to ascertain where the person with dementia would choose to be cared for. If they wish to remain at home, then a range of support options exist to facilitate this and help their family continue caring. A range of aids and adaptations are available to make the home a more dementia-friendly environment. These include the use of simple picture signs on doors to indicate specific rooms, for example, the bathroom, and more advanced technology such as alarms that indicate the person is wandering in the night. These come under the umbrella term 'assistive technologies (AT)', and a website specifically for people with dementia and ATs provides further information (www.atdementia.org.uk). The website 'dementia.com' is also very person-centred (www.dementia.com). Respite care, sitting services and day centres provide options for carers to have time for themselves.

28.4 Management of Behavioural Problems in Advanced Dementia

One factor that may influence carers' decisions to move a person with dementia into a care home is the onset of distressing behaviours. The vast majority of people with moderate to severe dementia will experience behavioural symptoms such as agitation, aggression and wandering. These may be initiated, or aggravated by, the onset of an acute illness such as an infection. However, whilst the risks from such behaviours are often not as great as carers fear, they can lead to high levels of carer stress and curtailment of the person with dementia's activities and may be the crucial factor that leads to entry into a care home. National guidance in the UK recommends firstly excluding a treatable cause such as pain, constipation or an acute urine infection; if there is no obvious case, then non-drug approaches are recommended as first-line management. In the community this may be difficult due to (i) a lack of access to specialist nursing and psychological services to enable an individualised assessment and determine the antecedents, behaviours and possible causes ('ABC' approach) and (ii) the limited high-quality evidence for the clinical and cost-effectiveness of some non-pharmacological treatments.

In the UK, a multi-disciplinary pathway for the optimised management of BPSD has recently been developed. This provides evidence-based guidance to primary, secondary and community care professionals, including care home staff, on the holistic management of these challenging behaviours (Alzheimer's Society: http://www.alzheimers.org.uk/). If the behaviour persists and becomes more severe despite the use of non-drug approaches, the GP can prescribe a short course of an antipsychotic drug, such as risperidone; however, prescribing of these drugs should be time limited (up to 6 weeks) and only reserved for severe and distressing symptoms. If longer-term drug treatment is considered necessary, there should be a careful assessment of the risks and benefits of the continued use of antipsychotics. There is some evidence for the use of other drugs for BPSD including antidepressants (citalopram; trazodone) and antiepileptics (carbamazepine), and these could be tried before an antipsychotic drug.

28.5 Palliative Care in Dementia: An Approach to Symptom Management

Palliative care is 'the active total care of patients whose disease is not responsive to curative treatment'. Control of pain and other symptoms and of psychological, social and spiritual issues is paramount. The goal of palliative care is to achieve the best quality of life for patients and their families. The NHS End of Life Programme highlights the importance of palliative care for all those with a life limiting illness. It promotes the use of specific tools – palliative care standards, advance care planning and care pathways for the dying – to facilitate good communication and proactive planning.

The principles of palliative care are largely grounded in a cancer care model but are potentially transferable to patients with other chronic illnesses. NICE (2006) guidance on dementia care recommends a palliative care approach in the more advanced stages of dementia: the GP and the primary care team are well placed to facilitate this, particularly as the GP will have, most likely, been involved from the point of diagnosis. However, in order to provide co-ordinated end of life care in dementia, effective teamwork is essential, with team members having a mutual understanding of each other's roles and responsibilities. The community nurse will provide general hands on nursing care, organise aids and equipment, offer emotional support and help co-ordinate and access other services such as respite care. Both the GP and nurse would liaise closely, if needed, with palliative care services, especially specialist palliative care nurses (often termed Macmillan nurses in recognition of the charity that supports their role), in order to access specialist advice and hospice-based services, such as day care and respite care. In some areas a 24 h community nursing service is available; a night sitting service may also be accessed, sometimes provided by Marie Curie nurses. Admiral nurses, as previously mentioned, will also play a key role.

In terms of practice organisation and palliative care provision, a new General Practice Contract was implemented in 2004 which defined core primary care services and optional enhanced services. It introduced a new concept; the provision of financial rewards linked to the achievement of clinical and non-clinical quality markers, through a Quality and Outcomes Framework derived from evidence-based care [13]. The Quality and Outcomes Framework for palliative care stipulates the development and maintenance of a GP palliative care register and regular review of all listed patients. Patients eligible for the palliative care register are those whose death would not be unexpected within the next year; consequently, patients in the advanced stages of dementia, especially those living in care homes, should be included on the practice palliative care register.

A major difficulty for GPs is prognostication. Due to the slow and prolonged dying trajectory in dementia, it may be better to honestly discuss such prognostic uncertainty with families. Despite this difficulty, there is a palliative care approach, which improves quality of life recommended to avoid unnecessary interventions. One common area of distress for family carers of people with dementia is the person's reluctance to eat or drink as the illness progresses. Families should be reassured that this is one of the signs of advancing illness. However, the GP should also exclude depression, swallowing difficulties or other gastrointestinal problems. If the person's prognosis is short, then good mouth care and oral hygiene is sufficient; if the patient is expected to live longer, then a discussion around subcutaneous fluids or PEG feeding with dietician input may need to be considered especially if the person is rapidly losing weight, although these are rarely needed in practice.

28.6 Managing Common Problems in Dementia Towards, or at, the End of Life

Many of the symptoms and problems faced by people with dementia at the end of life are common to older people with any terminal illness; the additional challenge for health professionals is that their communication skills are considerably impaired. Many are prescribed multiple drugs, which may cause side effects independently or in combination. It is important to be aware if the person has any renal or liver failure as this will affect the metabolism and excretion of some drugs. Regular medication review is essential; any non-effective medication should be discontinued and the number of drugs should be kept to a minimum. In dementia, the patient's compliance with medication and especially their ability to swallow is often a key issue and influences the form in which drugs should be administered. Transdermal patches, where appropriate, help to ensure patient compliance. Non-drug measures should also be considered, for example, could anxiety be helped by relaxation techniques or aromatherapy rather than benzodiazepines?

End of life care pathways, such as the Liverpool Care Pathway, were used to help doctors and nurses achieve better symptom control, but following a national enquiry, they have been withdrawn from use in the UK.

28.6.1 Management of Distress

An assessment of distress must be undertaken by asking carers who know the patient best to report key non-verbal signs such as grunting, crying and moaning. Pain/distress assessment tools exist but there is not one that is better than any other. In terms of treating distress/pain, the usual 'analgesic ladder' should be followed, starting with simple analgesia, such as paracetamol, and moving to second-level analgesia, e.g. codeine and finally opiates. One third of opioid naïve patients experience nausea for 7–10 days on commencing morphine, or other opioids, which should respond to haloperidol 1.5–3 mg od. Strong opioids will cause constipation; regular laxatives should be prescribed to prevent this. When titrating oral or injectable opioids against pain, increase the 24 h dose by approximately one third each time, e.g. increase from 60 mg bd to 80 mg bd to 110 mg bd. The prn dose of oral or injectable opioids is one sixth of the total 24 h dose and should be increased in proportion when regular dose is increased.

28.6.2 Nausea and Vomiting

A detailed assessment needs to be made as the choice of antiemetic depends on likely cause. If the oral route is not effective, the antiemetic should be given subcutaneously via a syringe driver for a few days to ensure absorption, before being prescribed by the oral route again. At the very end of life when the patient is drowsy, any regular oral antiemetic should be continued subcutaneously via a syringe driver.

28.6.3 Constipation

Constipation is commonly experienced by people with advanced dementia, exacerbated by poor appetite and fluid intake, immobility, and prescribed drugs, particularly opioids and antimuscarinics. Patients will often need a combination of stimulant (e.g. senna) and softener (e.g. docusate). Combination drugs are available (e.g. co-danthramer, co-danthrusate) which are more expensive but mean fewer tablets for the patient. If constipation causes discomfort in the dying phase, abdominal colic should be treated with hyoscine butylbromide subcutaneously (20 mg prn 2 hourly or 60–120 mg via syringe driver over 24 h).

28.6.4 Dyspnoea

The cause of the breathlessness needs to be assessed and treated if possible. However, the sensation of breathlessness can be partially relieved by a small dose of opioids given regularly (e.g. morphine solution 5–10 mg prn 4–6 hourly). If the patient is anxious or frightened, this is likely to exacerbate the breathlessness and can be treated with lorazepam 0.5 mg sublingually prn hourly. In the dying phase, opioids given subcutaneously (from diamorphine 2.5 mg prn hourly or 10 mg over 24 h via syringe driver) may help relieve the sensation of dyspnoea.

28.6.5 Terminal Agitation

This is commonly seen in the last few days or hours. The patient may appear distressed and unable to settle, although not in pain. This usually responds to midazolam given subcutaneously (2.5–5 mg prn hourly or 10–20 mg over 24 h via syringe driver). If the patient does not settle, higher doses may be needed, or as a second line, levomepromazine may need to be added.

In conclusion, research evidence confirms that people dying with dementia receive suboptimal care compared to those with terminal cancer. Good quality end of life care in dementia can be achieved. It requires good communication with open and sensitive discussions about future preferences for care; advice about Power of Attorney and other practical issues including support services and technology; continuity of care through a named lead GP/care home nurse; detailed observation for signs of distress once communication has been lost and referral to specialist services such as old age psychiatry for behavioural problems; and palliative care for end of life symptom management. Most importantly, the uncertainty of the dying trajectory needs to be clearly understood by health professionals and clearly explained to family carers to help them understand the slow and often prolonged pathway to dying.

28.7 Suggested Activities

Discuss with your colleagues whether your normal practice for identifying people in the terminal phase of dementia is adequate.

How do you support the family carers of people with dementia?

Clinical audit of patients with dementia who died in the previous year: Where was place of death? (And was it their preferred place of death?) Was symptom control adequate? Were family and carers involved in decision-making? What support was offered to the family carers after the death?

Key Points
- Prognostication in people with dementia is difficult; it is useful to communicate such uncertainty to families.
- Family and carers of people with dementia may require more support prior to the person with advanced dementia's death than after.
- Advance care planning discussions need to be carried out whilst the person with dementia has the capacity to ensure best ongoing treatment.
- Common problems such as pain and constipation need to be excluded prior to the commencement of treatment for behavioural problems on a background of dementia.
- GPs need to consider placing people with advanced dementia on their practice's palliative care register and ensure they have optimum community support from, e.g. Macmillan nurses or respite services for carers.
- Many of the symptoms attributed to end of life dementia care are similar to those in older people with any terminal illness and should be managed accordingly.

References

1. Brayne C, Gao L, Dewey M, Matthews FE, Medical Research Council Cognitive Function and Ageing Study Investigators. Dementia before death in ageing societies – the promise of prevention and the reality. PLoS Med. 2006;3:e397.
2. House of Commons All Party Parliamentary Group on Dementia. The £20 Billion Question – an inquiry into improving lives through cost effective dementia services. 2011. Accessed 02.09.2013.
3. Alzheimer's Society. Dementia UK: the full report. London: Alzheimer's Society; 2007.

4. Houttekier D, Cohen J, Bilsen J, Addington-Hall J, Onwuteaka-Philipsen BD, Deliens L. Place of death of older persons with dementia. A study in five European countries. J Am Geriatr Soc. 2010;58(4):751–6.
5. van der Steen JT. Dying with dementia: what we know after more than a decade of research. J Alzheimers Dis. 2010;22(1):37–55.
6. McCarthy M, Addington-Hall J, Altmann D. The experience of dying with dementia: a retrospective study. Int J Geriatr Psychiatry. 1997;12:404–9.
7. Mitchell S, Kiely D, Hamel M. Dying with advanced dementia in the nursing home. Arch Intern Med. 2004;164:321–6.
8. Sampson EL, Gould V, Lee D, Blanchard M. Differences in care received by patients with and without dementia who died during acute hospital admission: a retrospective case note study. Age Ageing. 2006;35:187–9.
9. Zwakhalen SMG, Hamers JPH, Abu-Saad HH, Pberger MPF. Pain in elderly people with severe dementia: a systematic review of behavioural pain assessment tools. BMC Geriatr. 2006;6(3):1–15.
10. Robinson L, Dickinson C, Rousseau N, Beyer F, Clark A, Hughes J, Howell D, Exley C. A systematic review of the effectiveness of advance care planning interventions for people with cognitive impairment and dementia. Age Ageing. 2011;41(2):263–9. doi:10.1093/ageing/afr148.
11. Sampson EL, Jones L, Thune-Boyle I, Kukkastenvehmas R, King M, Leurent B, Tookman A, Blanchard MR. Palliative assessment and advance care planning in severe dementia: an exploratory randomized controlled trial of a complex intervention. Palliat Med. 2011;25(3):197–209.
12. British Geriatrics Society. A quest for quality in care homes. An inquiry into the quality of healthcare support for older people in care homes: a call for leadership, partnership and improvement. London: British Geriatrics Society; 2011.
13. NHS Confederation. Revisions to the GMS contract 2006/7. NHS Employers and General Practitioner Committee, British Medical Association. 2006. http://www.nhsemployers.org/pay-conditions/primary-902.cfm. Accessed 31 Jan 2008.

Part VI
Conclusions/Summary

Enhancing Older People's Mental Wellbeing Through Research: A Case Study

29

Denise Tanner and Rosemary Littlechild

29.1 Introduction

This chapter is based on a research project looking at the experiences of older people moving into or between dementia services offered by social care agencies or the NHS [1]. The research was underpinned by a participatory research approach which included employing older people as coresearchers to work alongside academic researchers in different stages of the research process. This chapter shows how involvement in the research project can enhance the mental wellbeing of both older coresearchers and research participants.

We begin with a brief outline of the project itself. The remainder of this chapter illustrates the benefits of participatory research to, firstly, participants and, secondly, coresearchers, presenting the experiences of individuals who were involved in one set of interviews.

29.2 The Research Project

The wider project was concerned with the experiences of care transitions of older people whose needs are complex and not well understood and whose voices are rarely heard in research [2]. The research took place in four different sites in England. Here we focus only on the site that explored the experiences of older people with dementia and their carers. In recognition of the fact that the implementation of research findings into practice is often problematic, the project had two phases. The first phase comprised of two in-depth interviews (6 months apart) with

---

D. Tanner, PhD, MSocSc, BSc, CQSW (✉) • R. Littlechild, Msoc Sci, Bsoc Sci, CQSW
Institute of Applied Social Studies, University of Birmingham,
Birmingham, West Midlands, UK
e-mail: d.l.tanner@bham.ac.uk; R.J.Littlechild@bham.ac.uk

© Springer International Publishing Switzerland 2016
C.A. Chew-Graham, M. Ray (eds.), *Mental Health and Older People: A Guide for Primary Care Practitioners*, DOI 10.1007/978-3-319-29492-6_29

older people and their carers about their experiences of transition. The second phase involved working with local statutory agencies (social care and NHS) and the local Alzheimer's Society to identify and implement changes which arose from the research itself.

Older coresearchers were recruited who shared similar experiences to the intended participants, that is, they had experience of entering or moving between dementia services or were carers of people with dementia who had these transition experiences. The role of coresearchers included helping with the recruitment of participants, planning the interview process and designing research tools, carrying out interviews, discussing and analysing findings, planning and delivering feedback to local stakeholders and being involved in further implementation and dissemination activities. Coresearcher experiences and reflections were gathered as part of a semi-independent evaluation of the participatory element of the project, mainly through focus group interviews conducted during and at the end of the project.

29.3 Case Study: Research Participants

29.3.1 Philip and Penny[1]

Philip is in his mid-60s and cares for his wife, Penny, who has recently been diagnosed with dementia They live in rented accommodation in an isolated rural location. Philip and Penny have limited financial means and only just manage to 'get by'.

When Philip first became worried about Penny's memory loss, he struggled to get the GP to take his concerns seriously. He did his own research on the internet and contacted lots of agencies when trying to get help. He was often referred on and told to contact a different person or agency; he left messages, but his calls were not returned, or he was told that someone would be in touch later, but then heard nothing further.

At the time of the research interviews, Philip was very upset at the rapid decline in Penny's cognitive abilities, angry with himself for his lack of patience with her and disillusioned and frustrated at the lack of support from the services he had approached. By his own admission, he has 'a short fuse'. He has high blood pressure, gets easily agitated and has significant heart problems. The couple have two adult sons, but Philip does his best to protect them from the worry and demands associated with Penny's needs. There is a lot of conflict between Philip and Penny's parents. They will not acknowledge that Penny has dementia, so Philip is not able to discuss Penny's current or future care with them either.

Penny is much quieter than Philip, but friendly and smiley. She talked about how the support from her friends and family was helping her: 'They're all there for me, sort of enclosing me in this'. There are certain 'stories' from the past that she can

---

[1] All names are pseudonyms.

relay without faltering, but for questions about her illness, she looks to Philip to fill in the gaps or correct or extend her responses.

As part of the research, two interviews were carried out by Thelma (a carer coresearcher) and an academic researcher (DT) with Philip, and (on separate occasions) two interviews were carried out by Margaret (a service user coresearcher) and an academic researcher (DT) with Penny.

29.3.2 Benefits to Participants

Philip was 'at the end of his tether' at the time of the first research interview. He said that the people who were continually referring him on to other services should 'bat for England', as they were superb at batting away his requests for help. He felt that these people 'talked the talk', but they were just doing a job and 'did not really give a damn':

> Well I suppose … it's very difficult for people who've never been involved in it to comprehend or have a true understanding of what it is like; I mean, my life and the kid's lives have just been turned upside down, so dramatically, and there must be so many other people in the same situation, you know… and they're just dismissed or sent from pillar to post. (Philip)

Thelma had been in a similar situation of being passed 'from pillar to post' when trying to gain information and obtain support for her husband so she could relate easily to Philip's feelings of anger, frustration, exasperation and powerlessness. Philip was able to experience someone actively listening and empathising with his concerns and difficulties; he felt that Thelma understood his situation, shared similar feelings and experiences and cared about him as a person [3]. This contrasted markedly with his previous experiences of feeling that he was a nuisance, to be passed 'like a parcel' around the circuit of services. The significance for Philip of this sense of shared experience, personal connection and human compassion can only be fully understood in relation to the depth of despair he was feeling at the time:

> I am in a desperate situation, I feel it's, sort of, got to the stage where I feel, sort of, that I desperately need some help, and I just think if they listen to people and could say, well look, you know, this lady is desperate for help, or this guy really needs some help, something tangible. Nothing seems to be happening at all and, as I say, people talk a good story and oh great, you can get this and you could get that and you can do this and then people phone you up, and 'oh, let me send you another package'. And I say 'look, there's only so many hours in a day that you can read all these bloody leaflets, all this paperwork on dementia and Alzheimer's disease, you know, you get heart and soul sick of it'. That's why I said to the girl the other day, 'look, just don't send me any more packages'… There are times when Penny goes to bed at night, at quarter to nine, and she'll sleep a good twelve hours, and I sit here and I cry my eyes out and I just think, I can't cope with this anymore… I don't mean to be over dramatic about it, but I'm just digging myself an early grave and, to be quite honest with you, I don't care. There are times when I've said to Penny, 'I wish we both weren't here'…and, you know, I've said to her, I just think, oh let's just make a nice hot chocolate together with, you know, (put) a ruck of tablets in and just go to bed and frig 'em all. Sorry, I just get like that. (Philip)

As well as the emotional release from sharing his feelings and experiences, Philip was also able to gain some practical ideas from Thelma who had already travelled a similar path. For example, she was able to tell him about the level and type of support that he and Penny should be entitled to receive. This gave him greater confidence and clarity in his future dealings with services so that, rather than losing his temper very quickly, he could be both clearer about what they needed and more assertive (rather than angry) in expressing this. Although the aim of the research was to elicit older people's experiences of transitions, not to give advice or provide support, it is not reasonable to expect coresearchers to become 'the same as' professional researchers. Indeed, part of the purpose of involving them is because of their ability to form connections based on shared experiences [4]; it is therefore perhaps inevitable that the boundary between listening and supporting became more blurred than in a traditional research relationship.

Penny also benefited from her interaction with Margaret during the two research interviews. By the time of the second interview, Philip and Penny had been given information about the memory café run by the Alzheimer's Society, but Penny was reluctant to attend as she was worried that she would not 'fit in' and would have nothing to say to the other members. This loss of self-esteem and caution about interactions outside of the immediate family and friendship network is often experienced by people in the early stages of dementia [5]. When Penny was interviewed by Margaret without Philip present, she had to rely on her own responses, and this prompted her to be more forthcoming than when they were together. She was able to share her feelings about sensitive subjects, such as the impact of the dementia on her relationship with Philip:

> Well to be honest I know my husband struggles sometimes because he finds it quite hard and I suppose it's because he doesn't understand the things I do sometimes. Obviously I'm not the person I used to be so for him it's different. And he does get a bit, you know, why are you doing that and doesn't understand why I do things or, you know, the same as I used to be, and I just sort of think well I'm not like that anymore. I can't be that person. I sometimes get a bit sort of upset and think well why is he doing that? But he's very good. I mean he's done everything for me so, you know, I can't complain. (Penny)

The increased need to communicate and the 'safe' audience that Margaret represented prompted Penny to make efforts to use her communication skills, rather than leaving others to speak for her. Offering people with dementia opportunities for communication can counteract some of the social barriers that exacerbate 'symptoms' of dementia, such as social withdrawal and loss of verbal skills [6].

Penny was able to form a bond with Margaret during the interviews, including sharing humorous exchanges about having dementia. Their shared dementia diagnosis provided a focus for the relationship and served as a route to enhancing, rather than detracting from, their self-esteem. Their 'eligibility' to participate in the research and contribute their experiences rested on their dementia status; thus the shared acknowledgement of their dementia acted as a strategy for affirming a positive identity [7]. On a more practical level, the relationship encouraged Penny to attend the memory café, and this provided not only social benefits to Penny but also a regular break for Philip.

Both Philip and Penny were amazed at Margaret's cheerfulness, level of social skills and her status as a 'coresearcher' in a university-led project, despite her 6-year dementia diagnosis. This confounded their assumptions and stereotypes about what living with dementia was going to be like in the longer term, giving them greater hope for their own futures. Hope can itself sustain wellbeing for people with early-stage dementia [8] so this, too, was an important benefit of the research encounters.

29.4 Case Study: Coresearchers

29.4.1 Thelma: Carer Coresearcher

Thelma had been caring for her husband, John, for a number of years. It took a long time for John to receive a diagnosis, and even when he was diagnosed, Thelma felt that she was left to her own devices to find out about the condition and support services. As John's condition deteriorated, she faced new challenges, continually having to learn, adapt and fight to obtain the best care that she could for John in changing situations. They had to contend with a number of significant and traumatic transitions, such as when John was admitted to the hospital and his mental health needs were not properly catered for and when he received very poor quality care in a care home. When the research commenced, John was a permanent resident in a nursing home but Thelma still visited him every day. She felt that she had learned a lot 'the hard way' during her dementia 'journey' and she was keen to use this experience to help others.

29.4.2 Margaret: Coresearcher with Dementia

Margaret lives with her partner, Tom. She was diagnosed with dementia 6 years ago. She has always been an active and sociable person, who loves chatting and sharing a joke. She attends a memory café run by Alzheimer's Society every week, to which she can walk as it is only a short distance away. She is very open in talking about her dementia, and this approach is encouraged and supported by staff and other members at the café. Margaret believes that keeping her brain active is important in warding off further deterioration, and she welcomes opportunities that will help her to socialise and 'keep her brain ticking over'. She has significant short-term memory loss, but she and Tom have developed a range of strategies to help with this, such as writing short notes that Margaret can refer to during the day.

29.4.3 Motivations of Coresearchers

Coresearchers in the study were all motivated by the desire to see changes and improvements in services for older people with dementia. They believed that the research gave them an opportunity to use their experiences, as people who had dementia, or were caring for family members with dementia, to improve future services for those going through similar transitions. Talking about her experiences when her husband first became unwell, Thelma spoke for many carers when she said:

> We struggled at the beginning; we didn't know where to go for information or advice; we became really isolated and things were difficult; we were finding out things by accident talking to a neighbour or friend, just in conversation. I thought that by getting involved we could highlight gaps in services.

They saw their lived experience as a valued adjunct to what the academic researchers brought to the project. As Thelma commented:

> Here was an opportunity to be involved as an older person and be a voice for the older person. Somebody out there in the world of academia was placing a value on the experience of us older carers and giving us the opportunity to further the work of the academic researchers.

29.4.4 Benefits to Coresearchers of Participation

During the project, coresearchers formed friendships, some of which lasted beyond the duration of the study. The initial training allowed the coresearchers to share their stories and realise they had had many common experiences, including difficulties accessing services, a lack of continuity of staff, feelings of isolation and frustration and anxieties and embarrassment about the impact of dementia on the whole family.

The acquisition of new research skills of interviewing, analysing data, presenting the findings to audiences of service providers and participating in other dissemination events all added to the coresearchers' feelings of improved self-esteem and a more positive self-identity [9]. Margaret, presenting at a national conference, spoke with pride:

> I thoroughly enjoyed doing the interviews. I like getting out and meeting people and it made me feel like I was doing something useful. It was also interesting to hear about how other people deal with their problems – we can all learn from each other. Involving people with dementia in research has shown that people with dementia can take part in research and make a helpful contribution.

Being involved in the research enabled Thelma, too, to reflect upon her own life experience. After the research ended, she was asked to lecture on several occasions to medical students about her experiences of caring for a husband with dementia and also to social work students about her experiences as a coresearcher.

Involvement in the dissemination of the findings of the research gave coresearchers satisfaction that they could potentially influence important changes in the delivery of services [10]. There were both local and national feedback events where coresearchers read the actual words of the research participants. Thelma observed:

> The reaction of the managers was remarkable. It was obvious they felt most uncomfortable. It was so difficult for them hearing the emotive and powerful responses directly from the service users and carers. This had obviously not been presented to them in this way before. It made more impact than any written words could ever have done.

After the research had finished, the coresearchers found they had other opportunities to make use of their new skills and experiences. In addition to the teaching opportunities above, Thelma participated in several national conferences and gave three live local radio interviews about having someone in the family with Alzheimer's disease. Another coresearcher was part of research reference groups for a leading mental health organisation and has appeared in a training video for social care staff.

29.4.5 Challenges to Coresearchers

Some research studies identify disadvantages to coresearchers sharing similar experiences to participants whom they are interviewing [11]. These relate to both the stress interviewers may experience from hearing about difficult experiences and to the responsibility they feel in asking interviewees to relive potentially painful experiences. In this research study, there were no such drawbacks reported. As they perceived the experiences, coresearchers reported only positive benefits for themselves and for the participants.

However, this is not to say the interviews did not present challenges. Thelma found it hard not to be in a position to help directly some of the people she visited:

> The difficulty I found was in walking away at the end of the interview and to realise that I was not there necessarily to give answers as I had experienced. The point of the interview process was to explore the needs of the participants as they saw them.

29.5 Conclusion

The circumstances of both coresearchers and participants were very varied and the dynamics of each interview encounter unique. However, the benefits of involvement in the project, conveyed here through the experiences of Thelma, Margaret, Philip and Penny, are representative of the other carer and service user coresearchers and participants.

For the coresearchers, benefits included the formation of peer friendships and support mechanisms, a new layer of social activity and the opportunity to use social skills (this was especially important for the coresearchers with dementia), increased confidence and feelings of personal and social value and opportunities to become involved in other research and teaching initiatives. For the research participants, the benefits included increased emotional and psychological wellbeing through the empathy and understanding communicated in the research relationships, practical gains through sharing of information and introduction to new resources, enhanced self-esteem through having their views listened to and valued and a renewed sense of hope about their own futures.

Although the focus of this chapter has been on the benefits to the individuals directly involved in the research – the coresearchers and participants – the participatory approach also strengthened the outcomes of the project in terms of the changes in local policy and practice that it generated. These aspects are discussed elsewhere [12].

A key message from the project is that older people with dementia and who are carers of people with dementia can, with adequate support, take an active and meaningful part in research as both coresearchers and participants. This not only validates their personhood at an individual level [13] but also provides opportunities for them to make a valuable social contribution as citizens [14].

29.6 Points for Reflection or Discussion

- To what extent are older people with mental health needs involved within your own area of practice or research?
- How could this be promoted or developed?
- What potential challenges might you encounter and how could these be addressed?
- What benefits might there be for older people themselves, other key stakeholders and service/research outcomes?

Acknowledgements We are extremely grateful to the older people who participated in this research project as both coresearchers and participants and whose experiences form the backbone of this chapter.

References

1. Ellins J, Glasby J, Tanner D, McIver S, Davidson D, Littlechild R, Snelling I, Miller R, Hall K, Spence K and Co-researchers. Understanding and improving transitions of older people: a user and carer centred approach. Birmingham: University of Birmingham/ Southampton: National Institute for Health Research. 2012. http://www.netscc.ac.uk/hsdr/files/project/SDO_FR_08-1809-228_V01.pdf
2. Moore TF, Hollett J. Giving voice to persons living with dementia: the researcher's opportunities and challenges. Nurs Sci Q. 2003;16(2):163–7.
3. Cornes M, Peardon J, Manthorpe J. Wise owls and professors: the role of older researchers in the review of the national service framework for older people. Health Expect. 2008;11(4):409–17.
4. Miller E, Cook A, Alexander H, Cooper S-A, Hubbard G, Morrison J, et al. Challenges and strategies in collaborative working with service user researchers: reflections from the academic researcher. Res Policy Plan. 2006;24(3):198–208.
5. Langdon S, Eagle A, Warner J. Making sense of dementia in the social world: a qualitative study. Soc Sci Med. 2007;64:989–1000.
6. Killick J, Allan K. Communication and the care of people with dementia. Buckingham: Open University Press; 2001.
7. MacRae H. Managing identity while living with Alzheimer's disease. Qual Health Res. 2010;20:293–305.
8. Wolverson E, Clarke C, Moniz-Cook E. Remaining hopeful in early-stage dementia: a qualitative study. Aging Ment Health. 2010;14:450–60.
9. Tanner D. Co-research with older people with dementia: experience and reflections. J Ment Health. 2012;21(3):296–306.

10. Fudge N, Wolfe CDA, McKevitt C. Involving older people in health research. Age Ageing. 2007;36(5):492–500.
11. Staley K. Exploring impact: public involvement in NHS, public health and social care research. Eastleigh: INVOLVE; 2009.
12. Littlechild R, Tanner D, Hall K. Co-research with older people: perspectives on impact. Qualitative Social Work, 2015;14(1)18–35. doi:10.1177/1473325014556791.
13. Kitwood T. Dementia reconsidered. Buckingham: Open University Press; 1997.
14. Bartlett R, O'Connor D. From personhood to citizenship: broadening the lens for dementia practice and research. J Aging Stud. 2007;21:107–18.

Interprofessional Working

30

Jon Glasby

In 1942, the Beveridge Report on *Social Insurance and Allied Services* set out what came to be seen as a blueprint for the post-war welfare state [1]. Famously, Beveridge described 'five giants' (or serious social problems) which needed to be tackled: want, disease, ignorance, idleness and squalor. Although these social issues were described in very dated (and often pejorative) language, such themes are still with us and in many ways continue to shape how we respond to the provision of welfare. Thus, the 'giant' of 'want' might now be described as 'poverty' or 'social exclusion' and has traditionally been the responsibility of the social security system. Similarly, 'disease' was the responsibility of the newly formed National Health Service (and this initial focus on responding to disease perhaps helps explain why the health service has tended to view itself as a more of 'sickness service' that responds to ill health, one that one that necessarily sees its role as promoting health and well-being in a more positive sense).

The result was a situation in which a series of new state services were provided, often organised in a very top-down and silo-based manner (seemingly based on the assumption that it is possible to respond to each 'giant' in isolation) (see [2, 3] for an overview). Typically, there would be a central government department and then a series of regional bodies and a larger number of local delivery units (see Fig. 30.1 for an example).

Almost ever since that we have been learning the hard way that such structures do not do justice to the way most people live their lives: to the inherent 'messiness' of real life and the way in which different social problems interact (so that a family on a very low income might also live in poor housing, experience poor health and achieve less well educationally and in terms of future employment). As a result, successive governments have sought to encourage more effective joint working

---

J. Glasby, PhD, MA/DipSW, PG Cert (HE), BA
School of Social Policy, University of Birmingham,
Birmingham, West Midlands, UK
e-mail: J.Glasby@bham.ac.uk

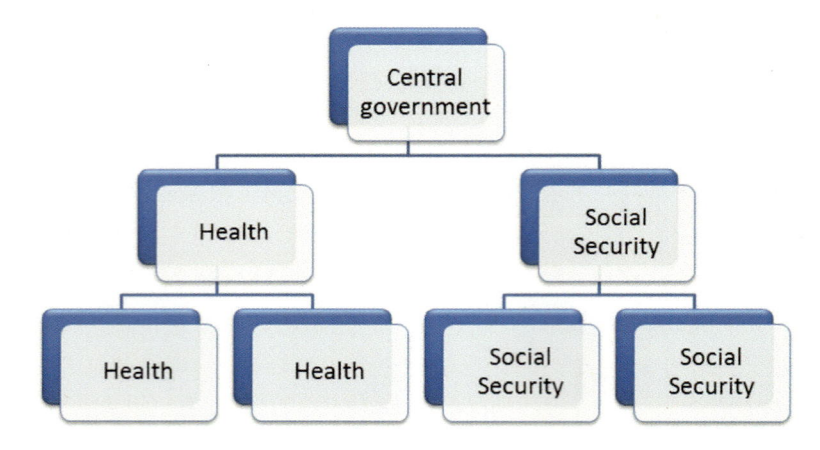

Fig. 30.1 Traditional, silo-based services

Table 30.1 Some key differences between health and social care

Health care	Adult social care
National	Part of local government
Subject to the Secretary of State for Health	Subject to locally elected councillors
Free at the point of delivery	Subject to means test and user charges
Boundaries based on GP registration	Based on local council boundaries (strictly geographical)
Looks to the sciences for its education and training	Looks more to the social sciences
Traditional focus on individual 'cure' and on medical treatment	Traditional focus on 'care' and on seeing the individual in a broader social context

between different parts of the system – particularly in situations where people have multiple and/or complex needs that could easily fall between the gaps in our existing structures.

Of all the different fault lines in the UK welfare state, one of the most important – but also the hardest to overcome – has been the relationship between different parts of the NHS and adult social care. From the 1940s onwards, these have been organised on the assumption that it is possible to distinguish between people who are 'sick' (who are seen as the responsibility of the NHS and receive care free of charge) and those who are 'frail' or 'disabled' (who are seen as having 'social care' needs which are met by local government and which are typically subject to means testing to often significant service user charges). The result is a situation in which the NHS and adult social care know they need to work together – but find it very difficult to do so given that they have separate legal frameworks, budgets, targets, geographical boundaries, accountability mechanisms, IT systems, approaches to charging, workforces and professional cultures (see Table 30.1). For one commentator [4], a fundamental 'law' of integration is that 'you can't integrate a square peg into a round hole' – and yet this is precisely what front-line health and social care workers are being asked/told to do.

When it comes to older people with mental health problems, health and adult social care often face additional barriers. Traditionally, the NHS has seen such provision as part of its mental health services, while adult social care has included older people's mental health as part of its generic older people's services. This user group has also often been seen as 'nobody's priority', with a national inspection from the former Social Services Inspectorate highlighting the dangers of this situation:

> The care of older people with a mental health problem... is a major cause for concern and presents a significant challenge for community care.... Social trends show that the number of very elderly people in Britain is increasing, older people are more likely to live alone, and the prevalence of mental ill health rises markedly with age. Therefore, the size of this group is growing and yet it is often forgotten. It is an easy group to ignore. Older mentally ill are reluctant to speak out, are rarely dangerous and are often sad, poor and confused. They may have no family to speak for them. In community care terms, they fall between traditional mental health and older people's services. Their care confronts different professional value systems as a balance is sought between protection and treatment, independence and risk. It requires typically a multi-agency and multi-professional response. Even so, older people with mental health problems are often nobody's priority. [5]

While this quote comes from a report in the late 1990s, the issues at stake feel just as important to this day – and indeed have grown in significance given recent demographic changes. All too often, older people with mental health problems will have a mix of physical health, mental health and social care needs that span traditional agency and professional boundaries, with scope for significant overlap/duplication, gaps, miscommunication and poor outcomes if care is not appropriately co-ordinated (see Marjorie's story, below).

30.1 Marjorie's Story [6]

Marjorie was admitted to the hospital with a suspected cancerous growth in her throat – which subsequently burst during a minor operation to remove and test a sample of the blockage. After an emergency procedure, she seemed to make a good physical recovery – but her family was concerned that her personality seemed to have changed significantly. To them, it felt as if Marjorie had aged 20 years. Always very sociable and fastidious about her appearance, Marjorie became very withdrawn and stopped washing, eating or cleaning her house. The hospital felt that it was relatively normal for someone to take a while to recover from the physical shock of such an operation and was not overly concerned.

At home, Marjorie had some minor home care support, but did not want the input of a social worker. Her GP wondered if she had become depressed and prescribed an antidepressant (which Marjorie did not want to take and so took out of the packet and hid down the back of her sofa). Over time, her family became increasingly worried – but felt that the different health and social care professionals were not listening to them. They also felt that Marjorie had in some way 'given up' and was deliberately keeping the different practitioners away because she did not want to live any more. However, the more they asked for help, the more they felt that services interpreted their concerns as guilt at not being able to do more for Marjorie as a family.

After several weeks, Marjorie was readmitted to the same hospital with dehydration/malnutrition and given 'build-up' drinks. She was discharged to a psychiatric hospital, but they could not find evidence of a diagnosable mental health problem and so discharged her back home. In a few weeks, she was readmitted to the hospital, given build-up drinks and transferred across again to the psychiatric hospital for another assessment. At this stage, she collapsed and was readmitted to the original general hospital (where it was discovered that the cancer had returned and was inoperable). Preparations were being made to transfer Marjorie to a hospice or to a nursing home when she died.

As Marjorie's story (which is based on a true story) suggests, providing non-joined-up care to older people with mental health problems can lead to poor outcomes – both for the person and their family, as well as for the health and social care system. While there are few easy answers, the case study illustrates the way in which front-line practitioners can be working really hard within the confines of their own agency/profession, but can fail to see the bigger picture or to provide an appropriate response if they approach the situation in too narrow a manner. Part of what is needed here is basic empathy – consciously viewing the situation from the point of view of the older person and their family to consider what the services we provide might feel like from their point of view (see also the reflective exercises at the end of this chapter). This sounds simple, but can be really challenging given scarce resources (which, if we are not careful, can force us to focus primarily on 'core business' and on the presenting problem, rather than taking the time to adopt a more holistic approach). Wherever possible, front-line workers also need to recognise the way in which their actions have a knock-on effect on the individual service user, their family and other professions/agencies. Sometimes this can be positive (where something we do prevents the need for another service or input from another professional). However, it can also be negative, where the stance we take leads to a poorer outcome than might otherwise has been achieved and makes the job of another worker even harder. Above all, Marjorie's story reveals the importance of drawing on the expertise of individual service users and their families – who are typically the only ones in the situation who know what life is normally like for the person concerned, what works for them, what a good outcome would look like and what the person was like before they came into contact with services. Anyone else (no matter how well professionally qualified and expert they are) typically only sees the person at a particular moment in time and therefore has a very limited insight. While individual service users and their families might disagree (as in this case study), we ignore such expertise at our peril. While health and social care can do much more to join up the services they provide, we will only truly deliver more integrated care when we all develop a more person-centred approach and wrap the support we can offer around the individual, their family and their unique circumstances.

30.2 Reflective Exercises

1. Think about an older person with mental health problems with whom you have worked:
   - To what extent was it possible to meet the person's needs by yourself and to what extent did you need to draw on the expertise of other workers?
   - How easy or difficult was it to contact and build a relationship with other health and social care professionals?
   - What were some of the barriers that got in the way of successful joint working?
   - What were some of the success factors?
   - If the older person was asked directly, what would they have said about the extent to which the different workers were able to co-ordinate their inputs?
2. Think of two situations where you have had to build a relationship with someone from a different background to yourself – one where things went well and one where they went badly! (This could be a health and social care example, but also could be an example from your personal life – meeting a new friend or partner, being part of a sports team, starting a new job):
   - Where things went well, what was it that contributed to a good process and/or outcome? Can you use this experience to draw out any more general lessons for what helps when working with other professions?
   - Where things went badly, what was it that caused the problems? Can you use this experience to draw out any more general lessons for what hinders joint working?

Appendix 30.1 Further Reading

For further details of the arguments in this chapter, see:

- Glasby J, Dickinson H. Partnership working in health and social care. 2nd ed. Bristol: The Policy Press. 2014.
- Glasby J, Dickinson H. A to Z of inter-agency collaboration. Basingstoke: Palgrave Macmillan. 2104.

References

1. Beveridge W. Social insurance and allied services. London: HMSO; 1942.
2. Glasby J. Understanding health and social care. 2nd ed. Bristol: The Policy Press; 2012.
3. Glasby J, Dickinson H. Partnership working in health and social care: what is integrated care and how can we achieve it? 2nd ed. Bristol: The Policy Press; 2014.
4. Leutz W. Five laws for integrating medical and social services: lessons from the United States and the United Kingdom. Milbank Memorial Fund Q. 1999;77:77–110.
5. Barnes D. Older people with mental health problems living alone: anybody's priority? London: Social Services Inspectorate/Department of Health; 1997. p. 1.
6. Glasby J, Littlechild R. The health and social care divide: the experiences of older people. 2nd ed. Bristol: The Policy Press; 2004.

Challenges and Opportunities

Carolyn A. Chew-Graham and Mo Ray

We have tried, in this book, to highlight areas of significant improvement in mental health services for older people through changes in legislation, policy and practice. Yet, despite many drivers for change, there is still substantial evidence that older people with mental health problems continue to experience stigma and discrimination. For example, common stereotypes and assumptions which often characterise old age (e.g. very old people are bound to be depressed, memory difficulties are a normal part of ageing, old people with complex needs cannot meaningfully participate in decisions about their support and care, older people of certain ethnic groups will be cared for by their families) interact with stigma about mental health and illness.

Changing attitudes to older people and mental health requires action across policy and practice areas. For example, refocusing attention towards older peoples' strengths and capabilities rather than a deficit model (Chaps. 2, 3, 6, 12, 21, and 25) would undoubtedly challenge practitioners within all areas of health and social care to consider how they worked with older people. Tanner and Littlechild (Chap. 29) demonstrate the positive and powerful impact of older people living with dementia as coresearchers on service development, the visibility of people living with dementia and the impact the project had on coresearcher's wellbeing and confidence. From a wider perspective, there is a growing interest in the social model of disability which rightly questions why older people living with dementia are more likely to experience structural and social barriers (Chap. 4).

C.A. Chew-Graham, MD, FRCGP (✉)
Research Institute, Primary Care and Health Sciences,
Keele University, Keele, Staffordshire, UK
e-mail: c.a.chew-graham@keele.ac.uk

M. Ray, PhD.
Gerontological Social Work and Programme, School of Social Science and Public Policy,
Keele University, Keele, Staffordshire, UK
e-mail: m.g.ray@keele.ac.uk

The Health Inequalities RCGP publication in 2015 [1] reflected on evidence from the 2010 Marmot Review [2], which concluded that in England, people living in the poorest neighbourhoods will, on average, die 7 years earlier than people living in the richest. The publication stresses that health inequalities are not simply a difference in health outcomes, but a difference in health outcomes *combined with* barriers to accessing the health-care system. In addition to physical barriers such as opening hours, location and transport, there are other barriers contributing to this exclusion, including perceptions of services and expectations of what will be offered if older people seek help, staff attitudes to patients and communication difficulties. We have highlighted in this book (Chaps. 4, 11, and 12) that inequalities across the life course create significant risks for mental ill health and challenges for mental health promotion.

The RCGP publication [1] made two recommendations that are particularly relevant to improving the care of older people with mental health problems:

Focus on incentivising ways of working that promote continuity of care in areas where patients would benefit most from a continuous therapeutic relationship with their GP – particularly areas where a high number of patients are living with multiple morbidities

Fund outreach programmes to help often excluded groups such as those with mental health problems, learning disabilities and the homeless to access general practice

We have demonstrated that older people with depression are an underserved group, with poor access to care (Chaps. 5, 6, 11, and 13) and who may find offered interventions unacceptable [3]. Newer models of care and intervention may help to address these problems [4] as well as ensuring that older people have access to a full range of supportive interventions including psychotherapeutics and counselling (Chap. 20).

Along with policy guidance and research initiatives, the publication of a number of evidence-based quality standards and guidance has focused on crucial areas for service improvement including the mental health and wellbeing of older people living in care homes (Chaps. 13, 18, 23, and 25). Milne (Chap. 13) and Phair (Chap. 24) demonstrate the continued importance of prioritising the mental health needs of older people living in care homes and the prevalence of depression amongst the care home population. Reductions in the use of antipsychotic medication (Chaps. 18, 19, and 24), improved recognition of the importance of primary care services for care home residents (Chap. 24) and a better awareness of the need to be appropriately occupied (Chaps. 13, 18, and 25) and the role of creativity and the arts (Chap. 12) in promoting mental health and wellbeing are encouraging developments.

Developing mental health policy and practice must be able to adapt responsively and flexibly to changing needs and priorities associated with growing diversity in population ageing and the new opportunities and challenges which accompany them. Taking a broader perspective, the importance and impact of good mental health across the life course is clear. The UK government strategy locates mental health and wellbeing as central to quality of life and fundamental to the success of the country's economic, educational, cultural and social activities. Clearly mental health promotion involves buy in, support and collaboration from all sectors, but there remains a need for greater public focus on and awareness of the importance of promoting good mental health across the life course and including in older age.

References

1. RCGP. Health inequalities. London: RCGP. 2015 (Online). Available from: http://www.rcgp.org.uk/Policy/RCGP-policy-areas/~/media/Files/Policy/A-Z-policy/2015/Health%20Inequalities.ashx. Accessed 15th Aug 2015.
2. The Marmot Review. Fair society, healthy lives. 2010 (Online). Available from: http://www.instituteofhealthequity.org/projects/fair-society-healthy-lives-the-marmot-review. Accessed 15th Aug 2015.
3. Rait G, Burns A, Chew CA. Old age, ethnicity and mental illness: a triple whammy. BMJ. 1996;313:1347–8 [Invited Editorial].
4. Gask L, Bower P, Lamb J, Burroughs H, Chew-Graham C, Edwards S, Hibbert D, Kovandžić M, Lovell K, Rogers A, Waheed W, Dowrick C, the AMP group. Improving access to psychosocial interventions for common mental health problems in the United Kingdom: review and development of a conceptual model. BMC Health Serv Res. 2012;12:249. doi:10.1186/1472-6963-12-249.

Appendix 1: GAD-7 Anxiety

Over the *last 2 weeks*, how often have you been bothered by the following problems? (Use "✓" to indicate your answer)	Not at all	Several days	More than half the days	Nearly every day
1. Feeling nervous, anxious or on edge	0	1	2	3
2. Not being able to stop or control worrying	0	1	2	3
3. Worrying too much about different things	0	1	2	3
4. Trouble relaxing	0	1	2	3
5. Being so restless that it is hard to sit still	0	1	2	3
6. Becoming easily annoyed or irritable	0	1	2	3
7. Feeling afraid as if something awful might happen	0	1	2	3
Column totals	___ +	___ +	___ +	___
	=Total score ___			

If you checked off *any* problems, how *difficult* have these problems made it for you to do your work, take care of things at home or get along with other people?

Not difficult at all ☐   **Somewhat difficult** ☐   **Very difficult** ☐   **Extremely difficult** ☐

From the Primary Care Evaluation of Mental Disorders Patient Health Questionnaire (PRIME-MD PHQ). The PHQ was developed by Drs. Robert L. Spitzer, Janet B.W. Williams, Kurt Kroenke and colleagues. For research information, contact Dr. Spitzer at rls8@columbia.edu. PRIME-MD® is a trademark of Pfizer Inc. Copyright © 1999 Pfizer Inc. All rights reserved. Reproduced with permission

Scores of 5, 10, and 15 are taken as the cut-off points for mild, moderate and severe anxiety, respectively. When used as a screening tool, further evaluation is recommended when the score is 10 or greater.

The GAD-7 originates from Spitzer RL, Kroenke K, Williams JB, et al; A brief measure for assessing generalized anxiety disorder: the GAD-7. *Arch Intern Med.* 2006;166(10):1092–7. GAD-7 © Pfizer Inc.

Appendix 2: PHQ-9 Depression

Over the *last 2 weeks*, how often have you been bothered by any of the following problems? (Use "✓" to indicate your answer)	Not at all	Several days	More than half the days	Nearly every day
1. Little interest or pleasure in doing things	0	1	2	3
2. Feeling down, depressed or hopeless	0	1	2	3
3. Trouble falling or staying asleep or sleeping too much	0	1	2	3
4. Feeling tired or having little energy	0	1	2	3
5. Poor appetite or overeating	0	1	2	3
6. Feeling bad about yourself – or that you are a failure or have let yourself or your family down	0	1	2	3
7. Trouble concentrating on things, such as reading the newspaper or watching television	0	1	2	3
8. Moving or speaking so slowly that other people could have noticed? Or the opposite – being so fidgety or restless that you have been moving .around a lot more than usual	0	1	2	3
9. Thoughts that you would be better off dead or of hurting yourself in some way	0	1	2	3
Column totals	___	+ ___	+ ___	+ ___
	=Total score ___			

From the Primary Care Evaluation of Mental Disorders Patient Health Questionnaire (PRIME-MD PHQ). The PHQ was developed by Drs. Robert L. Spitzer, Janet B.W. Williams, Kurt Kroenke and colleagues. For research information, contact Dr. Spitzer at rls8@columbia.edu. PRIME-MD® is a trademark of Pfizer Inc. Copyright © 1999 Pfizer Inc. All rights reserved. Reproduced with permission

Interpretation of total score

Total score	Depression severity
1–4	Minimal depression
5–9	Mild depression
10–14	Moderate depression
15–19	Moderately severe depression
20–27	Severe depression

Kroenke K, Spitzer R, Williams W. The PHQ-9: validity of a brief depression severity measure. *JGIM*. 2001;16:606–16

Index

A
Acetylcholinesterase inhibitors (AChEI), 235, 277
Action on Depression, 125
Acute organic brain syndrome. *See* Delirium
Adult attitude to grief (AAG) scale, 25
    audit opportunities, 25
    and comment sheet, 22, 23
    coping responses, 21
    CORE ims, 26
    key factors, 23
    palliative and bereavement care, adoption in, 25
    RRL model, concepts in, 21–22, 24, 26
    vulnerability, 22
Advance care planning (ACP), 320–321
Age Exchange, 135
Age-Friendly Cities movement, 138
Ageing population, 4
'Ages and Stages' project, 138
Agoraphobia, 83
Alzheimer's disease (AD)
    anxiety, 93
    dementia
        cost of, 204, 205
        sleep loss, 202
        UK, prevalence in, 200, 203
Alzheimer's Disease International, 303
The Alzheimer's Society, 34
Amalthea Project, 125–126
Amitriptyline, 95
AMP Programme, 126–128
Antidepressants
    adverse effects of, 99
    antidepressant discontinuation syndromes, 100
    antipsychotics, 96
    anxiety disorders
        in COPD, 110
        and depression, 110
        generalised anxiety disorder, 108, 110
        prescribing decisions for, 107–109
    beneficial effect of, 101
    benzodiazepines, 97
    buspirone, 97
    cardiac effects, 99
    classes of, 95
    depression
        with bipolar affective disorder, 107–108
        initial presentation of, 102–104
        mirtazapine, 105
        prescribing decisions in, 101, 102
        after previous deliberate overdoses, 106
        psychotic depression, 107
        recurrence of, 104–105
        referral to specialist service, 100, 101
        sertraline, 104
        St John's wort, 102
        after stroke, 105–106
        therapeutic dose and monitoring, 101
    drug interactions, 97–98
    hyponatraemia, 98, 99, 106
    lithium, 96
    MAOIs, 95, 96
    older patients, poorer response in, 94
    pregabalin, 97
    referral to specialist service, 100, 101
    risk of bleeding, 98–99
    SNRIs, 96
    SSRIs (*see* Serotonin reuptake inhibitors (SSRIs))
    TCAs, 95
    therapeutic mechanisms of action, 94
    younger patients, 94

Antipsychotics
    atypical, 96
    bipolar disorder, 96
    conventional and typical, 186
    psychotropic medications, 186–188
    schizophrenia, 96
    side effects of, 187–188
    sulpiride, 187
Anxiety
    agoraphobia, 83
    in Alzheimer's disease patients, 93
    antidepressants (*see* Antidepressants)
    avoidance, 83
    case-finding questions for, 48
    CBT and behavioural approaches, 83, 88–89
    collaborative care, 84–85
    in COPD patients, 45, 52–53
    in depressed patients, 93
    diagnosis of, 49–50, 93
    GAD (*see* Generalised anxiety disorder (GAD))
    health and social care services, increased use of, 45, 46
    hospital admission and discharge, 115–118
    losses, 21
    NICE guidelines, 80
    and pain, relationship between (*see* Pain in older people)
    panic and phobic disorders, 46, 82
    prevalence of, 45, 115
    risk assessment, 51–52
    risk factor for, 45, 46, 93
    stepped care model, 83–85
    suggested investigations for, 51
    symptoms, 47, 83
    third-sector organisations, role of (*see* Third sector)
'Art Lift' project, 136–137
Arts and creativity, 139–140
    audience participation, 134
    health care, role in, 133
    as non-pharmacological interventions, 133
    participatory arts
        ageing and mental health promotion, 138–139
        'Art Lift' project, 136–137
        'Arts in Mind' project, 136
        dance movement therapy, 136
        definition, 134
        'Good Times' project, 136
        musical activity, 135–136
        reminiscence therapy, 135
    'passive' engagement, 134
    psychotherapy, form of, 134
    as therapy, 134
    Women's Institute (WI), 133
'Arts in Mind' project, 136
Ascertain Dementia 8 (AD8), 232
Asset-based approach, 13–14
Assistive technologies (AT), 322
Atypical antipsychotics, 96, 101
Auditory hallucinations, 181

B
Beating the Blues, 124–126
Befriending, 122–123
Behavioural activation (BA)
    for anxiety, 83
    for depression
        benefits, 82
        diabetes, 90
        effectiveness in older people, 82
        functional equivalence, 87
        learning theory, 81
        negative reinforcement, 81
        rewarding and task-focused behaviours, 82
Behavioural and psychological symptoms of dementia (BPSD)
    CBT, 270–273
    formulation-led interventions, 269
    informal and formal carers, 269
    nonpharmacological, 269
Benzodiazepines, 97, 108
Bipolar disorder, 96
Black and minority ethnic (BME) groups, 36–37, 285, 313
Body language, 295–296
BPSD. *See* Behavioural and psychological symptoms of dementia (BPSD)
British Association of Art Therapy, 134
British National Formulary (BNF), 187
Bupropion, 107
Buspirone, 97

C
Care Act (2014), 5, 304, 306, 314–315
Care homes
    admission and death, 146
    delirium in, 170
    dementia, well-being and quality of life
        case study, 289
        common health problems, 286–288
        environment, impact of, 286
        impact on health and well-being audit, 289–290
        NICE guidance, 284

Index

physical activity, need for, 285
risk taking, promotion of, 286
technology, use of, 285–286
traditional approaches, 284–285
depression
   assessment of, 148–149
   care plans, 153
   case study, 155–156
   course and nature of, 146–147
   individualised interventions, 153
   mortality, 147
   policy issues, 153–154
   prevalence of, 146
   primary care support, 150–151
   research, 154
   risk factors for, 147–148
   treatment of, 149–150, 152
   well-managed transition, 152
   in UK, 145
Care in the Community, 29
Care Quality Commission (CQC), 151, 313
CBT. *See* Cognitive behavioural therapy (CBT)
CD-RISC scores, 13
Cerebral white matter disease, 94
Cerebrovascular disease, 202
Chronic obstructive pulmonary disease (COPD)
   anxiety, prevalence of, 45, 52–53, 110
   cognitive behavioural therapy, 88–89
Citalopram, 95, 97, 99, 101
Clinical commissioning groups (CCG)
   pharmacists, 277
Clomipramine, 95
Clouding of consciousness, 165
Clozapine, 186, 190–191
Cognitive behavioural therapy (CBT)
   for anxiety, 83, 88–89, 108
   dementia, 270–273
   for depression
      activity scheduling, 80
      age-related adjustment, 86
      'the Beckian cognitive triad', 80
      behavioural experiments, 80
      clinical effectiveness, 81
      cognitive distortions, 80
      COPD, 88
      diabetes, 90
      effectiveness in older people, 81
      homework tasks, 80
      relapse prevention plan, 80
      thinking and behaviours, changing patterns of, 80
   in third-sector self-help clinics
      Beating the Blues, 124–125
      Elderly Positive Thoughts Course, 125, 128–129
      Living Life to the Full, 125
Cognitive Function and Ageing Studies, 203
Cognitive rehabilitation, 236
Cognitive stimulation therapies (CSTs), 236
Cognitive tests for delirium (CTD), 168
Cognitive training, 236
Collaborative care (CC), 84–85
Commissioning for Quality and Innovation (CQUIN), 34
Committee on Safety of Medicines (CSM), 188
Community nurses, 5, 275, 302, 312, 323
Community singing, 135–136
Constipation, 325
CORE Information Management Systems (CORE ims), 26
Creativity. *See* Arts and creativity
Crisis resolution and home treatment teams (CRHTT), 189

D

Dance movement therapy, 136
DCM. *See* Dementia care manager (DCM)
The Debenham Project, 35
De Jong Gierveld Scale, 59
Delirium
   aetiology of, 167
   in care homes, 170
   case study, 173–174
   characteristics of, 164
   clinical features of, 165–167
   definition, 163–164
   diagnosis of, 167–169
   historical context, 163
   incidence and prevalence of, 164
   management of, 169–170
   morbidity and mortality, 164
   predisposing factors, 167, 168
   prevention of, 174–175
   primary care management in
      acetylcholine-dopamine imbalance, 172
      Intermediate Care scheme, 171
      non-pharmacological intervention, 171
      pharmacological treatment, 172
      polypharmacy, 171
   "Stop Delirium" project, 164, 165, 170–171
   symptoms of, 165
   terminologies, 163, 164
Delirium rating scales (DRS), 168
DelpHi trial, 275
Dementia, 115

ACP, 320–321
ageing populations and trends in health, 203–204
antipsychotic use in, 96
assistive technologies, 322
behavioural problems, 322
Care Act 2014, 314–315
care homes (*see* Care homes)
communication with people
    audit, 299
    body language, 295–296
    case study, 298
    diagnosis of, 297–298
    listening, 296
    memory problems, 297
    person, 294, 295
    physical and mental health, 294, 296
    physical environment, 294–296
    social environment, 295
    social interactions, 296–297
    speech patterns, speed, 296
economic impact of
    cost of, 206, 319
    estimation procedures, 205
    instruments, 205
end of life
    constipation, 325
    distress, management of, 324
    dyspnoea, 325
    Liverpool Care Pathway, 324
    nausea and vomiting, 325
    terminal agitation, 325–326
epidemiology, 198–199
identification and primary care management
    carers, 237
    case study, 231–234
    clinical assessment, 231
    cognitive assessment, 232–233
    DESs, 230
    driving, 236–237
    independent living in community, 238
    information provision, 234
    long-term management, community, 234
    MCI, 230
    memory assessment services, 233
    non-pharmacological interventions, 235–236
    pharmacological management, 235
    symptoms and clinical presentation, 230–231
impact of, 203
incidence of, 202–203
in Ireland
    differential diagnosis, 212
    incentivise general practitioners, 213–214
    National Dementia Strategy, 213, 215
    prevalence rates, 211–212
    Primary Care Education, 214
    primary care practitioners, 212–213, 215
    residential care diagnosis, 215
    YOD, 214–215
loneliness, 58
MCA (*see* Mental Capacity Act (MCA) 2005)
mental wellbeing, research project, 331–332
    coresearchers, 335–337
    research participants, 332–335
palliative care, 323–324
personal reflection
    change and uncertainty, 262–263
    diagnosis, 258–259
    integrated care, 260–262
person-centred care (*see* Person-centred care, dementia)
policy development for older people
    antipsychotic medication, investigation into, 33
    CQUIN, 34
    The Debenham Project, 35
    Dementia-Friendly Northern Ireland, 35
    Dementia-Friendly Wales, 35
    Dementia Strategy for England, 33
    dementia summit, 35–36
    'Dementia Without Walls' initiative, 34–35
    Design at the Dementia Services Development Centre, Stirling, 35
    Enhancing Healing Environments initiative, 35
    global policy action on dementia, 36
    ministerial conference on dementia, 36
    national awareness campaigns, 34
    national clinical leader, appointment of, 34
    national dementia plans, 36
    Prime Minister's 'dementia challenges', 34
prevalence of
    case study, 201
    global, 199–200
    populations, 200–201
    primary care, 201

subtypes, 200
prognosis, 319
psychotherapy interventions
    advice and strategies, 242
    case study, 244–245
    "Dementia–State of the Nation" report, 248–249
    Dementia Voice study, 242
    emotional impact, 241–242
    IAPT, 246
    LivDem (see Living well with Dementia (LivDem))
    QoL-AD, 246
risk and danger
    carers and risk, 304
    embodiment, 302
    hazards of, 302–303
    heat map, 305–306
    legal framework, 304
    wandering, 303, 304
school awareness curriculum
    case study, 254–255
    intergenerational activities, 254
    lessons, 254
    local networking, 254
    project, 253–254
specialist care
    geriatrician, 273–275
    mental health (see Mental health, dementia)
    pharmacy (see Pharmacy in dementia care)
    primary/secondary interface, 275–276
Dementia Awareness Week 2015, 225
Dementia care manager (DCM), 275–276
Dementia-Friendly Northern Ireland, 35
Dementia-Friendly Wales, 35
"Dementia–State of the Nation" report, 248–249
Dementia Strategy for England, 33
Dementia with Lewy bodies (DLB), 200
'Dementia Without Walls', 34–35
Depression
    aetiology of, 46
    antidepressants (see Antidepressants)
    in care homes (see Care homes)
    clinical features of, 47
    cognitive impairment, 87
    in COPD patients, 52–53
    diabetes patients, 45, 53–54
    diagnosis of
        antidepressant medication, addictive to, 47
        case-finding questions, 48
    dementia, 48
    older person, holistic assessment of, 50
    stigmatisation, fear of, 47
    suggested investigations, 51
    symptoms, 49
    therapeutic nihilism, 48
disease burden and disability, cause of, 45
health and social care services, increased use of, 45, 46
hospital admission and discharge, 115–118
losses, 21
and pain, relationship between (see Pain in older people)
Parkinson's disease, people with, 115
participatory arts (see Participatory arts)
physical illness, 93
prevalence of, 45
psychological therapy
    behavioural activation (see Behavioural activation (BA))
    CBT (see Cognitive behavioural therapy (CBT))
    collaborative care, 84–85
    NICE guidelines, 80
    stepped care model for, 83–84
recurrence, risk of, 46, 102
risk assessment, 51–52
risk factor for, 45, 46
third-sector organisations, role of (see Third sector)
Diabetes, 45, 53–54
Diagnostic and Statistical Manual of Mental Disorders (DSM-V), 184
Diazepam, 97
Direct Enhanced Service (DES), 230
Disability paradox, 10–11
Distress, 324
Donepezil, 235, 268
Dothiepin, 95
Driver and Vehicle Licensing Agency (DVLA), 236–237
Drug and therapeutic committees (DTC), 277
Drug-related problems (DRP), 275
Duloxetine, 96
Dyspnoea, 325
Dysthymia, 100, 102

E
Emotional loneliness, 58
Enduring Powers of Attorney (EPA), 320
Enhancing Healing Environments initiative, 35

F
Fear-avoidance model, 71–72
Fibromyalgia, 70, 71
Frontotemporal dementia (FTD), 200

G
Generalised anxiety disorder (GAD), 46, 50
  in Alzheimer's disease patients, 93
  benzodiazepines, 118
  buspirone, 97
  CBT, 110
  excessive worry about different events, 82
  pregabalin, 97
  stepped care model, 84, 85
General Medical Services (GMS)
  Contract, 5
General Practitioner Assessment
  of Cognition (GPCOG), 232, 233
2006 General Practitioner Contract, 237
Geriatric Depression Scale, 149
Geriatrician, 273–275
Gold Standards Framework, 275
'Good Times' project, 136
Grief. *See* Loss and grief

H
Hallucinations, 165, 166
Health and Social Care Act 2012, 6–7
Health care, 4–5, 342–343
Hyponatraemia, 98, 99, 106

I
Imipramine, 95
Impact on Participation and Autonomy, 61, 62
Improving Access to Psychological Therapy
  (IAPT) service, 246. *See also*
  Living well with Dementia
  (LivDem)
Independent Mental Capacity Advocate
  (IMCA), 311, 313, 320
Index of Multiple Deprivation, 136
International Statistical Classification of
  Diseases and Related Health
  Problems (ICD-10), 183
Interprofessional working
  case study, 343–345
  health and social care, 342–343
  traditional, silo-based services,
  341, 342
Irish Memory Clinics, 214

K
Keele Assessment of Participation
  (KAP), 61, 62
Knee pain, 70

L
Lasting power of attorney (LPA), 311, 312, 320, 321
Lewy body dementia (DLB), 172
Lithium, 96, 101–102
Liverpool Care Pathway, 324
Living Life to the Full, 125
Living well with Dementia (LivDem)
  Memory Matters groups, 243
  Minimum Data Set, 247
  NIHR-funded pilot study, 243–244
  primary care setting
  recruitment, 247
  support for carers, 248
  therapeutic material, 248
Loneliness, 46
  bereavement, consequence of, 21
  definition, 57
  dementia and cognitive decline, precursor
    of, 58
  depression, 21, 58
  emotional distress, 57
  emotional loneliness, 58
  losses, 21
  measurement of
    De Jong Gierveld Scale, 59
    three-item loneliness scale, 58, 59
    UCLA Loneliness Scale, 58
  morbidity and mortality, 21, 58
  negative consequences, 58
  prevalence of, 57
  social loneliness, 58
  social participation, 63
    community-based interventions, 60
    educational activities, 60
    family, friends and neighbours, contact
      with, 59
    group-based participatory activities, 60
    measurement of, 60–62
    television, 59
Long-stay institutional care, 29
'Look at Me' research project, 138
Lorazepam, 97, 172, 325
Loss and grief
  AAG self-report scale (*see* Adult attitude
    to grief (AAG) scale)
  ageing well with, 20
  depression and loneliness, 21

emotional support, 24
General Anxiety Disorder scale, 24
life course, 19–20
mental and physical health problems, 21
mental health care, access to, 24
Patient Health Questionnaire, 24
resilience, 24
RRL model, 21–22, 24
Low back pain, 70
Lower extremity pain, 70
LPA. *See* Lasting power of attorney (LPA)

M

Major depressive disorder, 69, 146
Medicines and Healthcare products Regulatory Agency (MHRA), 188
Medicines use reviews (MURs), 277
Memory impairment, 166
Memory Matters group, 243
'Men's Sheds' movement, 124
Mental Capacity Act 2007, 186
Mental Capacity Act (MCA) 2005, 304, 320
    advance decisions, 310
    decision-making, 310
    difficult decisions, 312–313
    MCA Code of Practice, 311–312
    mental health powers, 313
Mental health
    definition of, 137
    dementia
        BPSD (*see* Behavioural and psychological symptoms of dementia (BPSD))
        cognitive enhancer medications, 268
        communication with people, 294, 296
        generic medications, 268
        memory clinic, 268
        memory service, 268
        psychological approaches, 268–269
    losses, 21
    participatory art projects
        'Ages and Stages' project, 138
        benefits, 137
        'Look at Me' research project, 138
        Manchester, UK, 138–139
        'Music for Life' research project, 138
    policy development for older people
        active ageing, independence and self-responsibility, 37–38
        age-based discrimination, 30, 31, 36, 37
        asylum seekers and refugees, 37
        Audit Commission report, 30
        cross-government strategy, objectives of, 32
        dementia policy (*see* Dementia)
        detection and treatment, 37
        factors, 30
        low expectations, 30
        mental health services, modernisation of, 31
        National Service Framework for Older people, 30–31
        'New Horizons', 31
        organisational division, 31
        substance misuse, 36
        suicide prevention, 36
        Together for Mental Health, 32–33
Mental Health Act 2007, 186
Mental Health Strategy for England, 21
Mild cognitive impairment (MCI), 230
Mini-Mental State Examination (MMSE), 233, 235
Mirtazapine, 96, 99
Monoamine oxidase inhibitors (MAOIs), 95, 96
Movement disorders, 99
Multidisciplinary primary healthcare team, 4–5
Musculoskeletal pain and older people, 67, 68. *See also* Pain in older people
'Music for Life' research project, 138

N

Namaste care programme, 286
National Dementia Strategy, 153, 213, 215
National End of Life Care Programme, 320
National Institute for Health and Care Excellence (NICE), 185–186, 189, 284
National Service Framework for Older people, 30–31
Nefazodone, 95, 96
Nephrogenic syndrome, 98
Netherton Feelgood Factory, 125
N-methyl-D-aspartic acid (NMDA) receptor, 234
Noradrenaline/dopamine reuptake inhibitors (NDRIs), 95
Noradrenergic and specific serotonergic antidepressants (NaSSAs), 95
Nortriptyline, 95

O

Occupational therapy (OT), 236

Older age
  access to care, inequity of, 6
  ageing population, 4
  anxiety in (*see* Anxiety)
  delirium (*see* Delirium)
  dementia in (*see* Dementia)
  depression in (*see* Depression)
  Health and Social Care Act 2012, 6–7
  health care and, 4–5
  life expectancy, 4
  loss of independence, 3
  pain in (*see* Pain in older people)
  parity of esteem, 6–7
  physical frailty, increase in, 3
  social care and, 4–5
  social isolation, 3
  social transition, 3
Osteoarthritis, 67
Osteoporosis, 99
Over-the-counter (OTC) medicines, 276–277

P
Pain in older people
  chronic widespread pain, 68
  depression and anxiety, relationship
      between
    chronic widespread pain, 70
    expectations and modulation, 71
    fear-avoidance model, 71–72
    fibromyalgia, development of, 70
    knee pain, onset of, 70
    low back pain, onset of, 70
    lower extremity pain, 70
    lower quality of life, 69
    major depressive disorder, 69
    prevalence, 69
    primary care management, 73–74
    sleep disruption, 72
    stress, physiological response to, 72
  musculoskeletal pain, 67, 68
  pain interference, prevalence of, 68
  prevalence, 68
Paranoid delusions, 165
Parity of esteem, 6, 7
Parkinson's disease, 93, 115
Participation Measure for Post-Acute Care
    (PM-PAC), 61
Participation Objective, Participation
    Subjective (POPS), 61, 62
Participation Scale, 61, 62
Participatory arts, 140
  ageing and mental health promotion
    'Ages and Stages' project, 138
    benefits, 137

    'Look at Me' research project, 138
    Manchester, UK, 138–139
    'Music for Life' research project, 138
    definition, 134
  depression, older people with
    'Art Lift' project, 136–137
    'Arts in Mind' project, 136
    dance movement therapy, 136
    definition, 134
    'Good Times' project, 136
    musical activity, 135–136
    reminiscence therapy, 135
Pathways and Research of Dementia
    (PREPARED), 214
Patient Health Questionnaire, 24
PEACE documentation, 275
Personal Mastery Scale, 12–13
Person-centred care, dementia
  benefits of, 221
  comfort and security, 223
  communication, 222–223
  malignant social psychology, 220
  occupation, 223–225
  personally enjoyable and stimulating
      activities, 223, 224
  personhood, 221
  struggle for empowerment, 222
Pharmacy in dementia care
  community pharmacists, 276–277
  medication management dementia care
      pathways, 277
  specialist pharmacy services, 277–278
Physical exercise, 123–124
Positive Thoughts Course, 125, 128–129
Potentially inadequate medication (Pim), 275
Pregabalin, 97
Primary Care Education, 214
Primary care services, 4–5
Primary Care Workforce Commission, 5
Prime Minister's Challenge on Dementia, 253
Psychological resilience, 11
Psychosis
  case study, 191–192
  management of
    antipsychotic medication (*see*
        Antipsychotics)
    BPSD, 188–189
    CRHTT, 189–190
    NICE guidelines, 185–186
    psychological and psychosocial
        interventions, 190
    relapse and re-referral, secondary care,
        190–191
    return to primary care, 190
  patient assessment, 184–185

prevalence, 181–182
symptoms and classification
 delusions and hallucinations, 181
 early-onset schizophrenia, 184
 functional and organic psychoses, 182–183
 late-onset schizophrenia, 183–184
 primary psychotic disorder, 183
 risk factors for, 184
Psychotherapy
 anxiety, management of
  CBT and behavioural approaches, 83, 88–89
  collaborative care, 84–85
  NICE guidelines, 80
  stepped care model, 83–85
 dementia
  advice and strategies, 242
  case study, 244–245
  "*Dementia–State of the Nation*" report, 248–249
  Dementia Voice study, 242
  emotional impact, 241–242
  IAPT, 246
  LivDem (*see* Living well with Dementia (LivDem))
  QoL-AD, 246
 depression, management of
  behavioural activation (*see* Behavioural activation (BA))
  CBT (*see* Cognitive behavioural therapy (CBT))
  collaborative care, 84–85
  NICE guidelines, 80
  stepped care model for, 84
 procedural modifications, 86
 psychosis, 190

Q
Quality of Life in Alzheimer's disease (QoL-AD) scale, 246

R
Range of response to loss (RRL) model, 21–22, 24
Rating of Perceived Participation (ROPP), 61, 62
Reminiscence, 135
Residential care homes, 29, 145, 164, 215
Resilience and well-being
 areas of, 14–15
 asset based approach, 13–14
 critical approach to, 10
 definitions and dimensions of, 11–12

disability paradox, 10–11
implications, 15
levels of, 13
measurement of, 12–13
proliferation of interest in, 9–10
salutogenic approach, 10, 11, 13, 15
Resource utilisation in dementia (RUD) instrument, 205

S
Salutogenic approach, 10, 11, 13
Schizophrenia. *See* Psychosis
Schizotypal disorder, 183
Serotonin antagonist/serotonin reuptake inhibitors (SARIs), 95
Serotonin/noradrenaline reuptake inhibitors (SNRIs), 96
Serotonin reuptake inhibitors (SSRIs)
 adverse effects of, 99
 cardiac conduction abnormalities, lower rate of, 95
 cardiac effects, 99
 efficacy in older people, 100–101
 hyponatraemia, 98, 106
 risk of bleeding, 98–99
 sertraline and escitalopram, 101
 sexual dysfunction with, 107
 side effects, 95
 suicide, 95
 warfarin, interaction with, 97
Serotonin syndrome, 99
Sertraline, 97, 104
Six-item Cognitive Impairment Test (6-CIT), 233
Sleep disruption and older people, 72
Sleepwalking, 163
Social care, 5–6
Social Insurance and Allied Services, 341
Social loneliness, 58
Social participation, 58, 63
 community-based interventions, 60
 educational activities, 60
 family, friends and neighbours, contact with, 59
 group-based participatory activities, 60
 measurement of, 60–62
 television, 59
Social phobia, 93
Social resilience, 11
Social workers, 5–6
SSRIs. *See* Serotonin reuptake inhibitors (SSRIs)
Stepped care
 for depression, 83–84
 for GAD, 84, 85

St John's wort, 102
"Stop Delirium" project, 164, 165, 170–171
Stress, 72
Sun-downing, 166
Syndrome of inappropriate antidiuretic hormone secretion (SIADH), 98

T
TCAs. *See* Tricyclic antidepressants (TCAs)
Telephone friendship support, 123
Third sector
    arts-based activities, 122
    befriending, 122–123
    CBT in self-help clinics, 124–125
        Beating the Blues, 124–125
        Elderly Positive Thoughts Course, 125, 128–129
        Living Life to the Full, 125
    civic/societal sector, 121
    collaboration
        Amalthea Project, 125–126
        AMP Programme, 126–128
        Beat the Blues, 126
    debt/bereavement counselling, 122
    definition, 121
    physical activity, 123–124
    and pyramid of care, 121, 122
    voluntary/community sector, 121
    western societies, role in, 121
Together for Mental Health, 32–33
Tricyclic antidepressants (TCAs), 95, 97–98, 106, 149

U
UCLA Loneliness Scale, 58
UK Department of Health's Risk Guidance for Dementia, 305
UK National Screen Committee, 230
Unipolar depression, 96

V
Vascular dementia (VaD), 200
Venlafaxine, 96, 101, 105, 106
Voluntary sector. *See* Third sector
Vulnerability, 22

W
Warfarin, 97
Warwick-Edinburgh Mental Well-being Scale (WEMWBS), 136–137
Well-being. *See* Resilience and well-being
Welsh Government Intermediate Care Fund, 35
Women's Institute (WI), 133

Y
Young onset dementia (YOD), 211, 214–215

Printed by Printforce, the Netherlands